anisation.)

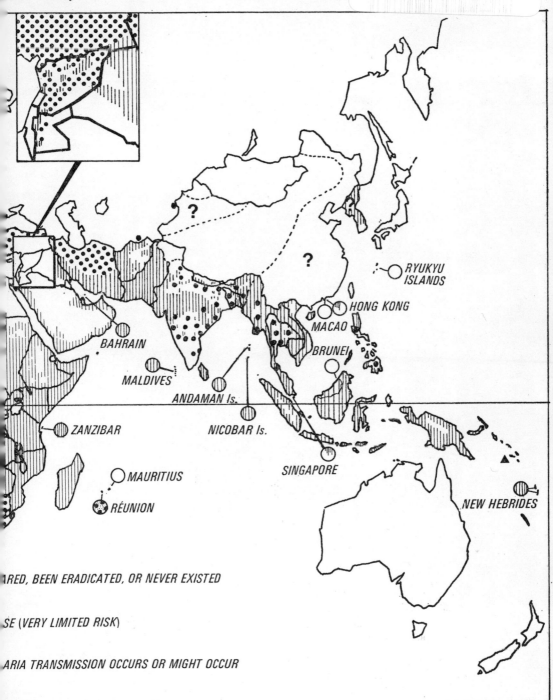

RYUKYU
ISLANDS

HONG KONG

MACAO

BRUNEI

BAHRAIN

MALDIVES

ANDAMAN Is.

ZANZIBAR

NICOBAR Is.

SINGAPORE

MAURITIUS

RÉUNION

NEW HEBRIDES

ARED, BEEN ERADICATED, OR NEVER EXISTED

SE (VERY LIMITED RISK)

ARIA TRANSMISSION OCCURS OR MIGHT OCCUR

World Health

World Health

Fraser Brockington
M.A., M.D., M.R.C.P., D.P.H., M.Sc.

Barrister-at-Law, Middle Temple
Emeritus Professor of Social and Preventive Medicine,
University of Manchester

Forewords by
Dr H. MAHLER
Director-General of the World Health Organization
and his predecessor
Dr M. G. CANDAU

THIRD EDITION

CHURCHILL LIVINGSTONE
Edinburgh London and New York 1975

CHURCHILL LIVINGSTONE
Medical Division of Longman Group Limited

Distributed in the United States of America by
Longman Inc., New York and by associated
companies, branches and representatives throughout
the world.

First edition, 1958
Second edition, 1967
Third edition, 1975

ISBN 0 443 01290 3

Library of Congress Cataloging in Publication Data

Brockington, Colin Fraser, 1903–
World health.

 1. Hygiene, Public. 2. World Health Organiza-
tion. I. Title. [DNLM: 1. Public health.
WA100 B864w]
RA425. B772 1975   362.1   75–4026

Printed in Great Britain

Foreword

It gives me great pleasure to introduce the third edition of *World Health,* a book that has long been held in high esteem by students and practitioners of public health.

Great changes have taken place since Professor Fraser Brockington completed the last edition, introduced by my predecessor, Dr M. G. Candau. At that time it was considered sufficient to provide health services *for* the peoples of the world, who were often not consulted about their own wishes in the matter and were allocated merely a passive role. The current trend is towards consulting each community and asking what sort of services it would like to see provided; also, and more importantly, communities are being encouraged to involve themselves intimately in the provision of services, which they then come to look upon as their own rather than as something foisted upon them from outside. In other words, a start has been made on the provision of health services *by* the peoples of the world.

The new outlook is being and will continue to be reflected in the policies and programmes of the World Health Organization. Professor Fraser Brockington shows how contemporary attitudes have gradually developed, and the third edition of his book will, I know, prove just as valuable to members of the health professions as did the others, as well as providing a commentary that is fascinating not only to those working in the health field but to everyone, professional or layman, who takes an interest in world health.

H. Mahler, M.D.

Geneva,
1975

Foreword to the Second Edition

Just over one hundred years ago, in 1851, the first effort was made to reach international agreement on a health matter. The subject was quarantine and the occasion the first International Sanitary Conference held in Paris, and attended by representatives of twelve European States.

At that time few people had any notion of what is now called public health, preventive medicine was scarcely dreamed of, and the principle of the responsibility of governments for the health of their peoples would have been considered impracticable.

Today almost all the countries of the world have formally undertaken to join in a common endeavour not only to protect themselves from the spread of epidemics, but also to attack communicable disease wherever it is found, and to raise the health standards of people everywhere. It is now a commonplace that health, like peace, is indivisible, and that it is in each country's interest that the peoples of other countries should live in healthy conditions. This common endeavour has its spearhead in the World Health Organization, which, with a membership of over 125 countries, is in 1968 celebrating its twentieth anniversary.

The disciplines of preventive medicine and public health have developed enormously in the last hundred years and particularly during the present century. They are, however, in their infancy compared with curative medicine, whose roots and traditions go back thousands of years. It is therefore not without difficulty that medical and administrative authorities are now coming to accept the incontestable need to integrate the curative and preventive branches of medicine and to introduce public health concepts into regular medical courses. Happily, the definition of health given in the Constitution of the World Health Organization – 'a state of complete physical, mental and social well-being' – is today being accepted more and more widely as an attainable, if distant, goal.

Professor Brockington's book attempts to present a clear exposition, based on historical, organizational, and practical considerations, of the public health approach and the world approach to some essential social problems of our times. Although students and public health workers will find here a treasure-house of information, this book is much more than a history. It aims at providing a synthesis of views current today on health questions, and as such it has great educative possibilities. It will also, I am sure, prove to be a guide and an inspiration to young medical men and others who may be thinking of

devoting their careers to a field which is full of promise for the future – that
of public health.

M. G. Candau, M.D.
Director-General, World Health Organization

Geneva
May, 1967

Preface

World Health involves more than a team of specialized workers; on the one hand, it is a matter for politicians, who must plan the building of services, and, on the other, it impinges upon national endeavours in agriculture, labour, education, insurance and other fields. Moreover, those who practise public health, doctors and others from so many different disciplines, versed in a variety of techniques, may fail for want of understanding of the deeper issues. This book, therefore, deals little with technicalities and much with values.

In the small compass of a single volume there has been little chance to explore deeply. Rather has the object been to bring together the chief characters who play a part in world health within a single diorama, in the hope that this will give the reader a better understanding of their relationships. Sources of further reading can be found through the bibliography.

The book has been written for all who are interested in the health of the world – now among the most important issues facing the world – and particularly for the workers in different countries who are directly involved, i.e., doctors, nurses, sanitarians, public health engineers, welfare workers, social workers, politicians, the many who give voluntary service, and others in allied disciplines whose work impinges upon public health.

The third edition has embodied experience gained since retirement from the chair of Social and Preventive Medicine at Manchester University, as a consultant for the World Health Organization in a number of European, Middle Eastern and African countries. I have been greatly helped in its preparation by colleagues in WHO at headquarters in Geneva and in the regional offices in Copenhagen, Alexandria, Delhi and Manila. To all these and particularly to Mr Sicat and Mrs Paganella in the WHO Geneva library I wish to express my deepest thanks. I am most grateful for advice and help on particular points from Drs Myron Wegman and John Westerman of the Schools of Public Health at Ann Arbor and Minnesota; to Dr Adelstein and his staff in the medical division and Mr Newman of the census division of the Office of Population Censuses and Surveys, London; to Dr Yellowlees and his staff at the Department of Health and Social Security, London; to Miss Bedford of the Manchester University Press; to Miss Joan Parrilla of UNICEF; to Mr Lal, deputy Registrar-General, India; to Dr Forendr Vongsfak, Ministry of Public Health, Thailand. I have had the greatest support and encouragement from Dr Candau and his successor Dr Mahler, Director-General of the World Health Organization, of which I am most appreciative.

Ballasalla   Fraser Brockington
Isle of Man
1975

Contents

Appendices

Part One: Introduction

1. The Meaning of Health and of Public Health

People talk of health today as of a known and measurable quantity. Yet even its meaning is elusive, and its wide use contrasts with any clear, distinct, or generally accepted definition. From its derivation, and in the picture which it presents to all our minds, it signifies a wholeness or soundness of body and mind. But when we seek to give this scientific precision, we are at once confronted with the difficulty of determining its relationship to 'disease'. Health and disease must be intimately related, for if disease did not exist it would be nonsense to talk of health. The two states are contrasted in our minds, as it were the two sides of a coin – so that when one is present the other is absent. The difficulty is to determine, as with light and darkness, at what point health and disease meet and whether they are mutually exclusive. If the most perfect functioning of the body is the light of the sun's zenith, and death the 'darkest hour', the point of distinction between health and disease can be anywhere in between. Health may be reckoned as beginning when there is light enough 'to distinguish between a light and a dark thread', or anything less than the zenith may be counted as disease.

Health and disease as distinct entities

If health is present only at the zenith – the condition of perfect equilibrium and perfect harmony, which Galen postulated[5] – then it is a final goal, and all that leads up to it is disease. Here positive and negative and other qualifying adjectives have no place. Health is raised to the level of an ideal, a blessed condition, to be attained only in rare moments of life, when the body is sound and the personality is reacting to a major challenge 'like a pale tenuous membrane stretched to its capacity' (A. Huxley).[6] Disease becomes all but universal. Thus we are, at once, forced to ask ourselves what is disease; for if we could define this might we not by elimination determine health?

Disease – a 'condition of the body, or some part or organ of the body, in which its functions are disturbed or deranged' (O.E.D.) – has by many been confined to those established pathological conditions which are clinically detectable. Disease is here what we see in the *pathological museum* – the results of invasions, toxins, degenerative processes, and accidents. Or it may include *sub-clinical conditions,* of which we may be unaware, detectable perhaps only by laboratory tests; or even a mere absence of *physiological reserves,* which in general parlance may be called poor health rather than established sickness. But over and above such distinctions there are more remote and more subtle deviations from normal which many include as illness. We now enter the realm of the body's reactions to stress, which play their part in the *milieu intérieur* of Claude Bernard.[2] The body may over-react to stress, or have an abnormal reaction to stress, or may simply be forced to react to too much stress. All of these may produce a condition of hormone overdosage. Certain anterior-pituitary and adrenal hormones may be produced in excess.[11] And there may be others, whose internal injections could cause damage to linings, resulting perhaps in peptic ulcers, ulcerative colitis, or cardio-vascular disease. We are now removing from the group of healthy people all those who suffer in a physical way from the tensions of modern life.

Ill-health so far defined, if much wider than gross physical destruction, is yet restricted to conditions in which there are somatic changes. There remains the possibility of ill-health without necessarily any disturbance of the soma even so remote as an upset in 'homeostasis'. Social or psychological disturbances may not have given rise to stress greater than the individual physique can withstand; but there is still a distortion of behaviour, which may be regarded as illness, now purely a psychological phenomenon – the neurones are healthy, but they are arranged in socially undesirable patterns. Thus we may have to add to the swelling flood of sick people all those individuals who are at variance with the social structure in which they live; among these are to be found the isolates, delinquent children, industrial misfits, problem mothers, and neurotics, and even those who think themselves to be ill, or who escape from unpleasant situations by presenting symptoms of illness. It follows that failure of personal relationships everywhere, in spite of the fact that they may be a potent cause of stress and hence of somatic changes, are by many regarded themselves as illnesses.

At this point we realize that if health is the absence of sickness in this very wide sense, we approach once again the concept of universal sickness – a situation from which statisticians, and no doubt others, including health administrators, instinctively shrink. As William Farr said:[4]

To accuse the human frame of perpetual malady is as ridiculous as to attribute, with some theological writers, unremitting wickedness to the human heart; but if every alteration of the multiplied parts of the human body, every transient tremble of its infinite movements, every indigestion in man and every fit of hysteria in woman, were reckoned, few days of human life would remain entirely clear; and if the same scrutiny were extended to the state of the brain, the world may very civilly be sent to Anticyra – *naviget Anticyram.*

Farr himself sailed in more frequented waters; and for his statistics of the health of the group he worked on the basis that 'in determining the amount of sickness, the attacks of disease, the slighter affections, are, therefore, passed over'.[4]

Galen, too, although considering that health in the abstract was an ideal state to which no one attained, was equally aware of the embarrassment of applying such a definition to the human race. He found difficulty in regarding as unhealthy all who do not function perfectly; as he said:[5]

If anyone should say that only those are healthy who function perfectly in all their parts, and that others who function less well are not healthy, let him know that he is undermining the foundation of the entire consideration of hygiene.

Furthermore, Galen maintained that it would in any event be impossible to maintain a constant state.[5]

For if ever the perfect constitution existed, it would not remain unchanged for an instant. So that it occurs to me to wonder at the opinion of those who consider that health and good constitution are one and invariable, and who can say that whatever departs in the least from this is not health; and introducing the concept of perpetual disease, they do not perceive that they are arguing about something which either never exists in the animal body, or, if ever it should exist, does not last any length of time.

Galen, therefore, like Farr, was prepared to overlook small ailments and to accept as constituting health a state of reasonable functioning and freedom from pain:[5]

that condition in which we do not suffer pain, and are not impeded in the activities of life, we call health; and if anyone wishes to call it by any other name he will accomplish nothing more by this than those who call life perpetual suffering.

He added the rider that he would exclude from ill-health all those conditions of impairment, or lack of vigour, which, as in ageing, are in accordance with nature.

Many believe that there is little to be added, eighteen hundred years later, except perhaps that health is not an absolute quantity, but a concept whose standards are continually changing with the acquisition of knowledge and with cultural objectives in different lands.

Health and disease as overlapping states

If, however, as has been cogently argued by Perkins (1950),[9] the dividing line between health and disease is placed in almost total darkness just on this side of death, then all life represents some measure of health. Even Falstaff on his death-bed, 'babbling o' green fields', will have had some health. In this concept not only does the absence of disease not exhaust the possibilities of health, but also health and disease can co-exist. It is attractive to think thus of health as a quality in its own right defined without reference to disease. We can then express it on a positive scale increasing to a point where there is not only a complete absence of demonstrable pathological conditions but an excess of physiological reserves, which is more than adequate for every potential stress (Stieglitz, 1949).[12] Furthermore, this permits of improvement in health and the building up of resistance in those who are not manifestly ill; it allows of the possibility of 'positive health' in which the individual glowing with health looks disdainfully at his merely healthy neighbour, as the very white looks at the nearly white in the soap powder advertisements. It was in terms of positive health that the World Health Organization framed the definition in its constitution that 'health is a state of complete physical, mental, and social well-being and not merely the absence of disease or infirmity'.[13]

Some have gone so far as to postulate that health in this setting is not an end in itself and that any definition must contain also the idea of purpose. Man is a social animal; he cannot easily live for himself alone. Health that exists for selfish enjoyment alone is in this concept an affliction – at least on the mental plane. Health must then be the result of a conscious attitude. To be truly healthy a man must find a synthesis of his animal and social imperatives; there must be a harmony. Health is here an adjustment with the environment – physical, mental, social, and cultural – on all sides:

Health is a state of feeling well in body, mind, and spirit, together with a sense of reserve power; based upon normal functioning of the tissues, a practical understanding of the principles of healthy living, a harmonious adjustment to the environment (physical and psychological); it is a means to a richer life of service.

The meaning of public health

Public health refers to the group as distinct from the individual. It suffers, like many phrases in common use, from double meaning, so that in this account of World Public Health we will sometimes be considering the *state of health,* but more usually the *body of knowledge and the machinery by which it is put into practice.* When we say that the public health is good or bad, we mean that the group or community is healthy or ill. Here we are in great uncertainty; even greater perhaps than with the health of the individual. What is health in a group? Is it the total of individuals' health or departure therefrom? Or is it that mixture of good and bad, which, reacting one on another, helps the group to grow and to prosper? Once again we are in the sphere of abstraction – not knowing, for example, whether to regard the neurotic as an asset or a debit. Can a community be healthy, we ask ourselves, without the creative ability of the neurotics, restlessly questing after strange sources of satisfaction?

We should voyage widely before reaching Anticyra in this search for a formula. Like William Farr we may decline the journey and follow Galen's lead in limiting our measurement of the public health to the sum total of 'human incapacity'.

In its other sense, the means to health, public health is the application of all scientific and medical knowledge for the preservation of the health of the group. The WHO Expert Committee on Public Health Administration, adapting Winslow's earlier definition (1923),[15] has defined it as:[14]

the science and art of preventing disease, prolonging life, and promoting health and efficiency through organized community efforts for the sanitation of the environment, the control of communicable infections, the education of the individual in personal hygiene, the organization of medical and nursing services for the early diagnosis and preventive treatment of disease, and the development of social machinery to ensure for every individual a standard of living adequate for the maintenance of health, so organizing these benefits as to enable every citizen to realize his birthright of health and longevity.

More simply Scheele said, 'Public Health is the basic institution created and maintained by society to do something about the death-rate and the sanitary conditions and many other matters relating to life and death'.[10]

In this sense it is both a body of knowledge and also a means to apply that knowledge. Here, at least superficially, we are on more certain ground. When society has determined what it means by health, and what it wants for itself, then Public Health is the way there.

Yet societies will ask different things of it in different parts of the world, and at different points of time. The recipe for health will not always be the same, since cultural values and beliefs differ. Mental health in one society may be ill-health in another. Public health in Japan and Thailand may be striving after objectives different from those it strives after in America or France. In Thailand time will have less meaning than in the USA, and the value which the culture places upon absence of friction in all human relations will be greater. Value systems will also affect the means to Public Health. The place assigned to women – leadership, partnership, or inferiority – in a complex of other factors, will often determine the course of events. In Burma or Bali the needs of religion will take preference, and in the USSR and USA, and Japan those of industry. Countries that hold nursing in high esteem will have an advantage over those that regard it as a menial task. Even the extent to which medical care will be wanted may be determined by the culture. Some nations, like Jane Austen's Mr Woodhouse, health conscious and hanging on the doctor's word, will want hospitals, medicine-bottles, and placebos; for others, asceticism and the inward fires of purposeful living.

Public health, whatever conditions it has to face, is pertinent to all times and places. It is a science and art capable of adaptation to the physical and social demands of any country anywhere in the world.

2. The Conflict of Living Matter

If words do not allow a precise definition of health, we can seek an intuition of its meaning by studying man in his origins and through his associations with other creatures. This takes us to the study of the interplay of different forms of life, which is one aspect of ecology first defined by Haeckel in 1869. So far we have been considering the meaning of health in the abstract and our account has been homocentric in outlook, with man and his illness as its focal point. But in the turmoil of living matter man is a peripheral figure. No longer the leading actor, but among the crowd, we are led beyond the drama of human life into 'earlier and other creation',[3] seeking the dominant features of life, and an understanding of man's submerged tendencies before they became changed by civilization 'into something rich and strange'. By finding man's place in the world of living creatures, we hope to learn what we can expect in health.

The biologist, who sorts out the chaos of living forms – not only in the animal and plant kingdoms, but also in the realm of single-celled organisms dwindling to the bacteria and the virus, almost molecular in size – defines the principal activities of life as growth and reproduction. Life proceeds in fits and starts with the cycle of generations; with each reproductive event there is an opportunity for variation in design; and through each period of growth that follows, the chance to test it. The slow development which we call evolution selects the designs which stand the stresses better. Growth depends on food gathering, which involves all organisms in an intense competitive struggle. The search for the materials of life is, therefore, the central problem which governs the interplay of living matter. No organism is an entity unto itself. The plants which manufacture their protoplasm from the air and soil, and thus make a real gain in living matter from the inanimate, are food for herbivorous animals. The flesh of herbivores is consumed by carnivores; these in their turn succumb to the attacks of others of their kind and bacteria. All flesh must die and feed the scavengers, when the multitude of small creatures, which seethe in rotting matter, return it to the air and to the soil.

In the confusion of this intense competition, life living upon itself and ever 'fire new from the mint', the delicate balance of species is poised, sensitive to new conditions which might favour one more than another. The geographical units, with their dominant vegetations, or biomes – tundra, taiga, deciduous forests, grass land, desert, or marine[1] – each have their own community, whose numbers remain roughly constant. Herons in Britain, storks in Germany, great tits in Holland, if undisturbed, fluctuate in all available censuses within restricted limits, the highest frequently only twice, and never more than ten times, the lowest. Rhythmical swings from high to low (as illustrated by the ten-year cycle of the snowshoe rabbit in Labrador, or the four-year swing of the lemming or vole in the Northern Tundra) is the general rule, involving both the species observed and its predators.[7]

Restraint on numbers, achieved by high mortalities, is the outcome. The robin has two broods a year, each with a clutch size of five; if all were to survive and breed, the population of robins would increase six-fold by the following year, and ten-million-fold within ten years. The robin has an infant mortality of 460 per thousand, the Michigan chipmunk nearer 900, and annual deaths of the survivors leads to extinction of the cohort within five years. Yet, kept in captivity, chipmunks live to eight and robins to the great age of eleven. If, for a time, the restraint on population breaks down, numbers begin to grow exponentially, until disaster overtakes the swollen herd – an epidemic of disease, shortage of food, a sudden climatic catastrophe, as drought follows a heat wave, or an irruption, as seen in the lemmings and the locusts. The original balance is restored.[7]

Such is the law of life as we see it, and as the ecologist describes it; but when studied biochemically or genetically, it can be seen to obey a simpler rule. Growth and reproduction depend upon nucleoprotein. This substance is present throughout the scale of life in the nucleus of the cells. The simplest organism consists of little else. The virus bacteriophage, which lives on bacteria, has 40 per cent by weight of nucleoprotein; and when it invades a bacterium, this is all that enters the host, since the tail, with its injecting device and the armour of protein, are left behind. Nucleoprotein provides the activator which turns the bacterium into a factory for manufacturing virus. It is life stripped down to its essentials.

A compound of this relative simplicity is responsible for the endless distinctions in living things which we see around us. Chemical differences in nucleoprotein hardly exist from virus to the anthropoids; yet this substance is a design for the mature organism, 'repeated' in the patterns of nucleoprotein in the nuclei of its cells. Chains of nucleoprotein, each with the possibility of variation greater in total number than the number of atoms in the universe, contain the secret code of human life.

In the biological estimation of living matter, nucleoprotein has overtopped all. It was present at the beginning of life, though perhaps in a simpler form; 750 million years ago, when there was less oxygen in the atmosphere and the intensity of ultraviolet radiation was greater, and when, on the mud banks by the shallow seas, conditions were favourable for the making of many strange new compounds, one of these became self-replicating and the spark of life was struck. Nucleoprotein is the continuing principle which has survived since the conception of life, and undergone countless modifications.

Since nucleoprotein is extremely unstable, and in imminent danger of disintegration under hostile powers of light, heat, and radiation, the central problem in the phenomenon we call 'life' has always been to survive. Had it not been so there would be nothing now for us to observe, nor ourselves to see it. Survival is the final value in nature. Nucleoprotein, under the menace of the physical world, has evolved endless accessory structures for protection, for the gathering of food, for reproducing itself by interaction with other nuclear protein, always with the strengthening quality of variation. In these terms the bulky intricate organisms, colourful, diverse, and untidy, exist only to serve the germ plasm and to ensure its survival. Thus there exists fundamentally an interaction of different patterns of nucleoprotein, each under pressure to establish its seed upon the earth, and to convert matter into its own substance. This ecological struggle, in which animals die young and violently, is one in which man must also participate.

Infectious disease as an ecological phenomenon

Many diseases may be thought of as an episode in ecology – expressions of strife between different creations of nucleoprotein engaged in the pursuit of food gathering. Thus, when ill with syphilis, tuberculosis, or poliomyelitis, man is an episode in the life of the bacterial world. Infection is a widespread manifestation of duels between species – all animals and plants suffer from infectious diseases; even the bacterium succumbs to bacteriophage.

Infection is of great importance to the animal world when there is a glut, or when drought or bad weather causes a massing of animals at the water pools, or in places of shelter. Botulism, and *Pasteurella multocida,* massacre the ducks in summer droughts, when as many as three million at a time have been counted dead on the shores of the Great Salt Lake.[7] But infectious disease is more important to human beings than it is to animals in the wild, since man, having escaped from other distempers and predation, lives long enough to succumb, or to reach a stage of overcrowding great enough to promote the spread of disease.

The human body is well equipped to meet the invasion of parasites as they occur. Defence mechanisms of various types exist. These can be interpreted, within the general ecological scheme, as devices for maintaining the integrity of one combination of nucleoprotein against the encroachment of another – the phagocytes (or amoeboid cells), the specific antibodies, bactericidal chemicals in the body fluids, and the inflammatory reaction which mobilizes the defences at the site of danger. The importance of these defences is thrown into relief by the plight of those who suffer from a partial lack of them. The patient with agranulocytosis may die because of his depleted store of phagocytes and the patient with agammaglobulinaemia because of his lack of immune bodies, despite support from the antibiotics, which man has recently enlisted.

Infectious disease is an ecological cul-de-sac – of advantage to neither species. The burden of all life is to survive, so that it is never in the interest of the parasite to kill his host which provides his living. The association of man and parasite tends, therefore, to follow a set course. A new disease due to an obligate pathogen makes its entry with a fierce epidemic, killing many, especially in the young adult age group. Gradually in the course of evolution, it seems, man and the parasite adapt themselves to each other, possibly moulding a mutually harmless or even beneficial relationship. Syphilis, now relatively mild, was, in the fifteenth century, when it came to the virgin soil of Europe from North America, an ulcerating pestilence, rapidly fatal. Measles, endemic to the greater part of the world, decimated in the early nineteenth century the islands of the South Pacific. Thus, in the twentieth century, man finds himself at various stages of adaptation and compromise with the obligate pathogens of the bacterial world.

But man has many associations with the bacterial world which could be described as peaceful, if not friendly, co-existence. Many of these organisms assist the body, manufacturing vitamins, for example, Vitamin B_{12} and other members of the B group, in the gut, and helping to digest the food and to keep out infection. The lactobacilli in the adult vagina ferment sugars and make an acid environment inimical to pathogenic organisms. Many other bacteria are harmless inhabitants of the human frame: the nose and throat harbours many harmless inhabitants – diphtheroids, *Streptococcus viridans,* neisseria, fungi, spirochaetes, fusiform bacilli, haemophilus; the gut has a bacterial flora so extensive that 50 per cent of the faeces is composed of bacterial protoplasm.

The existence of the truly potent pathogen is precarious. The addition of a single scientific weapon of defence is often enough to turn the scale. Smallpox and cholera, in many parts of the world, have been annihilated by simple remedies. Tuberculosis, in the developed world, is being extirpated, with a combination of science and social organization. The resistance is greater where the organism has second lines of defence upon which to retire; thus, plague kills man rapidly, but can continue in the rat, among whose numbers it smoulders, only occasionally irrupting into society; typhoid, quickly perishing in the acute phase of the 'disease', entrenches itself in the kidney and gall bladder, whence it can pass, for years, to the urine and faeces. Tuberculosis has owed its long success partly to resistance to the physical environment, and partly to the chronic nature of its processes which have aided dissemination. Much of public health can be seen as a struggle to escape from the conflict with bacteria and protozoa, aided by techniques which man's acquired wisdom gives him.

Technicological advance

Mankind has begun to extricate himself from the struggle for the perpetuation of germ plasm, in which all other species are so completely absorbed. This emergence from the primary biological issue has been achieved through the great development of his cerebral powers, especially those of communication, which has made possible the cumulative assembly of knowledge and technique, and the gathering together of individuals for mutual protection. Not only has man shaken off the marauding carnivores, and to a lesser extent the 'bacteria', but he has begun to alter the environment itself. Forests are turned into arable land, marshes into cities, buffalo into cattle, and yeast into protein. From agriculture to antibiotics, we find man changing the face of the globe, shaping it for his own comfort. But there is much to make us pause.

The discoveries which have lightened the load of human suffering have, until recently, been generally applied only to the few. The emergence of the masses remains precarious. Nor can it be said that man has wholly extricated himself from warring nature. Each problem solved uncovers another, as in the peeling of an onion. The turmoil of living matter is not easily quieted and its power to take charge of our destinies should never be far from our thoughts. Having upset the normal ecological balance, we live more and more in an artificial environment – a world of synthetic diets and values, of drugs and dust from the factories. More recently we have added radiation to the list of man-made hazards, and we know little of the effect which these innovations may have upon the body.

Upsetting the normal interplay of living matter also frees the underlying tendencies of unlimited multiplication and ageing of the population. Biologic-ally, ageing is a backwater in natural selection,[8] and ecologically, over-popula-tion is the signal for disaster. If living matter is not to provide its limiting factors, man must find his own answer.

Man has made of human life a sanctity. The value judgment of individual health finds little place in ecology, in which pain is an alarm to warn of danger and the individual is an experiment, an incident in the survival of the race. The pursuit of individual health is for many now an end in itself. This should call for much heartsearching.

Living matter has but one value – survival; man has many. These now obscure the primary goal of living matter; they are raised to an absolute level; in themselves legion, they shade like a spectrum from one opposite to another. Some are social in their impact, and call upon the individual to lead an 'honour-able' life in terms of the nation's ethos. Others encourage all kinds of inward-ness, from 'genuine' behaviour to the subtle quest for inner harmony. Each has its penalties for transgression. whether estrangement from society or self-division, and modern man is plunged into mental conflict. If the trumpet shall give an uncertain sound, who shall prepare for battle?

Thus, as we cast off the outward trammels of jungle warfare and become free to mould the ideals of our society, we should reconcile our conflicts in a common purpose – the pursuit of the health of mankind. Centrally the problem is one of replacing biological regulation as a means to further the health of the group, by human wisdom. Man, instead of nature, must become our loadstone. To this end, biology needs to be reinforced by social organization; and human wisdom to distil the best from the wide range of human values, and to find a truly human conclusion. This then is the great opportunity for world guidance which the World Health Organization has inherited.

Part Two: Health and Disease Throughout the World

3. The World's Mantle of Disease

The picture of health and disease varies almost infinitely throughout the world, so that a complete presentation of it is hardly possible. Even in massive volumes, only the more salient features of its kaleidoscopic patterns are presented. Here it would be idle to attempt any detailed description. Nor, should it be possible, would it necessarily help greatly in our understanding of world public health and its needs.

It is customary to distinguish four zones of the earth's surface: temperate, southern, Mediterranean, and tropical. The temperate zone stretches across North America and Europe to Japan and includes Australia and New Zealand; the southern zone is the lower half of South America and the lower segment of Africa, corresponding roughly to the Union of South Africa; the Mediterranean zone includes the countries which encircle the Mediterranean basin and the Near East, running out to Siberia, Manchuria, and North-West China. The tropical zone includes the south of North America, Central America, and the northern two-thirds of South America, Central Africa, South-East Asia, and the rest of China.[25]

Within this general framework we can examine the distribution of the four main groups into which the diseases of man fall – infections, degenerative diseases, nutritional disorders, and mental illness. These, if they do not cover every entry in the international list of causes of death, disease, and injury, at least help us to understand what problems face public health throughout the world. The outlines are imperfect and detail is lacking. For most of the world, the measurement of disease within each country, according to district, town, or social class, is too imperfect to permit of any true representation.

Infectious disease

Infections, parasitic, bacterial and viral, taken together are the cause of the greater part of human illness and death, although the exact extent of most, in the absence of proper recording, is little less than guess work (see ch. 22). The distribution and epidemiology can best be gauged by the data given in the annual productions of the *Demographic Yearbook* of the United Nations[7] and *World Health Statistics* by WHO*.[22]

Within the tropical and Mediterranean zones some diseases, like trachoma, yellow fever, plague and filariasis, appear to have natural habitats. Plague, if represented by dots, each dot indicating a thousand deaths, covers the whole of

---

* In a rapidly changing world scene, Simmons' *Global Epidemiology*[15] and the *World Atlas of Epidemic Diseases*[24] are somewhat out of date, but useful for general reference.

the Indian sub-continent in a mantle of black. Trachoma has a predilection for peoples in the Mediterranean zone; Spain, Italy, Greece, North Africa, the Near East, Siberia and North China. Sleeping sickness travels in Central Africa with the tsetse fly. Yellow fever stretches in a broad band across the middle of Africa and South America – ships have taken it, at some time or another, to Bristol in England and to the Eastern shores of North America, but never to India and other Eastern lands where it would naturally be expected to flourish. The schistosomas, causing the debilitating bilharzia disease, are limited to Africa, Asia and South America.

A great many specific infections tend to occur more frequently, and to be more severe, as we progress from the temperate zone through the Mediterranean zone to the tropical zone. Many severe specific infections, e.g. malaria, plague, cholera, leprosy, hookworm, are now rarely seen outside the tropics and parts of the Mediterranean. The plight of the tropics can best be seen in the devastating impact of malaria.

Malaria affects Africa, most of Asia, and Central and South America, involving 1900 million persons living in malarious territories. It is endemic in 145 out of the 209 countries for which data are available. Data provided by 30 countries of the African region, attending a conference at Brazzaville in 1972, indicated that 196 millions out of 201 millions were at risk and in 1974 it was said that 268 millions living south of the Sahara were exposed.[23] In eleven African countries, for which relevant data were available, in 1971, 12·6 per cent of patients were malaria cases. It is the cause of immense loss of infant and child life. In the world as a whole in 1973 some 140 million persons had clinical attacks of malaria and possibly 1·5 million died of the disease.[23]

The remarkable differences in the burden of infectious disease between tropical and temperate zones is further illustrated by comparing deaths from infective and parasitic diseases (abridged list, A 1–44, 1965) see p. 35 in the two parts of the northern hemisphere of the Americas. In Mexico, in 1970, infective and parasitic diseases accounted for 23·1 per cent of deaths from all causes; in the USA they accounted for only 0·9 per cent.

Intestinal infections covering, a wide range of conditions, are the cause of widespread illness throughout the tropical and Mediterranean worlds. In 1962, diarrhoea and enteritis (B 36, abridged list, 1955) accounted for a third of all deaths in Egypt (see also comparison of developed and underdeveloped worlds p. 35). Gastro-intestinal infections go largely unrecorded, unless leading to death, so that the real extent of illness is immensely greater. Cockburn has said very truly that 'when account is taken of the deficiencies in reporting cases or deaths from the infectious diseases it can be concluded that the weight of communicable disease in developing countries is vastly greater than it appears and indeed must be an almost insupportable hindrance to the improvement of social well-being and to economic improvement.'[4]

But it would be wrong to assume from this that the temperate zone, with all its development, necessarily has less infection than the rest of the world. Certainly deaths from specific infections cannot be looked upon as the only guide to an understanding of world distribution of infections. In England and Wales

(1971), there were 72,907 deaths (abbreviated list 1965, B 1–18, 24–5, 31–5) in which infections played a major role; this was 12·7 per cent of the total. Only 4,169 (0·4 per cent of total deaths) were caused by notifiable infectious disease (B 1–3, 5–16).[7] The chief difference between the two regions of the world lies in the nature of the infections; in the temperate zone they are predominantly respiratory and non-notifiable.

World wide differences are undergoing rapid change under the influence of development and public health. The effect of public health can be seen in the mortality from the common ailments of children – whooping cough, diphtheria, measles and scarlet fever. Taking the four together the mortality per hundred thousand had fallen in the decade 1961/2 to 1971/2 as follows: Netherlands 0·2 to 0·0, USA 0·3 to 0·05, Switzerland 0·3 to 0·05, England and Wales 0·4 to 0·1, Canada 0·6 to 0·1, France 0·8 to 0·1, Portugal 4·6 to 2·9, Mexico 33·8 to 10·9, Chile 39·0 to 3·5 and Guatemala 147·0 to 80·0.[15, 7]

Tuberculosis, a world wide infection which thrives in overcrowded conditions, has undergone remarkable changes in prevalence. It has long been the scourge of industrialized countries and of overcrowded eastern cities. The temperate zone, the scene of its greatest activity, has brought the disease under control with a shift of balance to Mediterranean and tropical zones. But even here, making allowance for under-reporting, the condition is markedly declining. Between 1950 and 1970/1, the death rate per hundred thousand for tuberculosis of the respiratory system fell from 58 to 7·1 in France, from 14 to 1·8 in Denmark, from 144 to 17·5 in Portugal and from 140 to 12·4 in Japan. In Hong Kong (29) and Chile (23·7) rates remain relatively high; in Jordan (7) and Costa Rica (5·7) there is little, perhaps because of the nature of the terrain, or peculiarities in living conditions; or maybe, as is often the case, deaths go unrecorded.

Similar striking changes have taken place in other diseases influenced by the discovery of new and effective preventive measures. Poliomyelitis, for years prevailed in the temperate zone, where hygiene had advanced sufficiently to prevent immunization by repeated subclinical doses in infancy probably conveyed by food or water. In 1949, cases reported per hundred thousand varied from 413 in Iceland, 37 in Sweden, 28 in USA, 21 in Australia, 14 in England and Wales, to 5 in France, 2 in Belgium, 1·6 in the Netherlands and 1·1 in Yugoslavia. By 1972 the picture had changed with a reversal of rôles. The temperate industrial zone had virtually eliminated poliomyelitis. In 14 highly developed countries the number of reported cases aggregated 76; whereas in 9 underdeveloped countries, with a much smaller total population, there were 1,386 cases. In 1970 Mexico, no doubt reflecting improvements in hygiene of food and water which will have lessened natural immunization in infancy, reported 2,043 cases, Zaire 584, Turkey and Mali 283.[4]

Thus the regions of the world with greatly differing climates present equally different pictures of disease and death. Nevertheless it is doubtful whether the climate, or indeed any other of the physical geogens, is significantly involved in these differences (see Ch. 5). Most of the differences are due to social and biological factors upon which development and the use of public health have brought their influence to bear.

Degenerative disease

The two main classes of degenerative disease, new growth and cardiovascular degeneration, are to be found the world over, although in markedly different patterns. Much of the difference is associated with ageing, which may be defined as 'an increased liability to dying under the ordinary stresses of life', but we are left to ask ourselves whether there is such a thing as ageing in itself, or whether every manifestation of it can be attributed to a process we normally call disease. Grandfather seems to be running down like a clock, but what is the underlying cause of his stiffness, asthenia, short-windedness, and loss of memory? Is it widespread intrinsic degeneration of his connective tissue, with an impaired capacity for repair? Or is it the hardening of his arteries, or chronic bronchitis and emphysema? The answer is not clear, but let us make a critical distinction: an intrinsic change in the vitality of the body cells, such as their capacity to multiply, or the hormonal environment in which they live, we will call ageing; a change caused by interferences from outside, we will call disease, even when this operates indirectly, as by lessening the supply of blood to essential organs by damaging the blood vessels. On this analysis, it seems unlikely that anyone dies purely from being old; disease is always a heavy ingredient, but clearly disease of a different kind from the ecological competition of nucleoprotein, which we have described in Chapter 2. It is not due to competition; it comes in late and slowly and does not involve the defence mechanisms.

Much of man's morbidity and mortality is now caused by degenerative diseases – atheroma, chronic bronchitis, high blood pressure – due, it would seem, to new ways of living, or to old ways now given a chance to produce long-term effects. Degenerative disease, the result of chemical, neurological, or even bacterial disturbances, may have its roots in the man-made geogens of modern life – stresses, diet, pollution of the air, and habits. It may also at least in part be the result of intrinsic processes in the germ plasm – the effects of genes, acting in the post-reproductive period of life, when the guns of selection are more difficult to bring to bear.[12]

Atheroma, due to the deposition to cholesterol and other fats under the lining of the larger arteries, is probably the end-result of several mechanisms, including the formation of small blood clots on the walls of arteries in response to repeated injuries and stresses, and the consumption of too much and the wrong sort of food. Chronic bronchitis progressing to emphysema and congestive heart failure is a slow destruction of lung tissue, the victim of repeated insults from mild infections, dust, tobacco smoke, and fumes from the factory ovens. High blood pressure, which contributes to atheroma, and to the deaths from cerebral vascular disease, although little understood, is almost certainly due to noxious influences related to man's environment.

In most countries the annual incidence of cancer per 100,000 population increases from about 100 cases at age 40 to 150 at age 50; thereafter it doubles in each decade to reach 1,200 at age 80.[16] In countries with a relatively young population, as for example Africa, where only 10 per cent are over 40 years of age, the incidence of cancer must be lower than in countries with greater proportions of old people. Inadequate diagnosis and reporting, themselves dependent on lack of medical and statistical services, play an even more important rôle than with infectious diseases. The calculation of absolute incidence and prevalence is generally not possible, and the usual method of comparison is still that of relative incidence, as a proportion of post-mortem findings or of hospital cases.

We do not know the cause of cancer, but the more we learn about 'the nearer causes' (Rous), the clearer it becomes that the main differences which occur in its relative incidence depend upon exogenous factors, chemical substances, radiation, infections, diet, sunlight, with long-continued provocation. Such factors themselves depend upon habits, e.g. circumcision, sunlight, and smoking, rather than upon matters intrinsically related to the physical and climatic character of the earth's surface; the Kangri warmer held next to the skin, or the excessive use of red Chilli peppers in the food; the eggs of bilharzia in the bladder, and a hundred other seemingly harmless episodes, may be playing a rôle in the production of different cancers. Circumcision is associated with a low incidence of cancer in the cervix and vice versa. Cancer of the cervix is incompatible with virginity; and it increases with declining economic standards.

In the great majority of human cancers, the aetiological agent is not known. Hepatic cancer is likely to be related in some unexplained way to diet, possibly to deficient protein or to frequent fluctuations in its intake, or to one or other of the spices most used in Africa and Asia; so too is gastric carcinoma, where the amount and character of the fat consumed, or the method of its cooking, may be the chief consideration in South-East Asia, if not in Japan. Cancers of the bucco-pharyngeal region are likely to be related in some way to the habits of tobacco chewing and such customs as chutta smoking, where the lighted end of the cigar is within the mouth – although the method of curing tobacco may well be invoked to explain discrepancies, such as the absence of cheek cancer in Indonesia. Some small amount of cancer depends on industrial practices. Chimney sweeps, workers in gas, tar, pitch, or creosote, and fishermen, get cancer of the scrotum through contact with soot and oil; aniline dye workers get cancer of the bladder; and at one time 50 per cent of Joachimstal miners died of cancer of the lung, due to inhalation of radioactive gases. Much exposure to radiation gives rise to leukaemia. Cancer in the form of 'sarcomata' has also been experimentally produced in animals by virus infection since Rous first filtered sarcoma in the Plymouth Rock Fowl (1910).

But behind the immediate causes of cancer, something even more fundamental can be dimly seen, something we may call a failure of ecology. Living species exist at the expense of one another, but on the whole they remain loyal to themselves, so too in the individual, dozens of organs and millions of cells remain controlled in the general interest of the germ plasm. Each cell, capable of rapid division, as seen in tissue culture, is held in check by some sensitive system of signals. Cancer cells no longer obey the signals. The germ plasm has lost its grip. Chemicals, radiation, body hormones, viruses, destructive genes, non-specific inflammatory agents, have produced an irreversible change in the cell proteins, and set the stage for a miniature evolutionary process which ends in the cancer cell.

Cancers in every crevice of the body, and of every type, occur in all peoples. The views which for long prevailed, that there are countries in which cancer is rare or non-existent, and that it is less marked in underdeveloped countries, is now recognized as false.[14] There is no evidence, for example, that primitive Africans have any lessened liability – rather the contrary;[6] that is to say when adequate consideration has been given to the effects of age.

The mapping of cancer is still highly imperfect. World maps resemble those of the cartographers who outlined the land masses in the fourteenth century. Apart from the local incidence and prevalence of certain cancers, including industrial forms, there are a few broad generalizations which can be made. The first of these is the remarkable prevalence of hepatic cancer in Africa and South East Asia. In Indonesia, Java, Sumatra, and among the Bantu miners, hepatomas have been reported as high as 80 per cent of the total cancers.[1] In Western countries in contrast cancer of the liver is no more than 1 to 2 per cent.

Second, cancer of the stomach prevails excessively in Japan, a large part of Western Europe, and the north of South America. Nearly half the cancers in Japan are in the stomach. In contrast in South-East Asia from India to New Guinea and in parts of Africa, the relative incidence is very small. Among the Javanese cancer of the stomach may hardly exist at all.

Third, cancers of the bucco-pharyngeal region, although the types vary much, overshadow all else in most parts of India; 40 per cent of all cancers in males are in this region of the digestive tract.[11] This distinction applies probably to most of South-East Asia, North Africa, to the Bantu, and in China and Japan.

Fourth, cancer of the lung, pleura, and bronchi is particularly marked among males in Western Europe, in the USA, and Australia. In Britain it is the chief cause of death from cancer among males. In contrast little or no lung cancer has been reported in Korea, Sri Lanka, India, Burma, Trinidad, and among the Bantu (Steiner).[16]

Fifth, cancer of the uterine cervix is relatively excessive in India and China, and relatively little-known in Western Europe, the USA, and Australia. There is commonly, but not always, an inverse relationship with the female breast cancer, which, for example, prevails excessively in some parts of Western Europe, in the USA, and in Australia.

Nutritional disorders

The first worldwide survey of the Food and Agriculture Organization (1946)[8] estimated that more than a third (38·6 per cent) of the world's people immediately before the Second World War consumed less on the average than 2,200 calories per head per day; a third (30·8 per cent) ranged between 2,200 and 2,700; a third (30·6 per cent) had enough (over 2,700). After the war the position was worse; nearly two-thirds took in below 2,200. Many lived on a diet of some 1,500 calories, near to the basal metabolic rate.[9] In terms of animal protein, the general picture was even more discouraging. Nearly two-thirds (59·0 per cent) of the world's peoples ate less than 15 grammes daily, little more than half the recommended requirements.

By 1963, the calorie content of the diet had regained the pre-war level, but the protein remained grossly defective throughout the underdeveloped and developing world, where 60 per cent of households derived more than 80 per cent of their calories from cereals, starch, roots and sugar.[10] In 1974, when 2/3 of the world's population still derived 72 per cent of calories from carbohydrates, the numbers estimated to be suffering from malnutrition were varyingly rated at between 400 and 1,500 millions; the true figure may well be not less than 800 millions.[18]

Dietary surveys of sample groups support these estimates. Where the calorie intake is most deficient the diet suffers from lack of balance, with excess of carbohydrate and too little protein, and is also subjected to wide fluctuations in amount, ranging from starvation to abundance, within relatively short spaces of time.

The areas of greatest deficiency are Central America, most of Asia, and some parts of South America, Africa, and the Middle East. Areas less affected include Southern Europe, three countries of Asia, some parts of Africa, of South America, and of the Middle East. A diet above 2,700 calories appears to be limited to the Western world, the New World, USSR, and three countries of South America.[9, 10]

In 1963, over half of the world's population lived on about a quarter of the world's food (made up of 19 per cent of the animal supplies and 44 per cent of the crop food); in Europe, Oceania and North America 29 per cent of the world's population consume 57 per cent of the world's food (comprising 69 per cent of the animal food and 38 per cent of the crop food).[10] It was then calculated that, if the world's population grew at the postulated medium rate, there would be needed, in 1975, 35 per cent more food merely to sustain the existing unsatisfactory diet; for a reasonable improvement 50 per cent more food and 60 per cent more animal products would be needed; in the developing countries the increase in total food might have to reach 80 per cent and of animal foods 120 per cent.[10]

This rapid expansion of food production has not materialized; in fact, an annual increase of only 0·5 per cent was achieved in the underdeveloped world and 1·5 per cent in the developed world; and even this shortfall was further exaggerated by rising consumption in the affluent countries. It now takes five times as much land, water and fertilizer to support the average citizen in Western Europe as it does the average Indian. In 1974, with food production further complicated by world crises of energy, economy and inclement weather, many countries faced famine (Chad, Mali, Mauritania, Niger, Senegal, Upper Volta, Gambia, Ethiopia, parts of Tanzania and Kenya); several were near famine (Bolivia, Syria, Yemen, parts of Nigeria) or on the brink (India, Sudan, Guyana, Guinea and Zaire.[18]

Among the most serious deficiency states now prevailing in many areas of the world are the protein-calorie deficiency diseases, kwashiorkor and marasmus.[20] Kwashiorkor, a syndrome associated with low protein consumption, affecting chiefly the age group 1 to 3, abounds throughout tropical countries, aided no doubt by parasitic infestations, and by the infections which destroy the blood and increase the metabolism during fevers. Protein starvation almost certainly aids the onset of cirrhosis, and, in association with wide fluctuations according to season, may play a part in the development of hepatic cancer, which is so prevalent in tropical regions. Yet so little protein is needed to stave off the worst effects of protein starvation. Kwashiorkor, with its retarded growth, depigmentation of the skin and hair, oedema, and liver damage, is absent among the Masai, who eat meat and drink milk; and among peoples, as in Thailand or Africa, within walking distance of the sea or lakes, who are able to eat fish. Nutritional marasmus, affecting chiefly babies under one, exhibiting extreme muscle wastage, loss of subcutaneous fat and very low body weight, is equally widespread.

Among the rice-eating countries, China, Malaya, Java, Japan, there is widespread disease due to lack of vitamin B_1, epidemiologically this affects half the total world population, perhaps a thousand million people. Apart from the final manifestation of beri-beri, which is found on a large scale only in South and East Asia, the ill-effects of a diet of polished rice are many and varied; in particular the babies of mothers starved of aneurin die in convulsions, paralysis, or heart failure, so that infant mortality tends to be high. In maize-eating countries, Italy, Spain, Portugal, Africa, Rumania, and Southern USA, there is pellagra, resulting from deficiency of nicotinic acid, associated with virtual protein starvation. Rickets occurs in Turkey, Yugoslavia, and other countries where infants are denied sunshine without the benefit of a good diet. Keratomalacia, due to avitaminosis A, is most frequent in South-East Asia, paradoxically in the tropical rain belt, where carotene, the precursor of vitamin A, abounds; in Central Java one to three per cent of pre-schoolchildren are said to suffer from acute deficiency with gross scarring of the cornea and blindness together with a high mortality.[3] It is also widespread in South America.[21] Iodine deficiency is still widespread (see p. 41); some 5 million persons in India alone may be suffering from goitre associated with cretinism, feeblemindedness, lowered educational ability, deaf-mutism, thyroid operations, and cancer of the thyroid.[3] Iron-deficiency likewise is everywhere common.[20]

These are but the highlights of specific nutritional diseases – the more obvious clinical manifestations of underfeeding. Poor nutrition predisposes to infections, particularly to tuberculosis; and to infestations, such as hookworm. It is perhaps the chief cause of high death rates from preventible diseases, low expectation of life, high mortality in infancy and early childhood, and disasters in childbirth, which afflict the majority of the human race, particularly those living in the tropical and Mediterranean zones. In 1974, it was said that 'more than

2/3 of 800 million children in the underdeveloped world were severely sick or disabled by malnutrition.[18]

For the Western world, with the lengthening of life that has followed the conquest of infections, an indirect result of technological development, high standards of feeding may have introduced other diseases, particularly diabetes, resulting from a high sugar intake, and the degenerative diseases of the vascular system, which may be related either to too much food in general, or possibly to some one or more articles which have come to play a predominant rôle in modern diet. The temperate zone tends to suffer, like other parts of the world, from less-well-defined iron and vitamin deficiencies in food, which may account in part for widespread secondary anaemias.

Mental ill-health

Little is known outside the temperate zone about the extent to which mental illness is present in different regions of the world. In the United States more than 550,000 persons are in hospitals for mental diseases; another 130,000 mental defectives are in institutions, and a further 100,000 under supervision – making a rate in all of 5·2 persons with mental disorders per thousand of the population.[2] This can be compared with 3·6 per thousand in England and Wales, where 30 per cent of the total hospital beds in the National Health Service are occupied by patients with mental disorders.* But smaller numbers in hospital does not necessarily mean a lower incidence. Hospital provision is probably a totally inadequate means of assessing the departures from normal mental health. Many factors have to be taken into account in such comparison. Hospital treatment varies with social customs and community organization. The liability to senile psychosis varies with the age constitution and the proportions of people with degenerative changes in the cerebro-vascular system – over 10,000 new cases of senile psychosis occur annually in the United Kingdom. In many countries mental illness also is absorbed, as it were within the community without special provision. Most of the mentally handicapped in all communities find a useful place to occupy unobtrusively; but the handicapped are increasingly prejudiced as the life of the industrialized community becomes more complicated.

The differential rates for schizophrenia, manic depression, and psychopathic personalities, and still more hysteria and anxiety, are almost impossible to gauge in the absence of detailed studies, which cannot easily be conducted, for most of the world, without medical and social services. Neurosis has been said to be more prominent in the highly developed world, as an accompaniment of secularization in an industrial society (see p. 112) – absenteeism, psychoneurosis seen in the doctors' surgeries, suicide, divorce, child delinquency, have all been given as examples. The rates for many of these conditions, in countries where reliable statistics are available, vary much; for example, for suicide per 100,000 of the population (1970/71): Switzerland 18·4, USA 11·1, Japan 15·6, Norway 8·4, Denmark 21·5 and Czechoslovakia 25·3.[7] But it is doubtful whether such

* Personal communication Dr Abe Adelstein O.P.C.S. London.

a comparison is of any value without examining the culture of the society in which suicide occurs. The Japanese scene may differ appreciably from that in the USA, and still more from that in Burma or Bolivia.

Most of the phenomena which we use to assess mental health are based on Western values and social patterns, which other countries may not have adopted. In the underdeveloped countries there is much which is of significance to mental health which we have not yet sufficiently studied. The tempo of life, where the drive for material advancement is less, may well be more favourable to mental health. Meditation, which plays an important rôle in Burmese life, and the absorbing ritual of religion as in Bali – in their present form and as they change with 'development' – are likely to be of the very greatest significance. When there are so many unknowns, we should withhold judgment upon mental health until measurements can be devised and epidemiological research undertaken.

4. The Developed and Underdeveloped Worlds

In the last chapter disease was seen to be distributed in a very varying pattern throughout the world. Here we see how much the world's picture depends on socio-economic considerations. In very general terms, the health of every country depends upon its state of development; by contrasting the picture presented by representative groups of countries in different states of development we can see, at least in its major considerations, what differences exist.

The world has been developing new ways of living ever since man was able to live in settled communities, if not before. But 'development' which is accompanied by social and technological changes affecting everything in the lives of the people, from the homes they live in to the chemicals they manufacture to protect them from major infections, was speeded up considerably in Europe some time in the middle of the seventeenth century; it became much faster when industrialization began a century later (see Chapter 13), and it has now spread so widely that every country in the world has been affected, in varying degree.

Development affects health and disease both favourably and unfavourably; favourably, by more or less unconscious changes in living standards, in diet, habits, housing, communications, literacy, social developments, etc., as well as by a conscious growth of public health designed to overcome particular hazards; unfavourably, by changes in the age structure of the population, by adverse aspects of industrialization (for example, smoke pollution), or by the acquisition of new harmful habits (for example, smoking).

Most people in developing countries live in villages where life, with a traditional organization and a hierarchical control, tends to be moulded by long-standing custom. The family, often extended, is a strong binding force. Life on the farm, and simple handicraft skills, in which men, women, and children take part, are based upon the home. Town living is limited to a few large cities. Such communities depend mainly upon agriculture, with as much as 80 per cent of subsistence farming. Husbandry uses hand methods, lacks fertilizers or any of the advantages of scientific practices, and makes poor use of manpower, as indicated by the large number (over 100) workers to the square mile of agricultural land; in contrast there is no mechanization, as indicated by the small number of tractors. Few manufacturing industries exist, so that whatever manufactured goods are available have to be imported, and little use is made of energy from coal, water, or petroleum. Capital and capitalized equipment are lacking, transportation systems are primitive, and inadequate use is made of the country's raw materials. Income per head, and as a percentage of world income, is low; so too is the level of literacy and of services of all kinds –

financial, organizational, professional, social – which ultimately depend upon it.

The peoples of these countries are subject in varying degree to uncontrolled hazards of famine, flood, and pestilence, so that the high birth rates are counter-balanced by high death rates, often with wide fluctuations. Diet is at, or below, 2,000 calories per head per day. The high infant and child mortalities, and a low expectation of life, leads to a characteristic population structure.

The picture presented by the developed world is the mirror image of the underdeveloped world. Famine, flood, and pestilence no longer occur; agriculture is generally second to industry; agricultural methods are highly mechanized and great use is made of scientific disciplines, including plant genetics. The number of agriculturalists per square mile is low (around 30), the tractor is greatly in evidence (UK, one to 57 arable acres), and farming is of a type designed to sell its products in the markets of the world, and not solely to keep the farmer and his family. The average diet is near to, or above, 3,000 calories per person per day. Great use is made of coal, water, and petroleum for power. Capital and capital equipment, transport, development of raw materials, income per head and as a percentage of the world income, literacy, and services of all kinds are at a high level.

Town life

The most characteristic sign of development is that of town living (see Chapter 10). In 1972, most of Europe had more than 50 per cent of town dwellers (Sweden 81·4, Denmark 79·9, UK 78·3, Belgium 86·7, Norway 44·9) as compared with the countries of the East, South America and Africa (India 20·7, Indonesia 17·4, Afghanistan 15·0, Togo 13·0, Sri Lanka 22·3), where urbanization is less than 30 per cent.

Urban life differs from that in the village by being more impersonal. Individuals and families tend to be more separated from the kinship group, and social organization in the form of traditional and local groupings is less in evidence. Women are economically employed to a less extent and in work of a different kind which takes them away from the home.

The lower death rates for developed countries are directly related to town living. In a group of 25 countries (in and around 1950) where town living exceeded 50 per cent, 12 had crude general death rates below 10 per thousand in contrast with 4 out of 29 where urbanization was below 40 per cent.[17] Infant mortality in 15 out of 24 countries with more than 50 per cent town dwellers was below 50 per cent; as compared with 4 out of 30 countries, where urbanization was less than 40 per cent.

Employment*

Striking differences exist in the nature of employment and in the extent to which women work outside the home. In the Congo, Botswana and Zanzibar, women constitute approximately half the working population, whereas in the USA they represent only about one third, as shown in the pi diagrams (Fig. 4.1).

* Comparability of economic activity is not easy to obtain owing to variable interpretation as to what this means. The Congo has been used as an example of countries recording 'unpaid family workers'. Botswana (49·95 women) and Zanzibar (47·4 women) gave similar proportions in the *Demographic Yearbook* 1972. USA. in 1972: women 37·2, men 62·8 per cent.

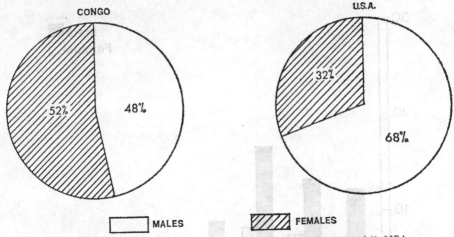

Fig. 4.1 Percentage of women in the working population of A. Congo and B. USA.

Economic employment begins earlier in the underdeveloped world. The proportions employed at lower ages, particularly of women, is greater and the reverse at higher ages. The employment of children (not recorded statistically) is greater in the underdeveloped countries (Figs. 4.2 and 4.3).

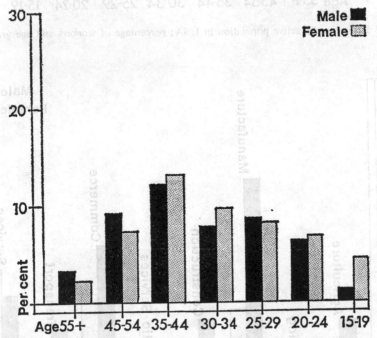

Fig. 4.2 Economically active population in Congo (1962). Botswana (1964) was: up-to-24, women 13·5, men 17·7; 25 to 34, women 11·7, men 8·7; 35 to 44, women 9·4, men 8·2; 45 to 54, women 6·7, men 7·1; 55 and over, women 8·2, men 8·3 (*Demographic Yearbook*, 1972[7]).

In the developing world, as represented by the Congo, the majority of the workers are in agriculture (Fig. 4.5); whereas in the developed world, as repre-

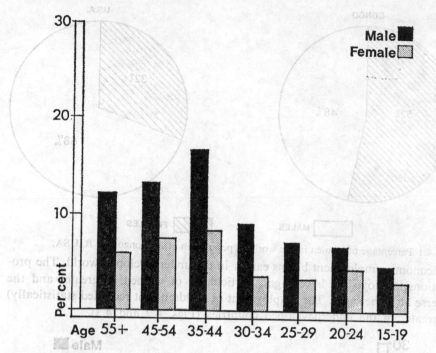

Fig. 4.3 Economically active population in USA; percentage of workers and age groups.

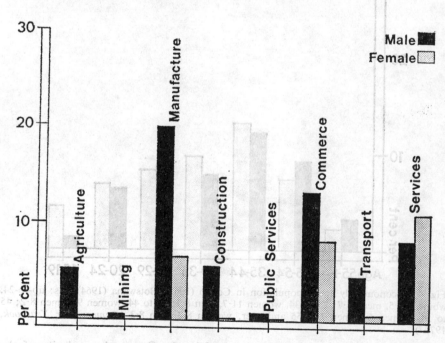

Fig. 4.4 Economically active population in USA; percentage of males and females at work in different occupations.

sented by the USA, employment in agriculture is less than in either manufacture or services and no more than equal to that in commerce (Fig. 4.4). The much higher proportion of women 'economically active' in the developing world is seen as a function of agriculture in which women act as unpaid family workers.

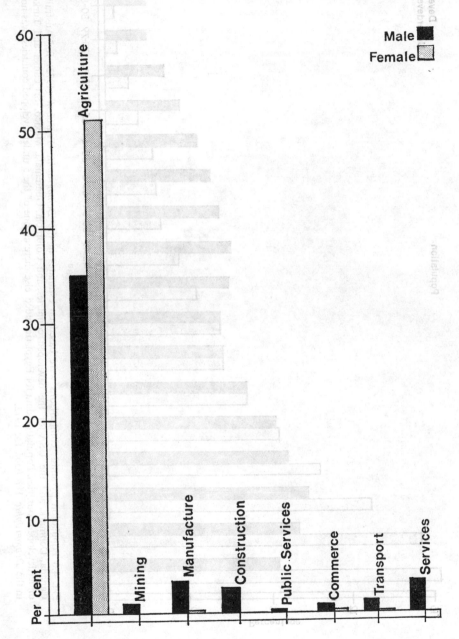

Fig. 4.5 Economically active population in Congo; percentage of males and females at work in different occupations.

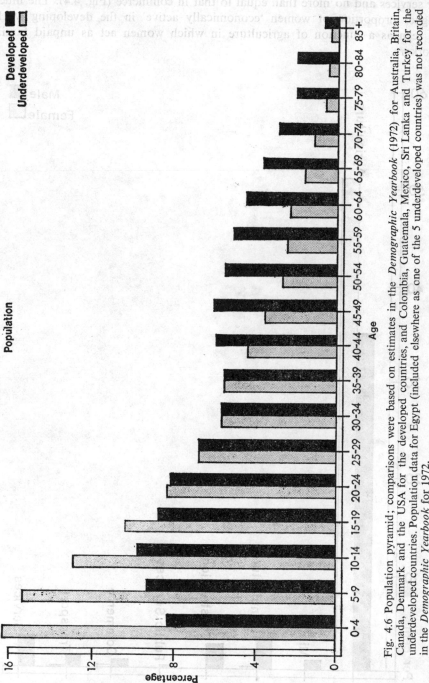

Fig. 4.6 Population pyramid; comparisons were based on estimates in the *Demographic Yearbook* (1972) for Australia, Britain, Canada, Denmark and the USA for the developed countries, and Colombia, Guatemala, Mexico, Sri Lanka and Turkey for the underdeveloped countries. Population data for Egypt (included elsewhere as one of the 5 underdeveloped countries) was not recorded in the *Demographic Yearbook* for 1972.

The population pyramid

In the underdeveloped world (Fig. 4.6), the population pyramid is broadly based, with a nearly uniform decline in numbers from childhood years until extreme old age. In the developed world (Fig. 4.6) the pyramid has a narrower base with greater uniformity from early adult life and through middle age. The proportions in the upper age groups gradually approximate.

The peoples of the developed world are older, in the sense that proportions in the higher age groups are greater at every age group up to 85 and over; 10·3 per cent are over 65 years and over in the five developed countries and 3·5 per cent in the five underdeveloped countries. In the UK, the percentage over 65 years in 1970 was 13, and in France 13·6. There is an excess of females in both types of country at higher ages, but substantially more so in the developed world; 6 per cent of females are 65 and over in the developed world as against 4·3 of males; in the underdeveloped countries, 1·9 per cent female as against 1·6 per cent male.*

The greater expectation of life and the greatly diminished child mortality in the developed world together markedly change the balance of the generations. In the five developed countries, out of every 1,000 persons, 266 were under 15 years of age and 110 were 65 years and over (in UK, 243 and 131). In the five underdeveloped countries, 444 were under 15 and 38 were 65 and over. In these respects, the underdeveloped world can be likened to Europe in the middle of the last century when, in 1841, England and Wales for example had 361 children and 44 persons 65 years and over in every thousand of the population.

Births and deaths†

The developed countries have much lower birth and death rates. The five developed countries had birth rates (1972) averaging 14·9 and death rates averaging 10·6; five underdeveloped countries had birth rates averaging 44·5 and death rates averaging 19·0. The infant mortality of the five developed countries was 15·8; only one of the five underdeveloped countries (Sri Lanka) had a recorded infant mortality (1972, 50·3).

The birth rate in the developed world is that of countries which have reached the low stationary phase on the demographic curve (see Chapter 8); the rate in the developing world, at or near the biological maximum, is that of countries in the high stationary, or early expanding, stage (see p. 70).

The low birth rate, together with a small infant mortality, reduces the strain of childbearing in terms of effective population production. One million women in five countries of the developing world in 1954 gave birth to 224,433 babies, of which 194,238 were alive at the end of one year, and 164,606 at the end of five years. One million women in five countries of the developed world gave birth to 136,032 babies, of which 132,437 were alive at the end of a year, and

* Sri Lanka had an excess of males (2·0 per cent) as against females (1·6 per cent).

† Comparisons of births and deaths were made on estimates in the Demographic Year-books 1954 and 1972 for five developed countries (Australia, Britain, Canada, Denmark and USA.) and five underdeveloped countries (Colombia, Egypt, Guatemala, Mexico and Sri Lanka).

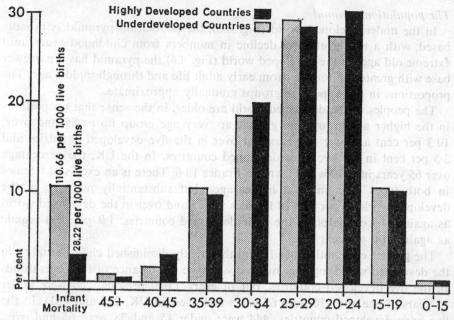

Fig. 4.7 Live births by maternal age.

131,867 at the end of five years. Thus with about 60 per cent of the gestations, the developed world after five years had achieved 80 per cent of population increase in the underdeveloped world.

The proportion of babies born to women in each group during the childbearing period reflects clearly the biological fertility of women in general, since it remains roughly similar in the two types of country (Fig. 4.7), despite the prevalence of artificial limitation in the one and its general absence in the other. Thus in successive five-year age groups from 15 to 45 the proportions are: underdeveloped, 10, 30, 29, 19, 9, 2·5; developed, 10, 27, 29, 17, 11, 1·5. The proportion of women of childbearing age, which is higher in the developed world at every age group from 15 to 45 (see Fig. 4.10), has to be taken into account.

Deaths

Vital statistics of countries with few doctors and poor recording systems are necessarily incomplete. The countries selected fell into the intermediate *Demographic Yearbook* classification (see Chapter 22) recording 'less than 90 per cent'; i.e., in advance of countries for which 'no specific information is available' (possibly half the world's peoples). Evidence of poor registration can be seen in the higher proportion of deaths certified as due to senility – in 1954, 14 per cent as compared with 1 per cent; and in Sri Lanka, for example, 24·4 per cent were certified in 1972, under B45 of the abridged list, as due to 'senility without mention of psychosis, illdefined and unknown causes'. This implies that the true picture of mortality in the underdeveloped world as a whole is worse than the recorded data suggests, since analysable statistics can be obtained only by countries already substantially developed.

The pattern of deaths in age groups differs markedly in the two types of country. A high proportion of people in the underdeveloped world die in early childhood. In 1970/1, 46·5 per cent of deaths in the underdeveloped countries occurred under 5 years of age as compared with 3·9 per cent in the developed countries. The comparison can be made with Europe a century ago, when England and Wales had 40 per cent of deaths under five years.

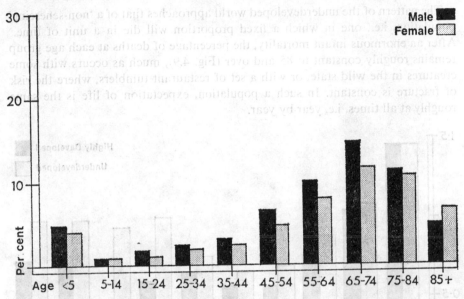

Fig. 4.8 Death by age and sex in highly developed countries.

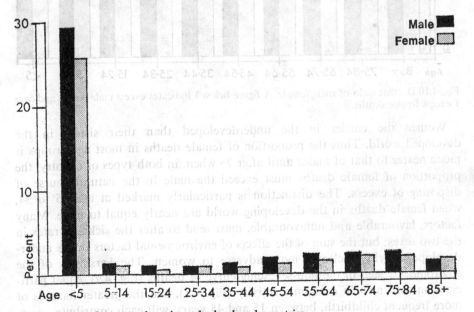

Fig. 4.9 Deaths by age and sex in underdeveloped countries.

The developed world (Fig. 4.8) shows the characteristic of a 'senescence curve'. From a relatively small mortality in younger years (excluding infancy), the percentage in each age group rises slowly to middle life, and then bulges out to a maximum at between 65 and 75 years of age. Most people live long enough for declining resistance, a biological event, to make itself apparent in a rapidly increasing death rate amongst later age groups. The life of man can, on the whole, be predicted.

The pattern of the underdeveloped world approaches that of a 'non-senescing' population, i.e., one in which a fixed proportion will die in a unit of time.[5] After an enormous infant mortality, the percentage of deaths at each age group remains roughly constant to 85 and over (Fig. 4.9), much as occurs with some creatures in the wild state, or with a set of restaurant tumblers, where the risk of fracture is constant. In such a population, expectation of life is the same roughly at all times, i.e. year by year.

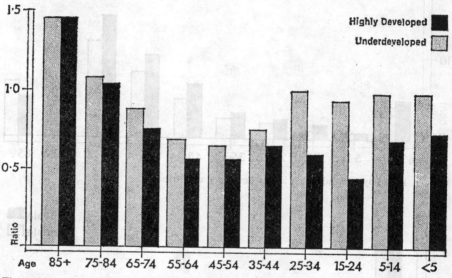

Fig. 4.10 Deaths: ratio of male/female. A figure below 1 indicates excess male deaths and over 1 excess female deaths.

Women die earlier in the underdeveloped than their sisters in the developed world. Thus the proportion of female deaths in most age groups is much nearer to that of males until after 75 when, in both types of country, the proportion of female deaths must exceed the male in the natural course of disposing of excess. The distinction is particularly marked at age 25 to 34, when female deaths in the developing world are nearly equal to male. Many factors, favourable and unfavourable, must tend to alter the sickness rates in the two sexes; but the sum of the effects of environmental factors in the underdeveloped world is clearly more adverse to women. The harshness of the environment, seen in the non-senescing curve of deaths (Fig. 4.9), equal participation with men in economic activity (Fig. 4.1), and the greater hazards of more frequent childbirth, between 15 and 45 years, will each contribute.

Causes of death

In the developed world, diseases of the circulatory system, together with cancer, account for the great bulk of the mortality. In 1954, diseases of the heart, intracranial lesions and cancer accounted for 66 per cent of all deaths, as compared with 8 per cent in the underdeveloped countries; and in 1970/1 66·5 per cent as compared with 13 per cent (Fig. 4.11). In 1954, heart disease and disasters of the circulatory system accounted for half the total deaths in the developed, as compared with five per cent in the underdeveloped, countries; in 1970/1, 48 per cent as compared with 8·9 per cent (B27–30 abbreviated list 1965).

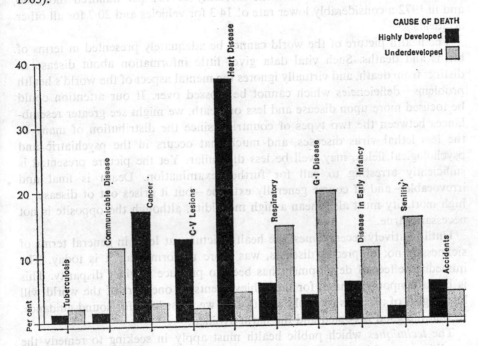

Fig. 4.11 Causes of death.

In contrast, the underdeveloped world succumbs enormously to infections. In 1954, conditions of an infective, or probably infective nature, caused 45 per cent of total deaths in the underdeveloped countries, as compared with 11 per cent in the developed countries, (12·7 per cent in 1971 (see p. 16); and 11 per cent of communicable disease, as compared with 1 per cent (cf. 1970/1, 13·6 per cent and 0·4 per cent). In 1954, gastro-intestinal disease represented 20 per cent of total deaths in the underdeveloped as compared with 4 per cent in the developed countries (cf. 1970/1, 8·7 per cent and 1·3 per cent). In 1964, the underdeveloped countries, with 98 millions, had 4,106 deaths from typhoid and paratyphoid fevers; and in 1970/1, with 129 millions, 3,509 deaths. The developed countries (1962) with 281 millions, had 26 deaths from typhoid and paratyphoid fevers; and in 1970/1, with 304 millions, only one death.[7]

Tuberculosis now seems to be a world wide scourge of something like the same proportions; at least as a recorded cause of death (in 1954, one per cent in the underdeveloped countries and 0·75 per cent in the developed; in 1970/1, 1·5 per cent and 0·23 per cent). But the true picture is almost certainly much underestimated, particularly in underdeveloped countries (see also p. 17).

The balance of advantage is certainly with the developed countries, but the end-result of such varying factors gives rise to a widely differing pattern in different regions, countries, and even districts. An example of this is the deaths from accidents which are dependent upon habits of driving, the state of industry, and the increase in old people; the result of this interaction not only differs, but is also subject to, variation as circumstances change; England and Wales in 1954 had an accident mortality of 107 per hundred thousand and in 1972 a considerably lower rate of 14·3 for vehicles and 20·7 for all other accidents.

The health picture of the world cannot be adequately presented in terms of births and deaths. Such vital data gives little information about disease as distinct from death, and virtually ignores the mental aspect of the world's health problems – deficiencies which cannot be glossed over. If our attention could be focused more upon disease and less on death, we might see greater resemblances between the two types of countries, since the distribution of many of the less lethal virus diseases, and much that occurs in the psychiatric and psychological fields, may well be less dissimilar. Yet the picture presented is sufficiently arresting to call for further examination. Death is final and irrevocable – and of course generally extreme – but it arises out of disease. A high mortality must also mean a high morbidity, although the opposite is not necessarily true.

Until relatively recent times, the health picture, at least in general terms of sickness if not of precise diseases, was more uniform than it is today. The immediate effect of development has been to produce a wider disparity. This is but a temporary phase, for the achievements of one part of the world will be the goal of all. It is to public health that we must look for sound guidance, so that the good is copied and the harm avoided.

The *techniques* which public health must apply in seeking to remedy the conditions resulting in ill-health in both developed and underdeveloped countries are of course many and varied, and beyond the scope of this book. But in successful public health we are involved not only in technology, but also in philosophical, anthropological, organizational, social, and economic considerations which determine the success or failure of technical procedures. It is with these wider issues – ecology, town living, occupation, industrialization, food, family life, hospitals, geography and climate, population, and beliefs and customs – that the next nine chapters will be concerned.

Part Three: The Pursuit of Health

5. Geography

The pursuit of health through the environment has fascinated medical writers ever since Hippocrates first described the effects of 'airs, waters, places'.[2] For 4,000 years, climate and season in relation to health and disease have been studied assiduously and commented upon voluminously. Geographical factors, or 'geogens', cover the whole gamut of influences that bear upon man's welfare – social, biological, physical – although it is not always easy to distinguish one category from another.

Social and biological geogens

Socially, the human being makes his own geogens, by population distribution and density, communications, beliefs and customs, habits of living, industrialization, occupation, and by the environment which he shapes for his daily life – housing, diet, clothing, and sanitation.

Biologically, the man is an incident in an ecological episode, in which disease is the result of aggression by other animal or vegetable organisms, or where ill-health results from tissue changes, some reversible, others irreversible, which are independent of other forms of life. The effective agents of disease, animal or vegetable organisms, can be introduced to the body *directly*, as with cholera, typhoid, or tuberculosis, by inhalation, ingestion, or through wounds – or *indirectly*, as with malaria, by means of a vector (carrier). For many, as for worms, an intermediary host is needed for the development of a larval stage; man may himself be the intermediary host. In some instances, as with plague, animals are the main habitat of the infection and man's involvement an incident.

The geographical patterns, and endemic foci, where specific diseases more or less regularly prevail,[6] and the variations within countries, districts, and classes are, as we have seen (Chapter 4), generally related most directly to social or biological, rather than to physical geogens.

Most of the difference in the picture presented by tropical and Mediterranean countries is due to diseases like cholera, small pox, enteritis and typhoid, which, if not prevented, might prevail anywhere; malaria, plague, cholera, leprosy, hookworm, bilharzia, etc., prevail, in the last resort, only because tropical peoples have not yet organized their lives in such a way that the chain of causation is broken; all have at some time, within the extraordinary and often inexplicable epidemic process, been distributed widely throughout the world. Small pox, which prevailed until recently in Africa, Asia, and South America, was one of the commonest diseases of the whole world during the eighteenth century. As late as 1754, a tenth of all mankind was crippled or disfigured by it,[7] and 50 years ago it was still widespread. Throughout the middle of the nineteenth century, outbreaks of cholera caused a heavy mortality in England and, in the view of many, were the real reason for progress in public health organization.

The same story of disease and death from diarrhoea and enteritis in Eastern and near eastern countries (see p. 16) could be told of Europe until well into the nineteenth century. Until 50 years ago diarrhoea was one of the most dangerous ailments of children under two years, accounting in some countries for over half the deaths. Today less than 0·5 per cent of total deaths within the Western orbit can be ascribed to it. The differences between the developed and underdeveloped worlds are often mainly due to control in the disposal of human waste. Many hold that the greatest single factor in world disease today is the common habit of indiscriminate defaecation. The manuring of land with uncomposted human waste also handicaps greatly, particularly through the spread of worms.

Much therefore that we see in the world's picture of disease is directly the result of man's failure to break the chain of causation. Insect transmission, in malaria or filariasis, for example, accounts for an enormous loss of life and debilitating illness. The whole of malnutrition is, in the last resort, preventable; so that the hundreds of millions who live in malnourishment, as well as the millions who have specific nutritional diseases, are suffering from man's failure to make an adequate adjustment between his social, biological, or physical geogens. Infection and malnutrition go hand in hand round one of the many vicious circles of which disease is the focal point.

Degenerative disease, when represented as black dots of 1,000 deaths, envelopes the continent of Europe and North America in a pall every bit as black as that of plague in India – although it may mean less to the community because it occurs in middle and later years, whereas plague kills young and old alike. India will exchange, in time, her mantle of plague and other infections for that of degenerative disease, unless, before then, the causes of degeneration have been discovered. The same forms of cancer may not be developed to excess, for much will depend upon the retention of old habits and the acquisition of new ones. If India, or any other tropical country, takes on the same pattern of cigarette smoking and pollution of the atmosphere with industrial waste, it is likely to follow England in the sharp spiral of deaths from carcinoma of the lung. The increase in mortality of lung cancer in Japan suggests that the spiral there has already begun. Burma, like the U.S.A., may abandon the cigar for the cigarette to her disadvantage. If, however, the near causes of cancer can be sufficiently determined, health education may be able to steer newcomers to public health away from dangerous habits.

But when all possible weight has been attached to social and biological factors, there remains much evidence for regarding physical geogens as as of importance to health, so that people who live in different regions and districts and under varying climates may be specially favoured or prejudiced.

Physically, the earth's surface is important for health, if we exclude height above sea level, mainly on account of the nature of the soil and because of the climate – temperature, barometric pressure, wind, sunshine and cloud, rainfall, humidity, and latitude. The physical characteristics of the globe, and its climate, must in the last resort have determined man's welfare and shaped his progress. By forming the soil, and indirectly controlling animal and vegetable life, they will have supplied him with the basic essentials of life, including clothing and food. By their responsibility ultimately for his diet, they will have determined his health, his propagation, and his civilization. The monsoons have favoured rice growing; the trade-winds have taken merchants and adventurers across the oceans, carrying incidentally the seeds of new vegetation from one part of the globe to another, and of old diseases to new habitats.

The cloudy atmosphere of the northern hemisphere, which keeps out the sunshine, must be counted as a sinner in depriving northern peoples of sun-made vitamin D, thus accounting for rickets which was an endemic condition of the temperate zone until cod liver oil and artificial vitamins were available. Both chronic bronchitis and carcinoma of the lung in Britain are, in some measure, due to the atmospheric conditions, which hold down the smoke and turn mist into 'smog'. Where cloudless skies prevail such disabilities hardly occur in the absence of cigarette smoking; but in contrast fair skins without pigmentation have an added liability to skin cancer. Rheumatism has long been related to damp and cold, with what precise mechanism we no longer claim to know.

Lack of trace elements in the soil does not apparently cause man, unlike animals and plants, much obvious harm.[1] Neither the cachexia and anaemia (pining), which is seen in ruminants on lands deficient in cobalt, nor the paralysis (swayback) of sheep, where soil content of copper is low, occur in man. Plants suffer in various ways from lack of boron, manganese, and zinc, but man rides above these difficulties of metabolism. Yet he is handicapped by lack of iodine in the mountainous regions of Switzerland, the Balkans, the Asian plateau, the Rockies, and Himalayas, particularly when living on older geologic formations or on sedimentations (see p. 22). Iron and copper deficiencies, which show themselves as anaemia, particularly in the temperate zone, may well also be determined by the soil.

The physical character of the soil or sub-soil also affects the ease with which water-borne infections occur, and it helps or hinders 'worm' transmission. Thus the soiling of land and waterways is a more serious matter in some parts than others. Hookworm is inhibited by dryness, so that in countries such as Egypt the soiling of land with human faeces is less likely to cause its spread; whereas a lightly moist soil, as in Thailand, Java, or Southern U.S.A., favours it. The chalky Dinaric Alps in Yugoslavia, once soiling of the surface land occurs, favour pollution of the wells. Excessive hydatid disease along the Dalmatian coast, and the Aegean shores of Turkey, may partly have depended upon this fact. The eggs of the worm *Taenia echinococcus*, which dogs excrete in large quantities, more easily gain access to man, and so give rise to the secondary stage of development as cysts in his liver and elsewhere. A similar phenomenon, before active artificial immunization, may have accounted for the relative freedom of Holland, Finland, and Yugoslavia from paralytic poliomyelitis – if, owing to the network of waterways, or to the porous character of the sub-soil, the virus is able to gain access to water supplies, and to immunize by repeated sub-clinical doses without paralysis, in early childhood.

What effect climate has upon bacterial pathogencity is unknown; but it is by no means certain that it is negligible. Amoebae, which devastate the East with abscesses in the liver and elsewhere, can be found in the gut of a high proportion of Westerners. Why do they not give rise to the same ill effects? Climate may account for the remarkable phenomenon of endemic cholera in India, for it is from India, over many centuries, that waves of infection spread across the world. Perhaps India provides the ideal conditions for the survival of the delicate 'vibro' outside the human body – low-lying lands and lakes, rich in organic matter and salts, sheltered from rain and sun.[5] Trachoma, resulting in much blindness – one of the oldest diseases known to man – has been called a disease of poverty and promiscuity; but this hardly seems sufficient to account for its relatively limited distribution in the mediterranean zone. It is not impossible that a climatic factor favours its propagation.

Temperature and humidity, the state of vegetation, and the abundance or otherwise of animal life, affect the vectors of disease, and so in turn the many members of the bacterial world which depend upon them to complete their life cycle, or otherwise to propagate themselves. Thus the mosquitoes, which carry malaria, yellow fever, dengue, encephalitis in many forms, filariasis, and other diseases, are affected, and their disease-carrying qualities altered, by a great variety of climatic conditions. The snails which are the intermediary hosts for schistosoma may find living conditions more to their taste in the waterways of Egypt than in those of Bangkok, or they may never have succeeded in finding transport for the long sea journey which intervenes. The African slaves, who took schistosoma to the New World, must have carried both 'haematobium' and 'mansoni'; and yet today haematobium, the typical bilharzia of Egypt, is hardly to be found in South America, where possibly the conditions for the intermediary host may have been less favourable. Similar influences may affect many other carriers, determining perhaps, at least in part, the distribution of malaria, yellow fever, and filariasis. Flies (African trypanosomiasis), ticks (Rocky Mountain Spotted Fever), and mites (scrub typhus) are all sensitive to climatic changes. And so, too, the rat may have found better living in India, and in turn have helped the bacillus of plague to maintain itself, so that when the great epidemics of plague slaughter him, the myriads of fleas could more easily transfer to man. The reason that plague occurs mainly in the rainy season is probably that the rat remains indoors, where, with the seasonal lowering of temperature and humidity to aid their propagation, the fleas increase in numbers.

Finally man's reaction to his environment – his output of work, his mental alertness, and his desire for change, and possibly many other attitudes and responses – may ultimately depend upon the meteorological conditions in which he spends his waking and sleeping hours. Both external and internal conditions are of importance. One basic need is for a measure of comfort – particularly in the home. Until the Greeks perfected the hypocaust, or hot-air system for internal heating of houses, all earlier civilizations were developed at or near to the 70°F isotherm. Moreover when Greece and Rome vanished, and the hypocaust with them, civilization returned temporarily with the Arabs to the same isotherm level.[4]

Yet it is certain that the more stimulating external conditions of the Northern climate, given good house comfort, have played a part in man's development. A mean temperature of 40°F in winter and 60°F in summer, with a relative humidity of about 60 per cent at noon, and high enough at night to precipitate dew, is the most stimulating for mind and body.[3] An area of *very high energy* runs through North-East and North-Central United States and North-West and Central Europe. A zone of *high energy* covers the remainder of the United States, except the deep South and the rest of Europe, excepting Southern Spain and Portugal and some sparsely populated northern parts of Scandinavia; it projects eastward into Russia to the borders of Siberia, and includes Japan. Few can doubt that energy takes its place among the complex factors upon which the health picture of the world depends and which this book sets out to examine. Much future progress may depend upon the use of technology, by air conditioning or other means, to create the conditions of maximum human energy output throughout the less favoured regions.

Public health with its modern armamentarium for speedy action against man's biological geogens is perhaps in danger of overlooking the influence of more long-term factors. Both the social geogens, of which much will be said in subsequent chapters, and the physical geogens, need to be closely studied. To be successful public health needs a balanced approach – in which social, biological, and physical geogens, and their many interactions, are under continuous pressure.

6. Beliefs and Customs

Science and superstition

The great majority of the human race lose their curiosity about the happenings of their daily lives early. The doctrine of Claude Bernard, 'to be of good faith and do not believe', is not usually easy to practise. For the ordinary mortal – if not for Abelard, Voltaire, or doubting Thomas – it is easier to accept the reasons for the phenomena which we daily encounter when these are given by those we respect than it is to doubt and discuss. Superstitious beliefs, therefore, abound throughout the world. In the developed world where there is a scientific background, superstitious beliefs may pass unnoticed; the myriads of bacteria may be identified with evil spirits, even if the aseptic ritual is adopted. Religious ritual may differ little in its superstitious content and less in its psychotherapeutic qualities from the Ghost Dances.[1] Science itself may play the rôle of magic and scientific routine can take on the character of rituals, so that in scientific societies, magic in the form of science has been made respectable; science has become the Sacred Cow. The greatest handicap of workers of one culture in the setting of another is their failure to appreciate the complexities of their own beliefs and the lack of objectivity which they themselves display.

The main difference between the magical beliefs held by different cultures can perhaps be looked upon as one of degree or of depth. The men and women of the Western world who still believe in luck, charms, talismans, and horoscopes do so a little apologetically.

Beliefs in the underdeveloped world, except the more recent accretions, have little connexion with science. The biology of infection in particular is quite unappreciated. Too often dressers, trained to boil instruments, have been known afterwards to wipe them on filthy rags; midwives, after swabbing their hands for an aseptic delivery, have run them through their hair. It is never safe to assume that people who wash will do so when hygienically it is most needed. Thus, in Indian villages one may bathe before a meal, but fail to wash the hands before attending to a childbirth. In this, the underdeveloped is perhaps less removed from the developed world than might at first appear. Water is regarded by most people as clean if it has no visible impurity or smell. Many who have taught first aid in Europe, for example to factory workers, will have realized how slight is the general understanding of the germ theory: the idea that bacteria can be undetectable except by laboratory techniques, and that they have life of their own in competition with man, is not easy to grasp.

Customs and beliefs take on incongruous patterns to outside eyes. Variations seem endless; some are practical, many apparently useless: some do good, others harm; some are deeply rooted, others of little consequence. Odd or curious as they often are, they all fit into the matrix of the culture. To understand them, and the psychological and social functions which they perform, we need to explore deeply. Health practices are based upon beliefs which penetrate into politics, philosophy, etiquette, religion, cosmology, and kinship.

Causation of disease

The concept of disease in the underdeveloped world falls, in very general terms, into three categories: conditions for which a cause has been empirically determined; those due to magic; and the psychological phenomena.[8] Natural diseases of which the cause has been ascribed include those due to cold air or to violations of hot and cold prohibitions. The commonly understood magical diseases in South America are due to 'Evil eye' (*ojo*), or to 'fright' (*susto*). Those due to psychological causes, in Peru for example, are shame (*chucaque*), disillusion (*tiricia*), anger (*colerina*), and jealousy (*caisa*).

In aetiology and in treatment the Hippocratic concept of disease can be detected in different guises. In its simplest form it postulates the existence of a balance of the four cardinal humours – blood, phlegm, black bile, and yellow bile – themselves endowed with elementary qualities, hot, moist, dry, and cold. Thus, in South America, to which the Spaniards brought Arab concepts of medicine, pneumonia is a cold disease and typhoid hot. The corresponding hot and cold food vary in each village of Latin America. In Xochimilco, for example, the hot foods include: sugar, honey, green Chilli pepper, and brandy, while cold foods include rice, meat, most fruit, and vegetables.[8] Galen's philosophy of disease as a lack of harmony with the universe can also be seen at work in many societies, where good thoughts, avoidance of quarrelling or aggressive acts are thought to maintain good relations with the universe, and, in consequence, disease is regarded as a punishment for sin, mainly against society.

Theories of contagion, generally far removed from our own, are firmly held. In Mexico, varying diseases, for example smallpox, venereal disease, and measles, are accepted as contagious, but chicken pox and tuberculosis are generally not.[8] Some regard intercourse during menstruation as a cause of venereal disease; among the Kgatla intercourse with a man with 'hot blood' engenders a condition known as 'hot hips'.[18] The agents of infection, and its routes, may differ widely. Excrement may be dangerous, but only when it comes into contact with another's excreta.[18]

Magic is commonly involved, both as a cause and a cure of disease.[7] Fears, expectations, and beliefs surround menstruation, childbirth, sexual relations, excretory processes, and foods. Thus a menstruating nurse in hospital can endanger a male patient. Excreta can give power for evil; many have told stories of the pathologist examining specimens of stools while the donors look anxiously on to see the material safely buried. Latrines in many places are regarded as dangerous, since sorcerers may collect faeces there (Uganda).[18] It may be safer to defaecate in a mountain stream (New Guinea).[18] Pregnant women can be dangerous to the community and must follow stringent regulations. The birth often has to take place according to tradition, sometimes in a special dwelling or in a special position – squatting, kneeling, or bearing down on a rope slung from the ceiling. The placenta may have to be buried under the house floor, because to put it elsewhere might blight the land (Kgatla);[18] or in contrast, where unity with the earth is strongly held, it must be buried under the appropriate tree or rock to maintain continuity. In Colombia it must be buried in hot ashes if the mother is to avoid pain. In rural parts of Japan it must be kept, if that of a female child, until marriage. Disposal of the lochial blood often causes anxiety because of the evil it may cause. Such magical beliefs are not fixed and immutable but capable of change.

Every known society has developed methods of preventing and treating disease. Most societies, today, have a mixed assortment of empirical, scientific, and magical remedies in their medicine chests. In a cholera outbreak in Yunnan, taboos, prayer meetings, placatory rites, injections, and hospital treatment were all tried.[6] Of the empirical remedies many are objectively effective: baths, massage, cauterization, splinting of fractures, inoculations against smallpox and snake bite, and an enormous pharmacopoeia which includes opium, quinine, and digitalis. Others without any obvious benefits, and often attended by harm, would no doubt have been found in Europe until recent times, and some persist today, including herbal remedies, the 'hot' and 'cold' qualities of foods, and strange poultices. The evil eye was believed in Europe to be a cause of illness, certainly in the thirteenth century and probably much later. The poultice of a live pigeon split open (Peru and Colombia) is not much different from that of the pigeon's fundament, which was a favourite remedy of Shakespeare's son-in-law, Dr Hall, as a cure for scurvy in and around Stratford-on-Avon.

All treatments, irrespective of their origins, including those from the scientific world and the useful remedies which primitive societies have independently developed, can be given in an entirely magical sense with spells, prayers, rites, dances, orations, and creeds. Where disease has resulted from a disturbance of harmony, it is common to restore equilibrium by ritual, as in the Ghost-dance, perhaps introducing psychotherapeutic techniques, which, in another setting, scientific medicine would itself accept.

Special days for treatment may be magically favoured (Tuesday and Friday in Peru). Special ceremonies are thought to have value in diagnosis as well as treatment, as, for example, the famous egg-rubbing ceremony for the diagnosis of *ojo* – the evil eye – which consists of passing a warm, freshly laid egg over the body of a child and then examining the yoke for a tell-tale spot.

Magical interference gives an apparently logical reason for disease and the success and failures of treatment. Belief in it certainly tends to close the mind to possibilities of effective action other than the rite and spell; and it may implant passive resignation to failure. But yet it would be wrong to assume that beliefs in magic are necessarily a hindrance to science;[9] it is much more the habits which hinder what we call progress. Certainly new ideas can be adopted, and given a magical flavour, more easily, for example, than most people can be persuaded to change their habits of defaecation.

Disease is so often seen as a product of culture and social background in the underdeveloped world that we may overlook the existence of this phenomenon elsewhere. Disease has its social content everywhere, as the modern exponents of social medicine have sought to show.[14] We no longer regard epilepsy, prematurity, mental subnormality, tuberculosis, and a host of other illnesses as entirely, or even mainly, medical. Doctors and hospitals everywhere are beginning to look into the social background of illness. How far this will take us no one now can foresee. Disease may also be regarded as a disturbance of equilibrium between the internal and external environments, and symptoms as evidence of attempts by the physiological and psychological systems of the body to regain an optimum state.[4] In this concept peptic ulcers, ulcerative colitis, and other chronic afflictions of the developed world, possibly multiple stress diseases, may be seen as the counterpart of the nutritional diseases and intestinal disorders of the rest of the world.

Disease is seen also as an escape phenomenon in most, if not all, parts of the world. This is made possible by the fact that it imparts privileges as well as disabilities – exemption from social obligations, the assurance of help, and freedom from responsibility. In this, psychological illnesses in South America, for example, resemble the chronic diseases in England; they can be an escape from conscious or unconscious difficulties. By *colerina* the South American can evade the embarrassing or unpleasant aftermath, and possible retribution, of a fit of anger; as in Europe the misplaced industrial worker or the soldier escapes from an intolerable psychological situation by visiting the factory doctor or appearing on sick parade.

So too in most countries there are reasons for doing nothing about illness until too late. Where chronic diseases are widespread, as with pinta in Peru or trachoma among the fellaheen, just as in Europe, when slighting references to malaria as the ague were in common parlance – the level of what is regarded as normal health is much lower. Thus the standard of health in many parts of the world includes a fair amount of disease. Disease may be an admission of weakness, and hence shameful. For these and other reasons help may not be sought.

The forces at work within society

The significance of beliefs and customs is increased in all societies by internal forces, which constitute a self-regulating mechanism. We may compare this with the *milieu intérieur* described by Claude Bernard; he discovered that the body maintained a steady internal state by self-regulating devices, which kept the activity of different organs – muscle, liver, lungs, kidneys – within bounds and in harmony with one another, and kept a stable background for the body's extraverted actions. Society, too, has its internal milieu and self-regulating mechanism for keeping its separate members in harmony. Each member feels the pressure of regulation. Such forces are many and varied, and a full description of them is beyond the scope of this short exposition; but perhaps the most important to public health are those which arise through the pressures of conformity, the systems of values and prestige, religious discipline, and social organization.

The pressure for conformity

In every society, in different ways, conduct is 'socially sanctioned'. We do what is expected of us in line with others. From our earliest days, for those who follow the rules, there are rewards; for those who transgress, penalties. Social ostracism, from the raising of the eyebrow to the ghetto, is a force of devastating power. It prescribes the goals to be sought, the code of what is done and not done and it interprets present and past experiences according to the culture from which it is born. Few can swim against the tide of public opinion. It is so much easier to subscribe. The well-to-do in West Town in Yunnan contributed to prayer meetings and rituals to fend off cholera, although at the same time supporting hospitals and modern treatment. To do otherwise would have been to defy custom and invite obloquy.[9]

Systems of value and prestige

A strong driving force in any society is the set of values which it has adopted and which it rates highly. The value system is a complex of many individual ingredients, which fit neatly together, each, as it were, in its proper place in one composite whole. Some of the components are to be found in religious teaching; others in writing or sayings of wise men; but most seem to have grown up over long years of usage, in response to the exigencies of the times through which the group has passed. The success motif of the people of North America can perhaps be seen developing in the long years of successful pioneering in the east-to-west trek across the north American continent. Its absence elsewhere, as in Burma, may be a by-product of religious beliefs. In so many places, as in England, industrialization has produced the cult of the ugly, while simpler societies have found contentment in adornment. Some look forward, and nothing is good that is not new; others look back and live in the past. Such values, whether religious or based on long-established custom, for the most part unquestioningly adopted, are taught to the young with little attempt at objective presentation. In every society the majority believes that its system of values is good and that to act according to it is the right way to live. Taken in, as it were, with mother's milk, this has an enduring quality.

Every society has a prestige system for rating individuals in terms of the culture: in most this is closely related to occupation (see p. 236), so that the more industrialized the greater the range of the scale. This often has little relationship to financial status – thus the learned Mr C., in Hsu's account of a cholera outbreak in Yunnan Province, ranked high on lists of subscribers, although his donation was small.[9] Prestige of groups within society can also be ethnological or religious, as in caste systems. But in whatever form they arise and are maintained, individuals act or react in accordance with the value which has been placed upon their status, or, if rebellious, they must pay the price.

Religious discipline

The pressure of religious teaching has been particularly strong in the field of hygiene, including the varying aspects of procreation and family life, which today are part of the teachings of social medicine. The emphasis upon impurity which is found in almost all religious teaching, sometimes carried to extremes and often quite meaningless, was designed to inculcate ideas about cleanliness and contagion which the group needed for survival. The sequestration of lepers, the destruction of houses in which those with contagious maladies had died, the washing of hands, and injunctions against indiscriminate defaection, were woven into rituals.[17] The owner of an infected house in the early Semitic societies was required to tell a priest, saying, 'It seemeth to me that there is as it were a plague in the house'. When the priest had visited the house and lent his authority, he was to cause it to be scraped within round about, so that the dust that was scraped off could be poured 'without the city into an unclean place' (Leviticus 14:41). The admonitions of Deuteronomy follow similar lines: 'And thou shalt have a paddle upon thy weapon, and it shall be, when thou wilt ease thyself abroad, thou shalt dig therewith and shalt turn back and cover that which cometh from thee' (23:13–14). So much has also been said in similar words for the Brahmins, Parsees, and followers of Islam.

The emphasis which the major religions have placed upon the sanctity of marriage, the proscription of illicit love and of sexual perversions, as well as the strictures on prostitution and the often brutal treatment of all concerned in procuring abortion, have all in different ways contributed to a virile society; so also has infanticide and other means of keeping the population controlled, manageable, and 'feed-able'.

Social organizations

Conduct also reflects the varying ways in which society is organized – internal groups, and chains of hierarchical authority give strength to the community, but they limit the freedom of action of the individual. In Japan, in earlier times, when it was divided for administrative purposes into local units, and these in turn into neighbourhood groups of households, all communications had to be made through the village official. In Arab society all important matters relating to the welfare of the community, such as those concerning land or marriage, are decided by the group in concert, including the church and all the families. The fellaheen rarely act as individuals. There are many such variations with differing emphasis upon the family, the village, the church, or the state.

The importance of beliefs and customs in public health service

The preference for folk medicine

Scientific medicine encounters many difficulties when it comes into contact with cultures that are different from that in which it was born. The medicine man, everywhere, from the Curandero in South America to the Inyanga in south-west Natal, has qualities in the eyes of the local inhabitants transcending those of the university-trained doctor. The medicine man seems so much more interested in you; yet he is not so foolish as to waste time and money on the

dying. He does not try to isolate you in hospital far from your friends and relatives, among apparently uninterested doctors and nurses, where, as like as not,
you will run into difficulties with the disposal of lochia or faeces, or where you
may be given food that you know is harmful. Neither does he laugh at you when
you ascribe your disease to a punishment for some emotion or to magic. He
gives you treatment with his own hand and does not send you to a pharmacist,
nor ask payment of you in advance of results. He does not reveal his ignorance
by asking questions, or by requiring elaborate tests. He does not take notes
which may have a magical hold on you. He never says he does not know what
is the matter with you.

The disadvantages of the hospital are likewise legion. How easily the evil
eye can get through its large window spaces, and how much better to remain at
home with a low roof and hardly any window. There may be someone overhead
to do you harm (Burma);[18] your talisman may be removed, or your body
immodestly exposed. If you are pregnant, you might come under a magical spell
by catching sight of a corpse (Burma and some parts of Africa). Hospitals are
places in which to die, and where movement is intolerably restricted and human
interest minimal.

Environment hygiene

Perhaps one of the greatest problems now facing the human race is the
disposal of human faeces. To the scientifically trained public health worker
it seems to offer little difficulty in its solution. And yet local beliefs and customs
are continually stultifying his efforts.

Defaecation in the open spaces, whether due to local beliefs, or, as in Siam
and Burma, for aesthetic reasons, is a major menace. The Thai selects a secluded
place behind a teak tree, with gentle breezes and a pleasant vista; but for himself and his fellows walking barefoot on the muddy ground there is daily
exposure to hookworm. The rains wash down the parasites from excreta into
streams; flies settle on the faeces, carry them on their feet, and regurgitate them
on to food. Dysentery and intestinal diseases follow.

Housing is similarly involved in beliefs of many kinds. Often people prefer
crowded quarters (Mexico). In Egypt the village resembles an anthill where,
at night, man and beasts are huddled together in a labyrinth of alleys.[12] The
world is an insanitary place, with water supplies almost everywhere polluted
and with little or no sanitation – largely because of these beliefs.

Mental health

The far-reaching effects of culture and social background upon mental health
have in three important aspects – the family, occupation, and industrialization
– been dealt with elsewhere in this book. Much remains to be learnt about the
distribution of departures from normal mental health throughout the world, in
particular the differences between the developed and underdeveloped worlds.[10]
The restrictions on human conduct, as well as the many supporting structures of
society itself, are certain to have deep implications for it. These must be studied
individually in each area. The effects of social pressure are also to be taken into
the account of public health. Pressure for conformity, particularly among the

naturally rebellious, is not likely to be without cost to the individual's peace
of mind.

Maternal and child health

The hygiene of motherhood and infant health is involved even more deeply.
A hundred different customs, some beneficial but many harmful, are at work.
The hygiene of infancy is less easy to teach when the value of a child is little,
as happens in cultures in which human values increase with living. Proscribed
foods for the mother before and after delivery can deprive the mother of essential nutrients. Delivery may take place in confined and unhygienic surroundings,
although often among friends in a mentally secure atmosphere. There are so
many reasons why mothers and babies die, and a dozen more to prevent the
development of family planning. How can a man be expected to use a condom
in his own marriage bed when this is practised with prostitutes (Puerto Rico)?[18]
The endless chain of cause and effect, for which beliefs and customs are
ultimately responsible, involves the public health worker so deeply that he
had better not begin his activities in maternal and child health than start in
ignorance. Very often it has proved a blessing in disguise that very little of what
he or she advocates is accepted.

Nutrition

Food is the subject of widespread beliefs – apart from hot and cold remedies
and the religious taboos. In Malaya, vegetables are thought to cause impotence.
In contrast reverence for rice leads to its misuse: 'whatever is eaten, unless
there is rice, there is no life in the body' is a popular Malayan saying.[3] In most
countries, food is a focus of emotional associations; its preparation may be
symbolic of love, discrimination, or approval. To change food habits is often
fraught with difficulty and danger. The religious attitude to livestock has been
a common cause of failure to use essential foodstuffs. Nutrition is also closely
bound up with many other aspects of life, so that to change it in almost any
way may have unfortunate repercussions. So great, indeed, is the range of
possibilities for nutritional disease to arise from alterations in human society,
that no one has yet fully comprehended it. Hardly any action to apply modern
public health techniques, or agriculture, or industrial development, can be
undertaken without boomerang effects upon the diet, which may result in more
harm than good. So delicate is the food balance in many regions of the world
that it can be upset by a visiting nurse, an agricultural expert, or the development of a nearby New Town. Change the tortillas soaked in limewater for
white bread in New Mexico and the children suffer from a calcium deficiency.
Cut short breast-feeding among Hopi Indian toddlers by sending them to
hospital and kwashiorkor may result later from inability to buy substitutes.

Syncretization

The culture of a society, although uncompromising and enduring, is yet in
constant change, taking in and absorbing to itself new ideas, when these do not
conflict with fundamental tenets, a process described as syncretization. The
beliefs and customs constitute the product of the past, like a coral reef slowly

built by accretion and fashioned by the friction of the waves. All new ideas are at first valued according to existing beliefs; those which have an affinity with something within the existing culture will be most readily acceptable. Thus it may be relatively easy to accept the germ theory if it can be interpreted in some traditional concept – as where the cleaning of vegetables was accepted as a purification rite, or where vaccination was regarded as a magic charm. On the other hand, those ideas that are intimately tied up with a sense of security will react with the strongest resistance to change. The rapidity and degree of change will depend upon many considerations. In general, when touching closely the interests of the community without impinging too greatly upon fundamentals – as with new methods of travel – they will be accepted.

Direct attacks on fundamentals may produce the opposite effect of giving them greater strength. This was the case with attempts to abolish female circumcision among the Kikuyu. Where, too, disease is thought to result from a failure to preserve equable human relationships, it may be dangerous to health to introduce new ideas too abruptly. We should also remember that people suffering from stress react negatively, thus a Zulu patriarch refused to allow his family to go to hospital until the doctor had retracted his suggestion that a married daughter had introduced tuberculosis to his family; to have believed this was to make her a witch. The process of grafting on to existing beliefs is generally much to be preferred to any radical operation. In Greece, where the humoral theory of contagion is very strong, it has proved best to allow it to take the place of infection in hygiene teaching. The object should always be to uncover misconceptions gently, and so allow people to find other and alternative means of security.

Beliefs about the nature of disease, generally stubbornly maintained, have changed in most societies over long periods of time. The Hippocratic description of disease, as developed by Galen, appears, eventually, to have reached most parts of the world, and in varying degrees to have been accepted.[8, 15] The adaptation of the Greek teachings to prevailing thought may have ben easier in some cultures than others; but most are likely to have welcomed a doctrine of such relative simplicity, which endowed the human being with easily understood remedies for a wide range of conditions – as illustrated in the principle of *contraria contrariis*, treating hot diseases with cold remedies. Yet it took 2,000 years for these to reach South America and complete the world tour.

Syncretization in the modern world increasingly involves the addition or assimilation of scientific ideas. This is, of course, easier for cultures which have acquired some scientific background, and correspondingly more difficult for those centring upon a nonscientific culture. But in essence the process is the same throughout the world. The amalgamation is largely unconscious. The individual in society does not stop to ponder the magical or scientific nature of the phenomenon confronting him.[9]

Beliefs and practices in relation to disease are certainly not wholly harmful; they may be beneficial or be capable of adaptation to good purposes. The taboos on a large number of vegetables in the Yunnan outbreak of cholera, although considered as part of the effort at pleasing the gods, or of avoiding abdominal cold, may well have helped in limiting the spread of cholera, since fruits were normally eaten unwashed and vegetables were often cleaned in streams and eaten lightly cooked.[9] The general idea of contagion also can help, while the impurity rituals, or patterns of cleanliness of the established religions, and many of the similar practices in pagan beliefs, have been of value to hygiene. These can form the basis of new teaching – providing it is understood that they may not be based upon any appreciation of the biology of infection.

Social anthropology in public health training

The practice of public health cannot be isolated or treated apart from the complexities of beliefs and customs; at almost every turn it involves adjustments, many trivial but some fundamental, in this cultural framework. Moreover, success in public health often depends upon modifications outside the purely medical field, so that a knowledge of the community in a wider sense is needed. The community should be studied for its folk medicine, its economics, its family structure, its politics and religion, and for its systems of value and prestige.[8] Such studies are just as important to successful public health as a knowledge of epidemiology and medicine.[13] Thus, it is of value in the South American village of Xochimilco to know that the married couple go to live in the husband's family and that the bride is dominated by the mother-in-law; or why, in the Pacific atoll of Yap, the women interfere with the cervix to terminate pregnancy and so avoid child-bearing before the age of 30.[11] The importance of such studies is well illustrated by the ill-effects of the attitude of doctors at one Latin-American health centre – an attitude found all too frequently all over the world. They were not consulted about magical or psychological diseases, since they had revealed their opinion of them by scoffing. In operating as if the folk medicine did not exist they had greatly reduced their power for good.[8]

Information about beliefs and customs is still woefully lacking despite the claim that the sociologists, anthropologists, and social psychologists have developed methods 'to a point where studies of society by competent scholars can provide basic information to assist all those practical men who struggle with the groups of problems we list under the head of human relations'.[5] But there is nothing to prevent practical men and women in public health from conducting their own studies. In any case, although the general cultural patterns facing public health are capable of being generalized, the details vary so much that local study is essential.

An understanding and appreciation of customs and beliefs can never be thorough at the outset, since the patterns in different societies are both intricate and varied. Generalizations are dangerous. But armed with the techniques of anthropology and perhaps even more important, with the correct attitude of mind, the public health worker can come to understand the significance of customs and beliefs, wherever he works. If he is to work effectively, he must not only see the world as the people do, but also understand the psychological and social functions performed by the practices and beliefs. It is only then

C

that he will be able to apply his scientific knowledge of public health to the best advantage. Understanding of beliefs and customs gives confidence to doctors, nurses, and others, which is essential to success, and it makes possible a sympathetic approach to public health problems, without directly attacking fundamentals. Health education and social anthropology must go hand in hand.

As the public health worker studies the community in which he is working he will also see how greatly the application of scientific knowledge can affect the daily life of the people. Someone has to be responsible for keeping the well in repair and to collect and burn the rubbish. Women have new duties – to light special fires for boiling drinking water, to wash babies' clothes, and to teach the children to use latrines. Getting children vaccinated and changing the diet are major operations.[12]

The main hindrance to the acceptance of scientific medicine is not that the scientific techniques themselves are unacceptable, this is generally far from true, but that the new ideas are clothed in a foreign culture. Public health must get out of its town clothes and put on a simple country homespun. Some have found that it is possible to fit scientific medicine into local culture without introducing irrelevant foreign values, as was the case in Kishan Garhi in the United Provinces.[11] We can at least avoid confusing hygiene with cleanliness, as illustrated by one African township where the maternity home gained favour once the restriction against spitting tobacco juice on to walls had been withdrawn.

Successful techniques are more likely to change ideas than teaching aimed directly at fundamentals. Nevertheless it must not be taken for granted that good results will immediately carry conviction.[11] Like Snow's contemporaries (see p. 145), people need a lot of proof. Also the often inevitable lack of immediate and clear-cut results tends to be taken as proof that the new method is useless. Misunderstanding as to the object of any measure can also produce unfortunate results. Thus when DDT spraying has been thought to be aimed at the flies, which everyone detests, rather than at the mosquitos, which no one minds, the appearance of 'resistant' flies in swarms immediately afterwards is taken as proof of failure. (Pampana and Russell, see Chapter 18).

In most public health practice, the systems of values and prestige can be turned to good account. Important individuals in the community can be consulted and given an opportunity to maintain their prestige by playing a useful rôle, and not like the influential Mr Chang in one agricultural extension scheme, left out to obstruct behind the scenes.[6] Popular acceptance of any programme is in direct ratio to the degree in which local representatives have taken part in the planning and conduct of it.[16] Local channels of communication can be studied; from the womenfolk gossiping at the well or in the fields, and the men in the coffee houses and on the threshing floors, to the teacher, priest, or headman. The clergy and others with vested interests may oppose change; but always when the desire for new methods is there, precedents can be found to allow it to go forward in tune with existing beliefs.

Finally, the changing of harmful practices will depend upon the gradual growth of understanding about science and its methods, which a general system of education should help to bring about. Lack of a common background and knowledge, which is the great obstacle, will slowly disappear. Great as are the difficulties which face public health in all parts of the world because men and women are so set in their ways and beliefs, they are not insuperable.

7. Family Life

Man's evolution forced upon him the acceptance of the family as the basic unit of society. The long process of gestation and relatively small number of offspring early required that the male should protect the female through the long years of her child-bearing period. Some form of 'elementary family', father, mother, and child, is universal in all human societies.[8] When and how this association developed is not known, or what part was played by group marriage, when the woman, as the indisputable parent of her children, occupied a commanding position. The male took the reins of control when trade, in which he could play an active rôle denied to the female, presumably transferred the seat of power – first under polygamy with several wives and a host of children, and later, forced by an increasingly complex economic system, under monogamy, with one wife and a steadily declining number of offspring.

The family is biological, as no other grouping – industrial, occupational, social – can claim to be; its ill-defined and amorphous structure with grandparents, parents, and children and collateral links through marriage, is a phenomenon of growth; and the characteristics of its members are largely the result of haphazard selection from a common pool of chromosomes. It is bound together by a mixture of economic and emotional ties, providing economic, social and educational services and pooling resources, with its own mores and government. Positive and compelling, it is recognized as an entity by all, including the many for whom government and community mean little or nothing. Families are to the community as individual bricks to a house; but infinitely more adaptable and enduring.

Families throughout the world vary greatly in internal composition and motivation. They live and act differently, have different kinship systems, and varying values and beliefs. They may be small and circumscribed, as in the Western world, or, as in the East, extended to include many relatives, and even strangers. Size and age composition vary with the population structure of the nation (see p. 30). The 'extended family' may live altogether in one dwelling, or a family compound, or it may be distributed throughout a rural community, or live within hailing distance from one 'turning' to another in an old-established industrial centre. Relationships of men and women, attitudes to children, and the respect and support given to grandparents, all vary. In some societies, children early work and earn; in others they continue in education until after manhood or womanhood has been reached (see pp. 26–29). In some the cult of lifelong marriage is very strong; in others, as new and more compelling ideologies are taken up, it is breaking down.

Family life reflects in a hundred ways the culture of the society of which it forms the fabric. Life in an extended family in Bali will have little in common with its counterpart in the USA, except the living together of man and wife and procreation of children. What poles apart are the sexual lives of the children after puberty; the Balinese slowly ripening into adults in a long sexual seclusion; the American satisfying the urge for success in a decade of petting.[14] In France working-class families may be fundamentally opposed to any change of their status, and so as it were fixed socially; in the USA they may believe implicitly in 'bettering themselves', although with less social mobility than is often imagined. In a Pacific atoll, the new wife may arrive to crouch in the corner of the tribal hut, a butt for the facetious remarks of her husband's relatives; in a Western city she may take the man she met in the Tube last week to the nearest Registry Office, unknown to any of their relatives.

Every society has its own family peculiarities, and most have great variations at different social levels; but in all the family is the most important unit – for the health of the community, as also for all major social needs. For good or ill, the home is paramount to public health.

The importance of the family to public health

The family and child care

The family has its most important influence through the rearing of children – the attitude of the mother, her skill in mothercraft, her biological dedication; the support of the father; and the physical and mental environment, which parents establish, are all involved. Customs of child rearing, which do much to determine the end-product, vary greatly; for instance, the two extremes of baby care, over-protection and active dislike, can both be seen in different tribes of New Guinea. But too few studies have yet been made in detail, even in the Western world. Nevertheless it is obvious that the considerable differences which exist in child care between different communities are of great importance.

Marriage is becoming increasingly monogamous, but where polygamy exists (in Chinese societies, Africa, Muslim areas, and the Pacific islands) and where there is polyandry (in Malabar, Sri Lanka, and Tibet) divided loyalties may complicate the relationship of parents with their children. Sometimes in China and almost universally in Malaya and other Muslim parts of the Indonesian world, the worst effects of this split in maternal discipline and paternal affection are avoided by having the wives in separate households.[8] But the more obvious distinctions arise out of different patterns of kinship, authority, adoption, and treatment.

The Western pattern of authority stresses the mother-and-child relationship to the almost total exclusion of the father; but in Asian-Pacific families, father not only shares equally with mother, but also plays an important rôle in education, by associating the child with his daily activities. The prevalence of adoption in underdeveloped countries has been said to reflect 'a very general attitude that to have small children about the place is a pleasant and good thing'.[8] No doubt it emphasizes also the greater economic and high social value of children, as well as the population pattern with unrestricted birth rate and the high risks of depletion of the family by death, particularly in childhood (see p. 29). One side-effect of widespread adoption is to reduce the problem of babies born out of wedlock to negligible proportions, since they are accepted and treated with normal care.

The treatment of children in West and East tends also to follow a different set of rules. In the West discipline is more rigid and, speaking generally, independence is less encouraged. In the East child care is more permissive, starting with the 'on demand' feeding at mother's breast, which continues throughout the long suckling period – a great safeguard, incidentally, against protein malnutrition in Fiji and Africa, until the white man 'knew better'. The excessive emphasis upon discipline in elimination of excreta, which is a feature of Western society, is much less marked in the East.

The West, as part of the process of industrialization (see Chapter 13), is much more nearly dependent on the elementary family; but in the East, as in under-developed countries generally, a much wider kin group is involved in child care. The child knows a wide circle of relatives, who participate actively in the family circle; with these he is intimately associated, in sleeping, suckling, feeding, and, in the early years, excretion, which takes place in the presence of others than the parents, without embarrassment to anyone. Hence, not only is the child's relationship with his mother more diffuse, but, correspondingly, he develops bonds of affection and authority with a much greater circle of relatives.

Western studies have emphasized the part played by the home in development of personality and character – the end-product of the interaction of the environment and the genetic make-up. Home moulds us like clay on the potter's wheel. Loss of the security, which is as necessary to the balance of the child's mind as an anchor is to a ship, and 'emotional deprivation', are the chief dangers. The broken home can give rise to behaviour disorders, or to faulty development, much as the tubercle bacillus may cause phthisis.

In the home that has foundered in disharmony, the children can become confused and unhappy, afraid, angry, distressed, and, less often but yet all too frequently, aggressive. They may do damaging things to people or property, probably as a relief to their pent-up feelings, or as a revenge for injustices which loom large in their young minds. Anti-social behaviour in the Western world commonly has its roots in the parents' lack of affection.[12] In some cases the result is delinquency: some anti-social act, which by chance puts the child outside the law. Some children become neurotic: restless, seeking attention inordinately and displaying affection indiscriminately. The very young, deprived for long of their mothers, can present a harrowing picture of misery and apathy. Failure of development may give rise to instability, or inability to make relationships, the so-called affectionless type for which the most important cause appears to be the lack of a continuing relationship, during the first few years of life, with one satisfactory 'mother'.

Most children from unhappy homes make useful adults; some, no doubt, much above average. The mother who gives birth to an abnormal child usually manages to steer his or her emotional development between the Scylla of rejection and the Charybdis of over-protection.[9] Men and women of great creative abilities have had unsatisfactory childhoods. Darwin produced the *Origin of Species* despite, or possibly because of, his father's stern repression. The mother's rôle can be played satisfactorily by others, as it was by Maria Millis as nanny to the young Shaftesbury, who was later to help to free the European child from the cruelties of a new industrial system. Much may depend upon constitutional weakness. But the broken home seems to have a self-perpetuating character, since its children appear more likely to reproduce the episodes in their own lives.[2, 6] We know too little of the life-histories of such children – much that we see in failure in the Western world may be part of the changing pattern of family and society, which development seems to entail (see pp. 26 and 108).

The family and sickness

The family also is the first defence in caring for sickness and in welfare. No system of social security, in developed and underdeveloped countries alike, would ever replace the family system of loans without interest, gifts in money and kind. Over large parts of the world, as in Thailand, the family supports relatives and often strangers in adversity; and it adopts and educates the children. In the three-generation family, even in an old-standing industrial slum, and still more, no doubt, in long-settled agricultural communities, the care of dependants at both ends of life, always one of the great and indispensable functions of any society, is a family concern. For the welfare of the aged and of the handicapped, the family shoulders more than 90 per cent of the burden.[17] Adolescents, particularly those who continue in full-time education, and adult workers, lean heavily upon it.

Sickness is always a family event; no member can be ill without affecting the others, so that, even when the doctor or the hospital is involved, the family must always be considered. The great problem in all families is what happens when sickness comes. When mother is ill or confined in old Bethnal Green, grandmother and relatives rally to her aid. In one form or another, given reasonable proximity, the family will devise its own aids to sick nursing.[20] Father has no need to stay away from work to nurse his family, except in the new housing estates, where the balance of the three-generation family has been disturbed. The family does more nursing than the hospital, even in highly-developed countries, and, according to sickness surveys, largely without the aid of the doctor.[18] Many consider that too much attention is given to hospital provision and that well-organized schemes of home care have much to offer – financially, socially, and psychologically (see Chapter 11). No form of national health service, in any event, can hope to succeed without the support of the family.

But the home can also cause illness. The human family is a happy hunting ground for the bacterial world; psychologically it suffers from tension; physically it may fail to keep pace with its own growth, with too little food or space; socially it may lack strength of purpose, or adopt unhealthy practices. Tuberculosis spreads within the family group – indeed for this reason it was long regarded as hereditary. Deaths from accidents to children in the home, in a developed country, exceed those on the roads. The problem family produces educational subnormality, as well as other forms of social disorder. Many social customs and beliefs about feeding during and after pregnancy, and other details closely associated with family life, are known to produce illness (see Chapter 6). There is also an important difference in the extent of illness in different types of home; premature birth, stillbirths, and infant deaths, as well as maternal mortality and morbidity, all increase as socio-economic standing of the home declines. The steady decline in infant mortality, which has taken place in the developed world over the past fifty years, has left intact the proportional difference between the rates for infants whose fathers are unskilled workers and of those whose fathers are professional men. Children of unskilled workers continue to be more likely to fall ill with respiratory infection, gastro-enteritis, and the childhood infectious diseases. Larger families, possibly because of overcrowding, have a greater chance of illness; the chance of dying is greater for the fifth than it is for the first in the family. Social surveys, the modern tool for gauging the forces at work in society (see p. 26), repeatedly focus attention on the home, as the main factor involved in important national considerations. Few examples of this would be more eloquent than the significance of the family to education – in Britain equal opportunity according to age, aptitude, and ability, may still be denied to those with inadequate homes (see p. 264).[15]

The forces at work upon the family

The strength and stability of the family, as an agent in public health, depend upon the interaction of many forces both from within and without – housing, social aspirations, psychological disturbances, kinship networks, and demographic changes. Social aspirations drive the housewife to home-making up to and beyond the limit of the budget. Demographic changes re-fashion the family; new housing estates tear it up by the roots and replant it far from accustomed habitats. The slum dwelling, so terribly destructive of ordered family life, must be viewed in the perspective of the friendliness and sociability of slumland.[20] Emotional conflicts and personality defects, the unbridgeable gap between unrecognized or fantasied expectation and actual performance on the part of the spouse,[16] can undermine marriage. Sexual relationships, which may themselves be dependent upon childhood experiences, may determine happiness and affect the atmosphere of the home. Lack of organization, poor homecraft, poor family planning, imposes a great strain upon it, as may in some respects the working mother.

Housing

Cave man, as his family grew, occupied more of the deeper recesses, unconcerned with the many refinements of twentieth century sociology. He was not concerned with risks of infection from overcrowding, which endangers the lives of the young and spreads the tubercle bacillus and other organisms in massive doses; nor with the hazard to mental health of house sharing for young married couples; nor with pure water supplies, the flush closet, seclusion for the secondary school child to do homework, the damp-proof course, light and air, labour-saving kitchen equipment, without which mental, physical, and social health may be unattainable. Today we know of these dangers, but we still, except for a very few, have not been able to meet them. Many families still live in slums where all the hallmarks of a healthy home are lacking (see p. 89).

The developed world is crusading to get rid of its industrial environment of slums. More and more slum-dwellers are going to suburbia and a few to new towns (see p. 89). Yet the paradox of the modern world has been the decline in housing standards, which has accompanied scientific understanding of what health – physical and mental – demands. Increase in numbers of people, and the world-wide demand for town living, are great obstacles. As families get smaller and split into larger numbers of household units, the difficulties increase. Lack of privacy 'helps towards less rigid forms of child discipline'. But as privacy becomes more valued for its own sake, the single-room house, which is all that so many countries now provide, is sadly wanting.

Social aspirations

For the so-called middle class of the industrial society, the quest for advancement is one main driving force, which builds up a different pattern of family life from that of the manual worker.[10] Non-manual workers – social classes 1 and 2 and the clerks and shop assistants of social class 3 (see p. 237) – centre their lives upon the family and plough back the greater part of the income into it; their conduct is a family concern. Thus the family is a self-conscious unit, bound together by centrifugal forces. It aims at bettering itself. The manual worker tends to centre his life more upon his workmates than upon his home; his recreational activities have a first call upon his earnings; his conduct is the concern of his colleagues. Resignation, rather than recovery, is the family attitude to all misfortunes, including ill-health.[11] In this setting, aspirations to social improvement are frowned upon.

Such relative lack of support by the male, which weakens the family, at least in terms of public health, is growing less. Bethnal Green[20] in London has changed much since the time of Charles Booth,[1] and still more from that of Mayhew[13] and the days when Dr Barnardo and Lord Shaftesbury poked under tarpaulins in dead of winter for homeless children.[3] The husband is more identified with the home; a new companionship between husband and wife is growing up with a rise in status of the young wife and children. An old Glasgow slum has recently been shown to have a much improved 'atmosphere'.[7] The old type slum dweller, irregularly employed and flitting from place to place, with a home only in name, has been replaced by a new breed of persons who live in slum property for want of anything better. Not that all slum dwellers want to leave the old friendly atmosphere – many, in fact, hesitate to take on the higher costs of a good home; but few fail to value the advantages of a good house as the basis of a sound home. In the new housing estate, to which many have gone from the slums of industrial Europe, the husband's identification with the home has gone a step further; he sacrifices his own luxuries to make possible higher standards.

The competitive spirit to which attempts to 'keep up with the Joneses' give rise is affecting family life all over the developed world. The window-to-window relationship of suburbia, in the new housing estate with its unexpected exclusiveness, helps to drive families into competition. The home now comes first in the family budget – curtains, carpet, kitchen gadgets, telephone, lawn-mower, car. Rising standards stamp their pattern upon all but the most independent and detached minds. 'Mrs Jones' is as censorious as 'Mrs Grundy'; she frowns upon the roof without the television aerial and the kitchen without the electric washer. Thus she drives women to work outside the home and helps to build up the load of weekly-payment purchases.

No one can dispute that the modern house is better than the 'family per bed' space in the half-demolished warehouses of Rangoon, the shacks in the Negro quarters of Atlanta or Johannesburg, or the underground dwellings in Moscow or one-time Liverpool. But there are losses as well as gains. The new equipment in the modern American home 'has led not to more leisure, more time to play with the baby, more time to curl up and read by an open fire . . . but has merely combined with other trends in making the life of the American home-maker not easier, but more exacting'.[14] Or, possibly, new standards lead to new demands and to changing values about the use of time.

Rising standards can also make demands upon the family budget which lead to sacrifice of essential needs. The biological expansion of the family must materially straighten the budget. 'Having a family was a guarantee of poverty for the working classes in the 1930s . . . poverty is concentrated on children, those with dependent children to support, and the old.' Many surveys have shown that the proportion of protective food declines as the family grows and that new housing estates have helped to exact this penalty. Anxiety, that ill-defined enemy of the public health, can get to work more easily where every halfpenny is already bespoken – another straw, and the camel's back may sag. The isolation of the new family units, from grandparents, friends, and acquaintances, also contrast, sharply with the old slum. The modern 'baby-sitter' tells a story.

We have yet to see whether these new ventures, physically so desirable, can build up the friendliness and helpfulness of the old slum. Unless this is done, some of the gain to health will be lost in the increasing strain of child-rearing and decreasing support in sickness. We have still to learn how to rebuild the three-tier family relationship in circumstances where the children are not permitted to take over their parents' house. The bulging schools of the first years of a new housing estate, or town, may be empty in twenty years.

The working mother

Women throughout the underdeveloped world work equally with men, but they do so from home (see p. 27). A phenomenon in most, if not all, industrial societies, is the woman who goes out to work leaving her young children to be cared for by grandparents, relatives, or child-minders, or in nurseries. The USSR is said to have half a million permanent places in nurseries and to make arrangements during the height of harvesting for up to 5 million. In Britain there are rather more than 50,000 such places (1973). We cannot here discuss the many issues to which this aspect of life in an industrial society gives rise.

Suffice it to say that 'The proper place for an infant under two years is at home. . . . Mothers with children under two years should be discouraged from going out to work. Day nurseries should be regarded as supplementary to nursery schools and classes'.*

Kinship networks and demographic changes

The strength of the family depends much upon kinship networks, however bizarre the patterns that these may exhibit in different parts of the world. The attachment of mother and daughter – a common finding in surveys in industrial urban life – is possibly an outcome of the Industrial Revolution, which detached the father as the wage earner. But something similar no doubt operates widely. Kinship, as we have seen, is the key to self-help systems and possibly to mental health. A nice interaction of length of residence and kinship makes for happiness and security in the old industrial slum, where the family does more than anything else to make the local society a familiar society, filled with people who are not strangers, where people are not lonely, where, whenever they go out for a walk in the street, for a drink in the pub, or for a row on the lake in the park, they know the faces in the crowd.[20] Familiarity breeds content.

When families get smaller, inevitably some of the power of the family is sapped. In Western Europe and the New World, this change has gone far. The sickening stream of infant funerals, although rationalized, and the deadly fears with which young lives are surrounded throughout nine-tenths of the world, have at last ceased in the Western world. No longer are 'the sufferings of the children thought of as inevitable, and even as reasonable'.[19] Children are no longer born to die. But, where the birth rate has fallen to a mere replacement level, uncles and aunts are fewer. More wives are left to carry their burdens alone. The increasing burdens of the aged fall upon too few shoulders.

The importance of public health to the family

However much it may vary in different parts of the world, the family should be the fulcrum of the Health Service. A sound public health service will make an ally of the family, seeking to understand the springs of its action and how to bring scientific knowledge to its aid; strengthening it from within and supporting it from without.

External supports may need to be medical, social, economic, and psychological. First, if we are to treat the family as a living and growing organism, it must logically have a family doctor – not, as so often is the case so widely throughout the world, a physician who looks upon sickness as a source of income. The family doctor should work, wherever national resources permit, with midwives, nurses, and social workers to promote the health of a group of families. One means to accomplish this is the Health Centre – the operative unit for family care within a larger administrative 'health unit'. Social work, like doctoring, should be on a family basis, and every effort should be made to limit the number and variety of social agents who handle separate and limited aspects of family

* British Ministry of Health Circular 221–45.

case work. Special measures will be needed, if possible within the public health scheme, to deal with problem families and illegitimate pregnancies.

Social and economic measures to support the family need to be specific in their action, if full benefit is to be gained. General measures of support, such as food subsidies, a national health service, unemployment payments – which are being developed as a means to vanquish the five giants, Want, Ignorance, Squalor, Sloth, and Disease – benefit the families incidentally rather than specifically. Family allowances, school meals and milk, reduced rentals, the cheaper purchase of clothing, and subsidized holidays can do much more to meet the biological stresses to which a growing family gives rise.

The solution to the problem of family housing will vary from Japan to Jamaica. But whatever slant the particular culture of a nation may have, or the climate or the kinship network, the fundamentals of hygienic living are the same. The single-room units of a family compound in Bali have the same need as elsewhere for light and air, for kitchen amenities, for pure water and sanitation; and those of Japan, with their paper partitions, must contend with the same frustrations as the one-family rooms of Moscow or the over-crowded two-up-two-down in Newcastle upon Tyne.[3] Public health is bound to put housing high on its list of problems; this is perhaps why the medical officer of health should be responsible for the health aspects of housing; nothing less than his unremitting efforts can remedy the appalling conditions which everywhere exist. The building of new towns and overspill suburbs needs to be undertaken with particular care, with the lessons of suburbia in the Western world in mind. The possibilities of reconstruction in old worn-out environments needs more study, as does that of re-establishing the three-tier family in new housing estates.

Internal supports for the family are less easily managed. Here we are involved in the spiritual, moral, and cultural life of the members, and of the society of which the family forms part. For the families at the bottom of the occupational ladder who present industrial societies, at least, with almost the greatest modern challenge, the first essential is an understanding of the motives which determine their lack of co-operation and unwillingness to 'progress'. Improvement in the health of unskilled workers and their families would proceed much faster if all doctors were aware of the extent to which their own attitudes and behaviour, as well as those of their patients, need to be modified.[11] Much the same indeed may be said for all the world. Only proper study can provide us with the information we need in any country.[8] Teaching is our only weapon, but it cannot succeed unless it is based upon understanding of the mental make-up of those being instructed. We must learn how courageous it is for the mother to 'break with tradition and the expectations of her group'.[4] Lack of knowledge of human biology, one of the great barriers to understanding, has also to be remedied. 'For the majority their knowledge is like confetti, little islands of disconnected information acquired from a variety of reputable and disreputable sources. This knowledge is set in a jelly of rationalization and beliefs derived from folklore and the more sensational theories of bygone days.'[5] Learning about these again often means learning about ourselves (see Chapter 6).

Finally marriage guidance can logically be looked upon as a part of public health – as a means to instil an understanding of the upbringing of the family which often comes only with years. The value of security and affection to the young child and the dangers of disharmony in the home are more easily grasped by grandparents than parents, but they can be taught. Teaching becomes all the more important as the need for family planning extends (see p. 74). When also the liberty of the subject and the right to advancement is enthroned, as in America, teaching the social and biological significance of the family becomes an essential support for family life, whose ties are weakening.[14] Teaching may do something to make the family a first call upon the resources of money and effort – without the blind acceptance of the philosophy of 'keeping up with the Joneses'. Marriage guidance may also do something to combat disharmony when the children find themselves in an atmosphere of warring personalities – it is better if possible to mend the home rather than break it, since love and security are hardly to be found elsewhere. Public health is involved in them all, from the kitchen to the marriage bed.

The world is on the move; migration, social mobility, industrialization, changing beliefs, the abandonment of old ways of living, all increase the strain upon the family and call for further measures to preserve it. For the protective care of kinship groups, tribal elders, and family councils we must learn to substitute wider social institutions.

Lastly, we need further studies of marriage and the family. The causes of marital disharmony are to be found in highly complex interactions of personal and social conditions. We need to understand them better, as well as the structure and function of families in different communities and their adaptation to a changing environment.

8. Population

The importance of population to health

Health in the group depends upon the dynamic relationship between numbers of people, the space which they occupy, and the skill that they have acquired in providing for their needs. Public health is, therefore, vitally concerned with population – the numbers of people, their distribution, their movements, the age structure, and the birth and death rates in specific age groups. The practice of public health will also vary, for good or ill, with the effects of man's activities, for as people multiply they create new opportunities for health and fresh perils; as they migrate such opportunities and dangers, new and old, go with them.

Over-population affects the health of the community, physically and mentally. It undermines physical health by increasing the risks of infection and by the more subtle, but powerful, influence of malnutrition; by shortening life; by disrupting the family through deaths of its younger members; by damaging the health of the childbearing population through frequent pregnancies without any corresponding gain; by denying the community many of the essentials of health. Mental health suffers because of the hopelessness of life in circumstances where there exist neither houseroom, food, well-being, nor any of the essentials which make a life of fulfilment and purpose possible.

World public health also has to take account of the strong feelings between nations to which population problems can give rise. Not only have means of communication brought all peoples into touch with one another, but to a large extent there is interdependence. The difficulties of living, and its opportunities, have become world problems; no longer can any people easily starve in isolation, nor can any enjoy the fruits of the earth unaffected by another's misery. The great differences which exist are sources of frustration and tension. Nations today disagree about the interpretation of population trends and also as to the proper course of action to be pursued.

Similar feelings exist within individual countries, where there are different ethnic groups, with varying economic, social, and intellectual developments. Thus the differential birth and death rate may be adding to the tension between whites and Negroes in the United States, the Union of South Africa, and erstwhile colonial territories, between Hindus and Moslems in India and Pakistan, and between Chinese and other peoples of South-East Asia. Such tensions are greatest where discrimination exists, but they are present in almost every community in varying degree, both in countries such as Canada where two national groups are treated on an equal footing, and also in homogeneous states where there are differential rates of propagation and survival in social classes.

Growth of populations

Slow growth until recent centuries

Man spread to most parts of the globe a very long time ago, and in every part his numbers increased. Little is known about them for certain before A.D. 1000, when the population was approximately 275 million. It then accelerated progressively until about the year 1650, when a total of some 445 million had been reached. Before this time the total population of the world probably fluctuated within narrow limits, but the range and extent of the fluctuations is not known.[1] Sometimes it advanced rapidly, sometimes slowly, and no doubt often, as is known for certain during the fourteenth century, the world total declined. The human race seemed to fare better in some regions than others. Thus in Japan up to 1750, and in the Americas up to 1500, the rate of growth seems to have been greater than in Europe, India, or South-West Asia. Some of this advantage may have been due to differences in the prevailing diseases, and much no doubt to variations in habits of life.

Since neither the capacity of the human female to bear young, nor her opportunities, despite slavery and polygamy, are likely to have varied greatly in human history, the even balance of numbers must have been maintained by deaths — before, during, and after birth — from war, disease, famine, disaster, and human interference. The average mortality of about forty per thousand, however it may have been built up, seems generally to have been offset by the addition of young at something like the same rate. The importance of each cause of death has varied at different times throughout the world. Deaths in war — the continual drain of persistent tribal incidents, as in Africa, perhaps more even than the massed slaughter of conquests, which occurred for several centuries in South-West Asia after 1258 — have played their part. Calamities including famine have been frequent and harrowing, but probably, as a total cause of restraint on population growth, they come a long way down the list. The extent of infanticide and abortion has varied with local circumstances and values. The peoples of earlier civilizations, Egyptians, Hebrews, Hindus, Chinese, Greeks, Romans, and Teutonic tribes, all resorted to them.[6]

The killing of female infants (always to be suspected when males much exceed females in the adult population) has been a deeply rooted custom among nomads and hunters, for example, in Africa, South-West Asia, and India; it was practised in England before and after the Black Death; it caused the cessation of population growth in Japan between 1750 and 1850 during the Tokugawa era. Abortion, by artificial interference and by medicines, has been widely practised; sometimes, as on the Pacific atoll of Yap in modern times, it has caused a heavy decline in population.[9] But both infanticide and abortion have been countered by religious sanctions, which have had their roots in the urge for survival, so that high fertility has generally been encouraged throughout man's history.

Yet it is to death from disease that we should probably look for the chief cause of population restraint — particularly to deaths in the young. Infant mortality must always have ranked high, since to the ever-present risks of infection have been added the hardships of life in primitive societies.

Expansion after 1650

After the middle of the seventeenth century (for the past 300 years) there has been a marked change in pattern with rapid growth and constant acceleration. After the lapse of 150 years, i.e., by the time Malthus[7] wrote, in 1758, the population had doubled, to reach 920 millions. By 1974, it had reached 3,800 millions. The population of the world increased between 1650 and 1700 by 20 per cent; in the half century from 1900 to 1949 the rate of increase had advanced to 52 per cent; the addition of people to the world between 1900 and 1949 was 800 millions – as much as during the previous 800 years.[1, 26] By the year 2000 the world's population could well reach 7,000 millions. The change in population growth since the middle of the seventeenth century was almost certainly due, not to any change in female reproductive capacity, but to a decline in overall mortality dependent upon new ways of living and new forms of society. Developments in commerce, in technology, in geographical exploration, and in political reform, none wholly new, now advanced so rapidly as to have the character of revolutions. Europe was the motherland of most of these changes and, in consequence, it was here that the swarming process began. After 1750 the Industrial Revolution in England (see Chapter 13) added further impetus. Then the whole character of life in Europe began to alter. The industrial areas became hotbeds of infection; infant mortality advanced alarmingly and pandemics of fever slaughtered young and old. But simultaneously living conditions outside the industrial belts were improved, a new agriculture produced more abundant and varied foods, and new amenities softened the harshness of life. The new public health, born at the end of the eighteenth century (see Chapter 14), played an increasingly important role.

Between 1650 and 1950, the population of Europe advanced from 100 to 541 million, and Europeans including those in other lands to 641 million; the 2 million in Oceania had become 13; 12 in Central and South America 162, and one in North America 166. The first advance in England, from 5 in 1750 to 25 million in 1850, was perhaps the most spectacular, but the whole of Europe and the New World was soon involved. Moreover, if Europe was first off the mark, the changes in living, which were at the root of this phenomenon, were not long in spreading to distant regions. The Far East had become involved certainly by the middle of the nineteenth century; the 339 million living in Asia in 1650 had become 1,320 million by 1950. The increase in population in Japan from 30 million in 1870 to 95 in 1957 is certainly as spectacular as that of England. India advanced from 255 in 1871 to 357 million in 1950; Egypt from 4·5 million in 1846 to 19·5 in 1947. In contrast, the supposed 100 million in Africa in 1650 had no more than doubled by 1950.

During the second half of the last 300 years, the impetus of population increase has shifted from West to East, or more properly from developed to underdeveloped countries. The rapid fall of death rate has been countered in the developed countries by a corresponding fall in birth rate – so that the population increase has everywhere markedly declined; in Europe and North America (1971/2), the birth rate lies between 13 and 18, with Australia and New Zealand higher at 20–30.[5] The net effect upon population levels is still subject to fluctuations and variations, as in the USA, since the Second World War, but in total the population of the developed world gives the appearance of a juggernaut, which has come to rest. Thus it is that, until 150 years ago, while the birth rate remained constant in Europe, changes in economic and social well-being were reflected in death rates. Since this time the death rate has declined to reach a more or less stationary lower limit of 8 to 11 in North, West, and Central Europe (as also in America north of the Rio Grande, and in Oceania). Population now fluctuates only with alterations in the birth rates. The decline in population has not been uniform in all sections of the population. It began with the professional and managerial classes and has spread slowly through the non-manual to the manual elements. Thus the gap between manual and non-manual groups has widened.

In the East death rates are now falling much as they did in the developed world after 1650, or more especially after 1750. Reductions have occurred in most parts, and in some these are substantial, if not spectacular. In Japan the death rate in 1971 was 6·6; in Sri Lanka it was 12·9 in 1951, only five years after the malaria campaign had been begun, 11 in 1955 and 7·6 in 1971; in Egypt in 1971 it was 13·1.[5] Such evidence as exists suggests that the changes have begun, as they did in the Western world, in the highest of the prestige classes.

The changes which have taken place in the birth rate in the developed world have hardly begun in Latin America and the East, where the figure remains high. Thus in Sri Lanka, despite the spectacular fall in death rate, the birth rate, 38 in 1951, was still 39·9 in 1971 – a natural increase of 3 per cent per annum. In a few instances at least, although not universally, the birth rate has a tendency to *rise* with the first impact of industrialization – as in the Belgian Congo, Honduras, Malaya, Nicaragua, South and South-West Africa.[6] A substantial fall has occured in some countries, as in Japan, where the birth rate was 31 in 1946–8, 19 in 1956 and 19·2 in 1971; smaller but noticeable falls have occurred in India (38), China (33·1), Puerto Rico (25·6) and Sri Lanka (29·9).

Considerable disparities now exist between the countries of the world in the extent to which the population exceeds or falls short of the optimum. Some countries, for example, India, Java, Egypt, greatly exceed the optimum density; others, no more developed, such as Turkey, Thailand, and Burma, could with advantage have more people; still others, such as Japan and the United Kingdom, maintain very high densities on the proceeds of highly-developed industrial systems. But every country which has not settled to a lower level of population stability, with a low birth rate to balance the low death rate, is in danger of finding its population greater than its resources, as modern developments begin to exercise their full impact. All the countries of the world, whatever the state of their population, are now in the same boat together, with the same stake in preventing it from becoming overloaded.

Technological advances and superior wisdom can perhaps overcome every existing difficulty. Certainly for many countries today in dire straits, where population has grown beyond the resources of the land, industrialization is looked to as the only answer to immediate difficulties – as in Egypt with its extremely high densities on all the cultivable land. All such changes are to be encouraged. Yet it is evident from our history that we tend to expand to the limit, and to make use of every gain to increase our numbers – new lands become filled and old lands are made to take more. To this process there must be an end. Malthus' contention that population must 'press upon' the supporting power of the land is true, even if food production be increased a thousand times.[3] In short, the growth of world population in the last 300 years does not express a trend, and it cannot be projected indefinitely into the future. Rather has it been a unique, unprecedented, and unpredictable phenomenon of limited duration.[26]

The demographic cycle

The history of populations since 1650 suggests that national growth takes place according to a cycle in which five stages can be arbitrarily defined. The first stage, from which each nation begins, is that in which population is stationary because a high death rate cancels out a high birth rate (high stationary). The second occurs when the death rate begins to fall while the birth rate continues at or near to the maximum (early expanding). The third is that in which the birth rate also begins to decline; the population continues to grow because the numbers born exceed those dying (late expanding). In the fourth stage the population again becomes stationary, with a low birth rate and a low mortality (low stationary); and in the fifth the population declines because the babies born are fewer than the deaths (declining).

Demographic cycles are likely to have evolved in previous civilizations. The Roman civilization may well have reached the fourth and fifth stages somewhere between the second and fourth centuries after Christ. In our own the cycle of population growth began, under the influence of development, at different times and places throughout the world. No known people now exists, however physically and culturally isolated, that has not been influenced, either directly or indirectly, by industrialization, or through contact with its products. Colonial influences, wherever they have occurred, particularly in the field of public health, are certain to have led to some decline in mortality. On this basis every nation should at least have reached stage two of the cycle – indeed must have, if we are to account for the world-wide increase in population since 1650. It is doubtful whether it is any longer possible to distinguish between countries in the high stationary and early expanding stages. China, conjectured at 74 millions in A.D. 1000, 150 in 1650, and perhaps five times this figure in 1957, is still arbitrarily placed by many in the high stationary phase, because, in terms of its great size, its population gives the appearance of a standstill; but in reality the death rate is already declining. Of the other countries which are generally placed in the high stationary phase, i.e., Afghanistan, Arabia, Ethiopia, Indonesia, Iran, parts of South America, and almost the entire African continent, except perhaps the Union of South Africa, it is hardly possible to say anything with certainty, in view of the almost total absence of vital records (see Chapter 22).

The regular sequence of cycles is not easy to follow, particularly since the great changes in death rates which have occurred in recent years. As late as 1952 many countries were placed in the *early expanding* phase – India, Pakistan, Burma, Sri Lanka, Thailand, Indo-China, Formosa, Korea, parts of the Middle East, Turkey, Madagascar, Mexico, Central America, and parts of South America;[2] many of these today would need to be placed elsewhere. In the case of some the margin of difference between births and deaths remains great. Sri Lanka, for instance, (1971) has a birth rate of 29·9 with a death rate of 7·6, India (1970) 38 and 16·7, Malaya (1971) 39 and 7·2, Thailand (1969) 42·8 and 10·4.[5]

In many countries, the Soviet Union, Japan, Argentina, Poland, Bulgaria, Rumania, Yugoslavia, Italy, Spain and Chile, where death rates are low and birth rates declining, the step to *late expansion* has already been taken. In the case of countries said to have reached the low stationary phase – western, northern, and some central parts of Europe, USA, Australia, and New Zealand – since the Second World War many have experienced a striking upsurge. The USA in particular has had a natural increase of about 1·5 per cent per annum (in 1972, birth rate 15·6, death rate 9·4), a rate higher than that of Great Britain in the period of rapid expansion in the second half of the nineteenth century. The final stage of declining births is, of course, hypo-thetical. Before, or at least soon after, it is reached, nations take vigorous measures to counteract it. Every nation tends to regard its own culture as the finest in the world, and none readily contemplates its extinction. A rigorous policy of support for the family, as in France, the only country so far to have experienced stage five in the modern era, redresses the balance.

Migration

The migration of peoples from their homelands, which tears up the family by its roots or disrupts it by the removal of cherished members, although age-old, has in recent centuries added enormously to the problem of public health. As a by-product of so many human activities – war, famine, disease, industrialization, religious persecution, over-population, and exploration – it has taken millions far over the high seas and across land masses, or perhaps no further than to the newly-built industrial areas, but always to a new environment, where customs and cultural ties differ and new hazards have to be met.

In past times, the overseas migration of perhaps 60 million from Europe – Spaniards and Portuguese to South America after 1400, Dutch to South Africa after 1700, and English and other Europeans to North America and Australasia, especially in the Great Resettlement between 1870 and 1920; the exodus of 15 million slaves from Africa to the New World, chiefly in the seventeenth, eighteenth, and nineteenth centuries; the nineteenth-century internal migration eastward in Russia and westward in North America; the uprooted millions from the villages of England during the Industrial Revolution (see Chapter 13); Chinese to Indonesia and Thailand, Indians to Burma or Africa; in more recent times, the influx to Israel, the displacement of Europe's millions after 1939, migrant labour in the USA, and the trek to industrial townships in

Africa and South America – all such movements of human beings from their accustomed habitats have features in common and all give rise to endless problems in public health, in epidemiology, in social disease, and in cultural assimilation. The ill-effects upon individual, family, and nation will vary with the extent of dispersion within the receiving nation, with the degree to which ties with the homeland are kept up, with the maintenance of separate ethnic groups, and with intermarriage, as, in earlier centuries, of Spaniards in South America, or more recently of Chinese in Thailand.

Insecurity is a common characteristic, manifesting itself in a dozen different ways in the congregation of ethnic groups, formation of minorities, and clashes between races. Anxiety is more prevalent, and also psychosis, if what has been found among New York immigrants can be more generally applied. Witch doctors have multiplied in urban South Africa. Cultural conflicts, between the first and second generations and of children and parents, disturb relationships. The population structure lacks balance, with few children and old people, and often less women than men. Living conditions are bad, with poor housing, overcrowding, and slums, and no knowledge of how to keep healthy. The habits of the old environment are ill-adapted to the new. Diseases, such as syphilis and tuberculosis, spread. Maladjustment and spiritual anarchy weaken the organic unity of the new society.

The future

The growth of the world's population, viewed as part of a complex of demographic cycles, seems to be a self-limiting process. Development, including industrialization, establishes a number of new and potent processes which tend to a decline in birth rate: rising income and consumption, improving education, emancipation of women and their employment outside the family, increase in physical and social mobility, improved security for old age, and the secularization of cultural values and institutions. The fundamental change is in the system of cultural values: the belief in high fertility gives place to a desire for other forms of fulfilment for the family. Mrs Jones, a less desirable addition to the system of values, comes to exercise her influence by raising the appreciation of success and the desirability of climbing the social ladder, for both of which too many children are an encumbrance. Many changes in a developing society also reduce the immediate economic value of children.

The assumption that population curves will eventually flatten out is therefore not fanciful. Some members attending the World Population Conference at Bucharest in 1974[25] stressed the need for the developed world to hasten with its help to speed up development, seeing in this a more effective means to population control than gratuitous advice about family limitation. But it is the time factor which is now important, since the advent of modern public health has greatly accelerated the decline of mortality. Cultural values change slowly and reactions against rationality are strong; meanwhile economic development may result in larger not smaller populations for an inconveniently long time. The underdeveloped world can aggravate its own problems, as indeed has happened in Puerto Rico, by concentrating all its attention on reduction of mortality alone.[9] Moreover, since the artificial limitation of increase in Western society has been the result of desires for economic and social advancement in a politically free regime, it is not certain that the same set of circumstances will be exactly reproduced elsewhere. The experience of Japan suggests that the traditional values of an agricultural society may be retained for a longer time after intense industrialization than has been the case in the Western world.[10] Colonialism may have done the same by different means, when it introduced foreign technicians and borrowed techniques, thus preventing the natural developments in social thinking which arise out of changes in the social order and which are necessary to a decline in fertility.[8] The spectre of Malthus, and of all the other bogeys of an overpopulated world, must therefore dog man's footsteps for some time to come, unless the stages in the natural cycle can be accelerated.

Limitation of the family cannot be imposed upon the human being; nor can the world community ever settle the actual numbers permissible to each nation, even if the necessary sanctions could be exercised. The hope of finding a solution to the world population problem rests upon the development of social movements, which enthrone the idea of a smaller planned family. This is the outstanding need of public health in the last quarter of the twentieth century everywhere in the world. Overpopulation has entered a new and dangerous phase, which is now capable of undoing all the benefits of public health. If we save life and lengthen it, and yet cannot control our exuberant fertility, we must set in motion a swarming process in which the inexorable forces of ecology are called into play to limit multiplication in the human, in ways so far encountered only in the rest of the animal kingdom (see Chapter 2). The spectre of biological suicide with human groups metaphorically charging like lemmings into the sea, or decimated by infections like ducks dying in millions along the shores of the Great Salt Lake (p. 10), may be ecologically possible, or even probable, but few will grasp the reality of such fearful happenings. Population growth is best seen as a danger to orderly development, which can swallow up advances in living standards. It must be seen in the context of the sort of society most suited to the enjoyment of the inhabitants of a country. Living space is not unlimited, nor is the enjoyment of nature's delights. Many countries need to ask themselves whether they wish to repeat the urban concentrations and sprawls, which now characterize the developed world. These are considerations within the grasp of most people.

The most natural vehicle for teaching the need for population control is public health, which not only regards the family as one of its mainstays, but sees in overpopulation the seeds of its own destruction.

Every means for population control, scientifically approved and culturally acceptable, should be considered; rhythm, sheaths, diaphragms, jelly, foam tablets, oral contraceptives, intra-uterine devices, sterilization, vasectomy and salpingectomy will all play a part.[2] Sterilization, as in India, Puerto Rico and elsewhere, and abortion, as in Japan, Sweden and Denmark may well provide the most immediate benefits and are appropriate to situations of great urgency;

yet they interfere most with personal choice and increase hazards for the childbearing population. Control of the family by contraception is preferable, taught as part of maternity and child welfare, and in marriage guidance. Instruction can be given by midwives, social workers, and nurses, and, as in Japan, awareness can be aroused through intensive health education of the public. The modification of public attitudes may be slow, but the means at our disposal, including wireless and television, are as great an advance in the technological field as any in public health. Moreover, we have reached a better understanding of how to further social movements through small groups and organizations.

Limitation of families, as seen in European society, tends to have begun among professional and higher business executives, and to have spread slowly down the social gradient. The disadvantages of this, genetically and socially, are only too plain. Yet this phenomenon may well be inescapable, and it can hardly justify delay in seeking to spread an understanding of family planning. The difficulties which face the world are sociological rather than technological; they are bound with habits of living, inadequacy of housing, poverty, and systems of values – just as are so many other problems in public health.

India, China, and Japan, among those countries where the need of population control is greatest, have already embarked upon such a programme, including field experiments to determine the best technique for action and teaching. Although birth rates as a whole have altered relatively little, yet a beginning has been made. Perhaps of greatest significance is the ready acceptance of this new teaching. The people are neither hostile nor indifferent, if perhaps a little slow to respond. A steady flow of scientific knowledge regarding contraception, and provision of facilities within the means of those wishing to adopt its practice, is urgent and will produce lasting results.[2] Much hangs on this prediction for India and the world.

Sociology can benefit from technological advance in this respect as in so many others. Technical developments in contraception, already studied over many centuries if not millenia, have in recent years given more hope of universal application. *Oral gestogens*, now taken by many millions, can be virtually 100 per cent effective[14] and *intra-uterine devices*, also used by millions, can protect '3 women out of 4'.[15, 18] *Periodic abstinence*, based upon scientific control data, with higher rates of failure, has much to offer.[13] We are at the beginning of a movement in which science and anthropology must go hand in hand to prevent man from biological suicide by overpopulation (see also WHO scientific studies[12, 13, 17-24]).

For the problems of migration, some of the answers will be found in the organized public health service, which is discussed elsewhere throughout this book. In this the medical officer of health, socially orientated and aware also of the psychological issues involved, will play an important role, as well as the general practitioner working in a team with other social workers. The health centre has much to offer.

9. Occupation

Occupation presented man with an early environmental hazard – perhaps the earliest, if we exclude the elements. The first arts of civilization depended upon the working of materials, which could not easily be undertaken without inhaling or ingesting harmful substances. The earth had to be mined for lead, copper, mercury, iron; the ores extracted in furnaces, and the metals worked; hides needed to be cured with alum; vegetable fibres had to be made into fabrics and these turned into garments; stone had to be dug up for building and cut to shape in the interests of art; clay had to be turned upon the potter's wheel, and glazed; simple chemicals to be compounded into paints. Where services to the public were established, once the centres of living had grown sufficiently in size, sewers had to be cleaned, bodies buried, clothing washed, and bread baked. Some occupations, which we think of as commonplace today, were slow to develop – glass making, although an early discovery attributed to the Phoenicians and known to the Egyptians, was little practised for many centuries; and it was not before 500 years of the Roman era had passed that the baker was known to ancient civilizations. Others came and went with changing customs – the purple factories, which scattered the Mediterranean seaboard, using immense quantities of the rock whelk, *Murex brandaris*, went out of fashion with the toga of the Roman patrician.

But the basic materials have differed little over many centuries, if, as in the art of making mirrors or gilding, new uses have been found for them. In all civilizations, presumably, painters have sucked lead and copper paint from their brushes, and masons have inhaled silica dust. The 'tremblings' resulting from the inhalations of mercury vapour and the paralysis which came from the ingestion of lead were probably as well known to the ancients as to Ramazzini.[11] The slaves and Christians, condemned to work in the mines, were short-lived, and so too were their successors in the Carpathian Mountains during the sixteenth century, according to the much quoted saying of Agricola in *De Re Metallica* (1556), that women were there found who had as many as seven husbands who had died successively in the mines. The extensive use of copper and bronze in Ancient Greece for buttons, medals, money, pins, and statues exacted a heavy toll among those who worked and fashioned it. The copper miners of Greece were short-lived, old and decrepit at forty, as they were in France in 1822, when Patissier[10] wrote.

Illness arising out of occupation has also probably always had a close relationship with social status. The labouring classes have suffered from higher mortality rates, and have lived shorter lives, than those who have not needed to earn their living by the sweat of their brow, although statistical proof, for obvious reasons, has been lacking until comparatively recent times. M'Cready, in the USA, in the early part of the nineteenth century, said that labourers were generally short-lived; for it was rare 'to meet with a laborer over 50 years of age', and they were generally broken down before they reached that period. In contrast professional men lived on the average over 60 years, lawyers 66, clergy 65·7, doctors 62·8, professors and teachers in schools 61, so that in all countries those in comfortable and affluent circumstances lived longer than the labouring population.[8] In France much the same was observed in 1840 and again at the turn of the century (1907–8) when there were marked variations in death rates between employers, salaried workers, and wage workers; in the age group 35 to 44, deaths per 10,000 were 82, 120, and 136 respectively, and at the age 45 to 54, 127, 203, and 232.[14] This has probably been true of all societies and not only those industrialized countries that we have come to regard as 'developed'. Certainly with industrialization, during the last two centuries, the margin of difference between the professional classes and manual labourers was at first widened and then began to narrow.

Much of the difference depends upon living conditions, housing, diet, and economic status, rather than on occupation. Yet, perhaps the most significant differences have been within the manual trades themselves. In France (1907), the mortality of plumbers, for example, was twice that of textile workers.[14] In the Registrar General's figures for England and Wales in 1931, the standardized mortality ratio of limestone workers was 72; the ratios for sandstone workers (132), ware makers, casters, and finishers in pottery works (135), workers in metalliferous mines (134), and slate workers (168), were twice as much or more.[1] Most striking of all has been the low comparative mortality of agricultural workers. In 1931 the standardized mortality ratio for the whole group of agricultural occupations in England and Wales was 73 for males, and for those employed in tending cattle and dairying 45. The agricultural labourer has probably never shared in the higher mortalities of manual workers generally; for angina pectoris in 1931, this class had the lowest S.M.R. of any group of workers, namely 32.[1] Small wonder that so many have extolled 'the advantage of spending days in the open air and in labours varied and good'. In 1807 data from all the hospitals in Paris showed that the mortality of occupations was greatest among the workers in the dirty trades and least among those who worked in the open air, and among workers in wood and iron, and lastly among butchers, who lived among the odours of fresh meat.[10] Good living, certainly in Europe, with a balanced diet, may have accounted for some of the advantages of country life. Butchers, and the slaughtermen, their wives, and their errand boys, Thackrah noted (1831), 'almost all eat fresh cooked meat, at least twice a day – they are all plump and rosy . . . cheerful and good natured.' 'But,' he added, 'longevity is not greater in them.' They lived too highly, in Thackrah's opinion, and developed a plethora, which gradually led to disease.[13] Modern statistics have also shown the truth of Agricola's observation that wives often do not share in the occupational risks of their husbands.

Many factors enter into the hazards of the manual trades which such figures depict; dust in the air, specific poisons, accidents, excess of moisture and temperature, infections, long hours, and cramped postures. The disadvantages certainly do not all lie with labouring, for to the hazards of the work itself must be added those of the habits of living which accompany it, habits which work engenders, but which are not necessarily part of it. While the potter has damaged his constitution through the centuries with silica dust, others who have never been subjected to such risks have done as much harm by simple neglect of physiological principles of healthy living. Thackrah's descriptions of harmful habits in Arts, Trades, and Professions were no doubt particular to the early nineteenth century when the commercial traveller, dining at the traveller's table, drank his pint or bottle of wine, then took negus with several of his customers; and at night had a glass or two of brandy and water. The result was disease: 'first an affection of stomach and head – frequently a variety of nervous and hypochondriacal feelings; subsequent congestion of the abdominal veins; finally organic disease of the liver. And if . . . not suddenly taken off by apoplexy . . . he merges into dropsy and the bloated mass sinks into an early grave.'[13] Innkeepers too were addicted to unnecessary drinking, and they ended with 'apoplexy and dropsy closing the scene', and shopkeepers were 'too engrossed in keeping the shop, standing behind the counter all day or sitting in a small back parlour, wanting the inclination for exercise or for recreation and amusement . . . breathing an atmosphere contaminated and adulterated . . . pale, dyspeptic, and subject to affections of the head.'[12] Too many mercantile men had a disposition to have their house and warehouse within a stone's cast, so that five or six days a week they took scarcely any exercise. Of all Thackrah's perspicacious observations, those which reflect upon the importance of exercise touch most closely the weaknesses of the twentieth century. Like M'Cready in the USA, he also deprecated haste at meal time:[13]

The way in which men of business take their meals is also injurious to health. It is far too hasty. They seem to be travelling by the stage, and expecting every moment the summons of the coachman. The Arabs say, that 'he who does not care to chew his victuals hates his life'; and the adage is too often verified in this country, by the gastric disorders which result from a want of mastication.

The evils of which Thackrah observed, neglect of exercise, too great concentration on the acquisition of wealth, and addiction to the pleasures of the table, are the concomitants of occupation in all cultures and all parts of the world, and probably will remain so. The present-day rise of incidence of coronary disease in developed countries, and its social gradient 'from labourer to gaffer', may reflect them.

The growth of public health in occupation

Concern of the worker may well have been one of the earliest forms of public health. In Rome, public baths were available to everyone. 'The workers after having worked all day, went there in the evening to wash and to undo the fatigues of the day; they were less subject to illness than the workers of our own century'.[11] The founders of great cities and kingdoms took particular care of workmen and tradesmen. The colleges and societies of artificers, to which Plutarch refers, like the guilds of a later European civilization, helped to protect the interests of the worker. Ingenious devices, including masks to put over the mouth and nose and extraction conduits sucking out the foul vapours of the workshops, were early inventions.

Workers themselves, as Patissier remarked in 1822,[10] have been so little jealous of their health that they have disdained to surround themselves with means of preservation; it is much the same today. But the dangers of many occupations, and the heavy mortality and distressing sickness which have followed their practice, exerted strong pressures for reform. It was the mercurial poisoning of the gilders that caused a distinguished merchant of gilded bronzes to finance research through the French Royal Academy of Sciences into the means to avoid the dangers of inhaling mercury vapour – which resulted in the *fourneau d'appel*.[10] Likewise in devising means to work the mines without the worst of risks, the inhabitants of the British Isles have often set the pace. 'The Saxons and the English, from time immemorial, the one in extracting metals, the other in mining coal, have become our masters in this type of improvement'.[10] We have little means now of knowing how effective were the measures of protection in the mines and workshops, and other dangerous occupations, throughout the centuries. There was, no doubt, a growth of technical knowledge, which was practised with varying thoroughness by enlightened employers and intelligent workmen.

Occupational disease has been a challenge to medicine, but only in relatively recent years. Bernardino Ramazzini was the first to throw down the gauntlet, when in the preface to his account, *The Diseases of Artificers* (1700), he wrote : [11]

Must we not in fact agree that many occupations are a danger to those who engage in them, and that the unhappy workers who fall ill when they looked to be able to support themselves and their families, die cursing a thankless job. . . . It is but reasonable that medicine should contribute its share for the benefit and comfort of those for whom the law has been so tenderly careful, and display itself in a particular manner (a thing hitherto neglected) for the safety of tradesmen, that they may follow trades without injuring their health.

Medicine has since displayed itself to good effect. Doctors, in the quiet of the study and by painstaking observations in the field, have examined the dangers of following various trades. Mortality statistics have done much to compel attention. As Patissier sagely observed:

When it has been established that the procedure in some occupations occasions great mortality . . . government will appeal to the learned and require them to modify the work or discover a healthier form. Doctors, for their part, will point means to preserve health . . . then, too, we will have the possibility of advising children about the choice of a profession according to their constitution, physique, temperament, and disposition.[10]

Patissier, like Ramazzini, who 'thought it no indecency to step some times into the meaner Sorts of Workhouses, and View the Secrets of Mechanic Arts',[11] may have been hitching his waggon to a star; but these early pioneers were helping to set our thoughts in the direction of world health. Many have followed in their footsteps, through the workshops of Europe and the New World. Greenhow's pilgrimage through the factories and workshops of England, 160 years after Ramazzini, examined the effects of industrialization in causing pulmonary disease in a wide range of occupations. Greenhow indicted dust:[4]

Grinders of cutlery, needles, and other steel articles; miners, quarrymen, stone masons china scourers; potters, turners of earthenware, makers of plaster-of-Paris moulds, hacklers of flax and Mexican fibre; sorters of wool, alpaca, and mohair; operatives employed in the manufacture of waste silk, and in the carding-rooms of cotton factories; wool-combers; workers in bone, ivory, horn, and mother-of-pearl, and makers of walking-sticks and wooden handles for cutlery, umbrellas, and parasols.

In all these trades, the atmosphere became loaded with fine dust of metal, stone, clay, soot, flax, or woollen fibre. In mining and wool-combing, flat-pressing, and in the potteries, there was damage to the lungs by inhaling fumes and from an over-heated and highly dried atmosphere.

Hot and exceedingly moist atmospheres, ill-ventilated and over-heated factory rooms, extremes of temperature, stooping and constrained postures, long-continued sedentary work, and ill-ventilated and over-crowded rooms, all played a part in pulmonary disease. This added many more trades: straw-plaiting, silk-piercing, glove-making; slip-making, and flax-spinning; lathe-making; decorating and 'throwing' of earthenware; welting and finishing of hosiery.

What occupations remained to which men might engage without the danger or likelihood of succumbing to pulmonary disease? The risk certainly was high. The mortality from pulmonary diseases among the male inhabitants of Sheffield (1848–54) was an average rate of 8·39 per thousand – and this at a time when the use of fans to suck away the dust had been widely adopted. But as Greenhow so acutely observed:[4]

Although the introduction of fans has produced such beneficial effects, the occupation of needle pointing is still attended with injury to health. A small quantity of fine dust, only perceptible when the sun shines brightly, escapes the indraught of air . . .

For 250 years, doctors in Europe and the New World have sought to unravel the tangled skein of disease in industry by the study of industrial processes, the workshops in which they occur, and the workers themselves. But the truths about occupational hazards, although they stimulated interest, provided no automatic remedy – it still remained to apply them to the vast and ramifying industrial patterns of rapidly expanding societies; and without public health organizations there was little chance of enforcing measures of protection. Patissier[10] asked that occupations which were a danger to health should be prohibited; that dangers be diminished by machinery to supplement manual labour and prevent gases and vapours from poisoning the environment; that public baths be established as in Roman times; and that those who were injured and whose health was damaged by occupation should be helped by the State and by insurance schemes. It was a beginning. Systems of factory inspection, notification of industrial diseases, special rules for dangerous industries, medical supervision of workers, institutes of hygiene, and public health action of all kinds have grown from it.

Thus, largely as a result of Ramazzini, M'Cready, Patissier, Thackrah, Greenhow, and others, a small team of medical pioneers, the industrial workers became the first of the so-called vulnerable groups to be the subject of organized public health, when Europe and America, in the middle of the last century, took the first hesitant steps in the supervision of the factory worker's health; France sending circulars to the *Préfets* in the *départements* (see Chapter 14) and England appointing factory inspectors under the Shaftesbury Factory Act (1833). An early step was the medical examination of new entrants to industry and the exclusion of women and young children from the mines. Provisions for ensuring safety and a reasonable working environment, cubic capacity per head, temperature, humidity, ventilation, sanitation, and regulations covering dangerous trades, have required special codes and systems of inspection by skilled technicians in a wide range of ever changing processes. Increasingly the industrial health service has been concerned with problems in social medicine – the psychological and social problems of the worker (see Chapter 13).

In these developments doctors have played a large part both in central government departments and locally. Nationalized industries in Britain and elsewhere have provided their own medical service. Large private industrial concerns have appointed whole-time medical officers with the duty to advise on all matters affecting the health of the worker, to study sickness, absenteeism, and industrial disease, to examine workers for occupational risks, to carry out periodic health checks, and to educate the worker in health matters. In the UK by 1950 nearly 5,000 factories had provided their own health service.[1] In Russia, industrial health is supervised by public health doctors working from the industrial policlinics (health centres); a high proportion of workers in industry are given annual health checks by a team of policlinic specialists (see p. 134).

The problems of factory health, particularly in old industrial societies, are complicated by the large number of small factories for which so far it has not been possible to organize the same measure of health cover. In the UK, of some 250,000 factories and workshops, four-fifths have less than 26 workers; only 12,000 have more than 100, and less than 5,000 more than 250 workers. The small factory has much to offer in sympathetic management, of importance to psychological and social health, but it often lacks much in the hygiene of the environment.

For occupational health outside the factory, in shops and offices, hotels, catering establishments, the home, and the professions, much less has been done. The protection of health for these occupations will depend upon further research into the risks involved – into coronary disease, for instance, which affects most of the professional classes, particularly doctors and business executives.

The future of occupational health

Throughout the industrialized countries, hazards to health in factory life have been much reduced, particularly those due to inhalation of dust through the introduction of mechanical devices to draw away the dust or to prevent it from rising; so that wherever organized public health operates successfully, the dusty occupations have lost most of their terrors. No longer can we point at the metal filers, where no instance was known, in 1833, of a working filer exceeding the age of 50; nor to the mason whose 'chippings from the stone occasioned serious and often fatal injury of the lung'; nor to the lead miners who 'rarely work more than six hours a day, yet . . . seldom attain the age of 40'; nor to the fork grinders 'who use a dry grindstone and die at the ages of 28 or 32'.[3]

The workers into whose systems poisons have entered by other means, manufacturers of lead and painters 'sallow and thin' and 'soon broken in health',[3] and paper stainers, poisoned by arsenic or white lead, have been protected, following the discovery of substitutes and the prohibition of materials. But new discoveries continually introduce new hazards. The manufacture of new chemicals has already done so on many occasions. Many of the newer metals, for example, cadmium, platinum, and beryllium, have proved harmful when absorbed into the body, and their use has given rise to new dangerous trades, such as the coating of tubes for fluorescent strip lamps with beryllium compounds, the smelting of cadmium ores, and the welding of its alloys.[6, 7] White phosphorus gave mankind the inestimable advantage of a 'strike anywhere' match, and the terrible malady of 'phossy jaw'. Phosphorus poisoning, of which the first case was reported in Vienna in 1838, was finally rendered unnecessary when a satisfactory substitute in sesqui-sulphide of phosphorus was put into operation in France in 1898.[6, 7] Chronic benzine poisoning, taking the form of aplastic anaemia, is more recent; and, since benzine is used as a solvent in great quantities, and in a variety of industries, it remains a danger.[6, 7]

Arsenite of copper, named 'Scheele's green' after its discoverer, began to be used extensively in the middle of the nineteenth century in colour printing and in the preparation of ornamental wrapping paper, wallpapers, and artificial flowers. The arsenic poisoning which resulted was brought to public notice by one of the first medical officers of health (Dr Hillier in the Parish of St Pancras, London), and the study of its disastrous effects upon the health of this new occupational group was brilliantly undertaken by Dr Augustus Guy, one of the earliest epidemiologists to use statistical methods.[5] Now that aniline dyes have displaced Scheele's green as a colouring matter, paper and flower making is no longer hazardous, but arsenite of copper is still manufactured as an insecticide for preserving fruit trees; and it is an ingredient of sheep dip. More recently it has come under suspicion as a cause of epitheliomatous ulceration in those engaged in its manufacture. The twentieth century has introduced the hazard of radiation in mines, factories, and medical work. Various occupations add small numbers to the swelling total of lung cancer (see p. 20).

New hazards come and others go with the changing patterns of life. The chimney-sweep with his cancer of the scrotum is no longer seen; but other occupations have had the same effect (see p. 20). The cattle driver who walked '20, 30, or 40 miles a day' and the gentleman's coachman who 'filled up his time by filling up his stomach' were specific to an age now past.[13] The chaise drivers, postillions, stage coachmen, and guards of coaches who suffered from 'irregular living and the habits of frequent potation' have come and gone.[13] But the hazards to which they were subjected may well have been no more than that of the long-distance lorry drivers today. For many, the risks of unphysiological living, particularly lack of exercise, have increased with changing customs. The commercial travellers are no longer 'riding from town to town' as in 1831, nor does the practice of medicine and surgery today require 'that a considerable portion of time be daily devoted to study and the rest to professional visits . . . which afford exercise in the open air, and thus tend to invigorate health'.[13] Whatever was the virtue of travelling by horse in the open air has gone; and for it is substituted travel by motor car, whose hazards are not yet fully understood.

Thus, occupation remains one of the main hazards to health throughout the world; it leaves no room for complacency. In the form of industrial accidents it is a major cause of incapacity – among roughly 20 million insured workers in England and Wales during 1961/62 accidents caused nearly three-quarters of a million spells off work. Accidents in mining and quarrying, as from time immemorial, constitute a particular danger. They accounted for over a third of the total, and, when taken together with accidents in the engineering trade, for about half the total of spells off work of all the working population.[9]

In many occupations, such as coal mining and working in the carding rooms of mills, dust is still causing illness, although it is less immediately obvious than that produced by mercury, lead, and copper. We encounter bronchitis of the flaxman, which Thackrah described so meticulously, and which was rediscovered 125 years later.[12] Many occupations, such as tailoring, shoe-making, or laundry work, are still carried on under harmful conditions, although without any specific or noxious agent involved. The cross-legged tailor, of whom Thackrah wrote, 'his body bent for thirteen hours a day' and 'sitting all day in a confined atmosphere'[13] is still to be found in all too many parts of the world. Jewellers and workers in gold confined 'to a leaning posture, with the head much depressed and the elbows generally forced to the sides of the trunk, for ten, fourteen, or sixteen hours a day'[13] are not entirely unknown. Stone masons, as in Jordan, tap endlessly, like woodpeckers, and inhale siliceous dust. There remain many occupations where the temperature and moisture, and most recently noise, is excessive. As Greenhow said, referring to the cutlers of Sheffield, lead miners of Alston and lacemakers of Macclesfield in 1858, 'it is probable that a careful examination into the nature of these employments and the manner in which their hurtful results are produced would show that such results are not inevitable consequences of the several industrial occupations'.[3]

The road to health in and through occupation, with no end in sight and with constant changes of direction, has been long and tedious. All nations travelling along it are driven at different paces, but inexorably, by the increasing demands of technical development. The protection of the worker as a vulnerable group in society, with supervision of his environment and of the effects of technical processes upon him mentally and physically, is therefore sound public health. Such public health measures may be based upon institutes of hygiene as in Yugoslavia or upon health centres as in Russia; they may be part of a health unit as in France or an independent service as in Britain. The organization must suit the circumstances and philosophy of each nation. But for all, irrespective of the details of the plan adopted, greatest advantage will come through the integration of occupational health with other public health work and with the general medical care of the worker in his home setting.[1]

Finally, occupation is an essential ingredient of health. Since man is a social animal, he must have an object in life, otherwise 'he is like a tree without a leading shoot' – he dissipates his strength in irregular pursuits or decays from listlessness. Man's difficulty has been to seize the benefits of occupation without taking on its dangers. Work in itself should not cause illness, but rather health. As M'Cready said:[8]

In reviewing the various employments by which man obtains his bread by the sweat of his brow, we are struck by the fact that various as is their nature, there is nothing in the great majority of them which is not compatible with health and longevity.

10. Town Life

Man's desire, as a social animal, to play his part in groups has exerted an important influence on public health. When man was a forest or cave dweller, thinly scattered across the surface of the globe, we can be certain that, although he had much to withstand, there were many dangers that we have since endured of which he knew little or nothing. In leaving behind his nomadic life, perhaps in the neolithic period, to live in villages, his epidemiological history began afresh. The web of his social obligations was woven into new patterns, his environment developed new hazards, and his long battle with bacteria began in earnest. Then came the towns, 'a living personality, expressing and cherishing the instincts, tastes, beliefs, and corporate pride of the citizens, widely and richly pictured'[7] and, of course, bringing with it fresh hazards as well as new opportunities for health. What has been the influence of the town upon world public health? Has it improved health or worsened it? Has man seized the new opportunities or fallen prey to the hazards?

The shattering epidemics, which have smitten cities during the past twenty-five centuries, and of which the memories live with us for their effect upon history, such as the plague in Athens in 430 B.C., of which Thucydides told, or the pestilence of A.D. 543 which Gibbon reconstructed, are to be accounted, but not too seriously judged. They may well have been isolated events. For the health of a town we should look equally, if not more, to the long intervening years and to the diseases which prevail at all times. As John Graunt (1662) said:[6]

> Upon the proportion of chronical diseases seems to hang the judgement of the fitness of the country for long life ... in countries subject to great epidemical sweeps men may live very long, but where the proportion of chronical distempers is great, it is not likely to be so ...

The extent of the 'chronical' disorders, as a measure of the balance between good and ill, is, of course denied us. Until late in the sixteenth century when the Bills of Mortality began to be kept in London, there was little to go upon except descriptive writing and archaeological remains.

The early civilizations in Crete, Egypt, Greece, and Rome, all at some time, if not immediately, designed and built model towns, clean and spacious with pure water supplies and well sewered. The latrine and the flush closet were invented, not as some have said during the European Renaissance, but in Crete, perhaps 3,000 BC or earlier. No sight is more remarkable than that of the water-pipes and sewers, still intact in the foundations of the Aesculapian hospital where Galen once walked at the foot of the acropolis of Pergamum, with the modern city, lying adjacent, devoid of sanitation. The cities of Rome and

Greece had internal heating to their houses by means of the hot-air system and their city dwellers may well have enjoyed a greater measure of comfort than at any time until the nineteenth century was well advanced.

The ancients practised hygiene in the sense of basic sanitation in their cities, as assiduously as Edwin Chadwick was to do in those of Britain two millennia later – and probably with as little understanding of its basic principles. Galen knew that phthisis was contagious. Avicenna, a thousand years later, in his *Qanun,* is said to have recognized the spread of disease by water.[9] But did the Greeks and Romans understand, or even suspect, that infections might be water-borne? More probably they were influenced by aesthetic considerations.

Hygienic practices, which in any event may not have been universal or even general, in ancient Rome and Greece and in the Arabian and other civilizations, are not likely to have been wholly satisfactory, with the ever present risks of contamination of food and water. We ourselves in the twentieth century with all our scientific understanding have prevented the worst of the water-borne diseases for only about one-eighth of the world's population. Without any exact understanding of the mode of transmission, it is more likely that the ancient civilizations suffered considerably from water-borne diseases.

Most ancient cities (once they had outgrown their early lay-out) seem also to have harboured slums, so that the poor, not to mention the slaves, may well have lived in overcrowded and unhealthy quarters.[21] We need to look behind the Greek cult of physical fitness, the public amenities, sun-bathing, soap factories, and aqueducts of ancient Rome. Ramazzini, quoting Lucilius, paints a dismal picture of the slaves occupied day and night in the baths, subject to many ills, dropsy, ulcers, abscesses, pale, sad, puffed-up, cachetic, and often attacked by the maladies of those upon whom they attended.[14] The life expectancy, calculated from burial inscriptions, of about thirty years (400 BC), certainly supports the belief that there were many adverse influences at work.[20]

When the barbarian hordes swamped the Roman Empire and the Goddess Hygeia suffered the fate of other deities, town life for most of the European continent became increasingly inimical to health. But the Islamic civilization continued and extended the hygienic practices of Rome and Greece, adding to the understanding of contagion by descriptions of smallpox, anthrax, measles, and scabies. Hospitals became centres of learning, and medical schools, under such men as Al-Majusi, taught that the first art of medicine is keeping health in the healthy. The cult of personal hygiene occupied large sections of their many textbooks. Cities employed sanitary inspectors to have oversight of the preparation of food.[9]

But, as with the Greeks, the towns must have carried many risks which only a deeper understanding of bacteriology could have avoided. The running water from the River Tigris, introduced into each department of the Adudi Hospital built at Bagdad in AD 981, may well have been heavily polluted. Elsewhere in Europe, with the exception of Spain, the world no longer practised the art of sanitation. The aqueducts lay in ruins and the massive drains remained with the foundations of the cities for later generations to unearth. The opportunities for health which the town provided were ignored, and the hazards mounted.

This state of affairs is said by many historians to have continued until relatively recent times. Shattuck, writing his report of the Sanitary Commission of Massachusetts in 1850, said: [17]

> It does not appear that any sanitary regulations existed from the seventh to the fourteenth centuries. In those dark ages people lived without rule of any kind; and consequently frightful epidemics often appeared to desolate the land. Although so ancient, few subjects have since made so slow and so little progress, as the science of public health.

Not everyone can agree with Shattuck about medieval Europe. The medieval city had much to commend it. It was small and circumscribed and set in a countryside to which everyone had easy access. There were gardens and open spaces, municipal baths, hospitals, and often water pumped from the river in wooden conduits. Here, where 'if the ear was stirred the eye was even more delighted', townsmen took joy in their civic life.[11] Overcrowding and the horrors of insanitation have been a later development, dating from the sixteenth or even early seventeenth century, when the call of the town and the increase of the population generally began to have its effect, and when open spaces were built upon, the shallow wells became polluted by seepage and 'the pestilential heapings of human beings' began.[18]

The New World waited until the nineteenth century before towns passed the medieval stage. In the early eighteenth century the Americans were of constitutions so sound and robust as to be rarely exposed to the shocks of any disorder.[8] A century later M'Cready commented that his countrymen had so far enjoyed 'good and peculiar advantages'. But he went on to doubt whether this could continue with 'the increased size of towns, the diminished price of labor or fluctuations in demand for it . . .'.[10]

Nevertheless, it is likely that the balance of disease has been against the town in all stages of its development, with few exceptions throughout history. Towns have tended to relax restraints on conduct and have tempted to excesses harmful to health. They have fostered prostitution, spreading gonorrhoea, at least, in the centuries before the world pandemic of syphilis. They have encouraged alcoholism. In the seventeenth century, London's half million people drank 1·5 million barrels of beer, or 3 barrels per head, per annum.[2] This may well be a near record. But if not one thing, it was usually another. Rickets, which John Graunt did not find 'among the casualties' in the Bills of Mortality until 1634,[6] and no doubt bronchitis, have been the plagues of London, ever since the sea coal came down from Newcastle in quantities sufficient for its foul fumes to blot out the sun and fill the lungs. The inhabitants of seventeenth-century London were highly subject to 'stuffings of the Head, Hoarseness, Coughs'.[8] Rickets began to flourish in the country town of Hallamshire in South Yorkshire, later to be the steel city of Sheffield, as it did in London under the smoke pall that the new iron furnaces produced. Hippocrates is said never to have mentioned atmospheric pollution. But in the sunshine and clear atmosphere of Rome and many other Mediterranean cities, which never knew smog, there was malaria. Towns have also had their occupational hazards. The metal-men whom John Graunt described, 'men being long sick, and always sickly', were town dwellers.[6] However gracious we may suppose the medieval town to have been in its outward form, it is certain that the workers in ill-lighted and ill-ventilated work-shops of Europe died earlier and suffered more than their contemporaries on the land.

Much will have depended on their geographical situations. The citizens of all the northern towns, as they outgrew their slender vegetable supplies, will have been generally on the verge of scurvy, a disease which must have been unknown to the Mediterranean civilizations. Rome was unhealthy because of malaria, and 'in Hispania, Lusitania, and Cisalpine Gaul the expectation of life was far higher than in the capital'.[4] Carthage in North Africa, besides enjoying 6 million gallons a day of pure water through an aqueduct built in Hadrian's time, was situated in a dry desert air, altogether free from malaria.[4] The con-federation of city states of Pamphylia, now Antalya, in Southern Turkey, lapped by the waves of the Eastern Mediterranean, cannot have suffered the half of the 'chronical diseases' of the Londinium of Roman and Saxon times.

The extent of the ill-health occasioned by town living began to be studied scientifically only in the seventeenth century. Since Captain John Graunt, FRS, wrote his *Natural and Political Observations on the Mortality* (1662), towns have generally been regarded as places of higher mortality. As Graunt pointedly said of London:[6]

As for unhealthiness, it may well be supposed that although seasoned bodies may, and do live near as long in London as elsewhere, yet new-comers and children do not; for the smoaks stinks, and close air, are less healthful than that of the country.

The Parish Clerks' Bills of Mortality, in fact, show clearly that from 1593 to the year 1800, i.e. over 207 years, the deaths invariably exceeded the births, and often to an enormous extent, the maximum being reached in the memorable year 1665, when the deaths were 87,339 as against 9,967 births. Between 1603 and 1644 there were 363,935 burials and 330,747 christenings. Throughout the eighteenth century, deaths exceeded births by 6,000 a year or in total by 600,000 for the century. Only the steady migration from country to town, sup-ported by the higher birth rates of village life, sustained the City of London and caused it to grow:

The streets were filthy without, the houses filthy within. The rooms of the poor were more like pigstyes than human habitations, unventilated, and strewn with rushes, which were seldom changed; and the wretched inhabitants closely packed in these miserable hovels must have become very prone to suffer from infections of all kinds . . . There were no underground drains, and the soil of the town was soaked with the filth of centuries.

This description[13] would have applied widely throughout Europe in the fifteenth, sixteenth, and seventeenth centuries and, with modifications to suit the cen-turies, cities everywhere in course of rapid growth. Thus M'Cready describes New York in 1836:[10]

One great source of ill-health among laborers and their families is the confined and miserable, apartments in which they are lodged. In the rapid growth of our city (New York) in particular the number of buildings has by no means increased in a manner corresponding to the great influx of strangers . . . large buildings . . . have been divided into numerous small, dark rooms, every one of which is tenanted by a family . . . narrow alleys with small wooden tenements, which costing but little, and being let to numerous families, yield immense profits. The alley is often not more than six feet wide . . . apartments . . . underground.

So it is with much of the world today. Hostages are thus given to fortune.

The factors which produce disease and death in town life, poverty, insanitation, occupation, habits of life, atmospheric pollution, etc., are not easily distinguishable one from another. Yet each can be individually considered and remedied. Poverty, for example, can be distinguished, as Edwin Chadwick said in the report of the Royal Commission into the State of Large Towns and Populous Districts in England and Wales, 1845:[16]

It is too commonly supposed that the evils above adverted to are the inseparable concomitants of poverty; and doubtless, so long as the inhabitants of the most neglected and filthy abodes in crowded cities are unable to provide for themselves better and healthier dwellings, sufficient light and air, more open situation, effective cleansing and drainage and adequate supplies of water, their vigour and health are undermined, and their lives shortened by the deleterious external influences consequent upon the want of efficient arrangements for securing the above objects.

High mortalities and excessive disease continued to prevail throughout Europe and the New World until well into the nineteenth century.[20] All was not due to the insanitary state of the towns, but much was. Estimates of life expectancy in various European towns between the thirteenth and seventeenth centuries ranged from 20 to 40 years; for example, in Geneva, it was 21 years in 1561–1600 and 28 years in 1601–1700, and in Breslau 33·5 years in 1687–91. The expectation of life at birth of the Swedish population as a whole in 1755–76 was only 33–40 years.

The mortality rates prior to the twentieth century were everywhere greater in the cities than in the country. Thus in Brandenburg (1739–48) the crude death rate was about 25 per 1,000 in rural areas, 31 in small cities, and 36 in larger cities like Berlin. In Stockholm, 1755–76, life expectancy at birth was about 14 for males and 18 for females; while the figures for all Sweden were 33 and 36 respectively. In the United States, in 1830, mortality conditions were far worse in the large cities than in small cities and rural areas. In Glasgow in 1837 the death rate was 41, of which 8·6 was due to 'fever'.[3]

But gradually, as Europe and the New World have developed, the rates of mortality for town and country have approximated. Social reforms, environment sanitation, rising economic levels, and the application of new knowledge to public health practice have all played a part. The reported death rate for Vienna (24 per 1,000) was already below that for Austria as a whole (29 per 1,000) before the end of the century (1886–90). In Sweden the death rates of urban areas have been below those of country since 1911–15. Infant mortality in Swedish towns fell below those of the country for the decade 1920–30, and in the USA in 1930.[19] Around 1910, males in Zurich could expect to live 1·7 years longer than all Swiss males. Finally, among 26 countries in 1948 and 1949 for which crude death rates appear in WHO publications, the principal cities had lower rates in 10 and equal rates in 3.[20]

In most of the towns of Central European countries and in the United States of America, the infant mortality is now lower than in rural districts. Among the more advanced countries, Britain, except for London, remains partly an exception to this rule; here the chief excess begins after the neonatal period, when the adverse influences of the environment come into play. Town dwellers after 'childhood', however, have age-specific mortalities higher than in country districts particularly after 45 years, when atheroma and chronic bronchitis, (much less prevalent among country dwellers and particularly agricultural workers) begin to have their main effect (see p. 76). The excess of degenerative disease, aided by pollution of the atmosphere and the more sedentary life, is likely to grow with the ageing of the population.

But towns are an important influence mentally and socially, as well as physically, and in these they have much to cause misgiving. Overcrowding, house sharing, lack of household amenities, are severe handicaps to mental and social health, straining family relationships and adding to neurosis by psychosomatic diseases. In 1951 Britain, after 6 million new houses had been built in 30 years, had 3 million households, holding 13·5 million people, living at an average of more than one person per room – the maximum for healthy living prescribed by the Royal Commission on Population;[15] nearly 60 thousand households lived at more than 3 per room. Over 2 million dwellings were shared between two families, including the high proportion, up to 75 per cent in one city (Aberdeen), of mothers having a first baby – a situation giving rise to worry, unhappiness, and insecurity. One in five households were without exclusive use of a water-closet and twice this number had no exclusive use of a fixed bath; one in ten were without exclusive use of both kitchen sink and stove. Twenty years later conditions had improved. But on census night 1971, there were still nearly 7·5 million households containing 1·25 million persons living at an average of more than one person per room; 10,250 households containing more than 3 persons per room (not counting households with less than 10 rooms, or less than 10 persons); 5·2 per cent of households had no exclusive use of WC, 12·3 per cent no exclusive use of fixed bath or shower, and 0·86 per cent no exclusive use of both sink and stove.[1]

For many in such conditions in the slums of Europe and the New World, in the last quarter of the twentieth century, the term 'living' is an exaggeration. The effects of the ill-considered building of the Industrial Revolution and its aftermath have not been easy to eradicate, particularly when the idea of what a good home should include has steadily advanced. To think in terms of persons per room is often to ignore the meaning of family life. The modern prescription for a home includes good insulation, space heating, and a room for the children to study in, as well as internal plumbing, sanitary conveniences, bathrooms, and technical aids to housework from food mixers to clothes washers; except for the older folk and single workers a minimum of three bedrooms is needed. In an attempt to escape from the outworn environment of the industrial towns Europe and America have spread out in successive overspills into the countryside – leaving large areas in the centres of the towns culturally desolate and dead. The question which William Cobbett (1762–1835) asked, 'What is to be the fate of the greatest wen (London) of all?' (*Rural Rides*), might now be applied widely to the towns of the developed world.

Town living altered little in extent during many centuries, when the world's population grew only slowly (see Chapter 8). Ancient civilizations had relatively greater concentrations than anything today – perhaps a million people lived in a dozen or more cities of antiquity, Nineveh, Babylon, Memphis, Thebes – but then and later the bulk of the people were rural dwellers.[21] Europe, too, was mainly rural throughout the Middle Ages, when, moreover, towns were also small; London in the fourteenth century contained only 35 thousand people. But from the sixteenth century in England, and in the rest of Europe from the eighteenth century, or at varying times during the nineteenth cenury, there has been a steady growth of urbanization.[21]

It is difficult to compare urban living because of the varying definition of a town; in some countries this is determined by arbitrary administrative divisions, whereas in others it depends on size with varying lower limits. On the basis of two thousand inhabitants as the lowest level, Britain, a hundred years ago, was over 50 per cent urban-dwelling, while France (26), Denmark (21), USA (15), Norway (12), Sweden (10), were mainly rural. In 1972,[5] Western Europe, North America and Oceania were predominantly urban – Britain 78, Australia 86, Denmark 80, USA 73, New Zealand 81, France 70 Sweden 81, Norway 45; while countries of Asia, Africa and much of South America were mainly rural – Kenya 10, Sri Lanka 22, India 21, Paraguay 36, Turkey 38.

The growth of towns in many parts of the world is now proceeding fast. The annual rate of change in recent years has been in Egypt 1·79 per cent, in Venezuela 2·75 per cent, and in the Union of South Africa 3·16 per cent, as compared with England and Wales where the rate of increase has fallen to 0·04 per cent.[19] Urban living in Japan increased from 38 in 1954 to 72 in 1970 and in Colombia from 29 in 1954 to 62 in 1972.[5] Outside the developed world, people are crowding into the towns, often to live in circumstances of great discomfort and dangerous congestion and adding to the problems of public health in countries that already have too many. Here they are reproducing again the effects of industrialization from which Europe and the New World have only recently escaped. What can be said of the cities and towns that now abound where it is not a question of one person or even one family to a room, but of many families and even a family per bed space, without water or sanitation? As the Hammonds said of England when the Industrial Revolution had done its worst, 'the idea of the town as a focus for civilization, a centre where the emancipating and enlightening influences of the time can act rapidly and with effect, the school of social arts, the nursery of social enterprise, the witness to beauty and order and freedom that men can bring into their lives, had vanished from all minds'.[7]

The Industrial Revolution has left the world with a legacy of outworn towns, sprawling suburbs, and disfigured countryside. The towns of Europe no longer stir the ear and delight the eye; they have been dragged at the heels of the giant industry during two centuries of agony. Physically now more healthy, except for their smoke clouds and fumes, they have lost their identity, ever sprawling farther into the countryside. As industrialization spreads throughout the rest of the world, towns everywhere may well have to undergo the same trial. Yet the world needs good towns. The town should be a pleasant place in which to live and a joy to visit; it should shelter the good life, making social activities easier and cultivating the arts. It should be a centre of intellectual stimulus and a place where the products of organized effort and combined wealth increase the pleasures of the senses – and where public health has not only removed the hazards but increased the possibilities of health. Once again it is to public health that the world must look for a lead.

11. Hospitals

Herodotus may well have been misinformed, as Sigerist suggests,[19] when he made a statement that has rung down the ages, that the Babylonians lacked physicians. The sick were placed in the market-place to have the benefit of the observations of all passers-by; but physicians there were, although probably many less than in Egypt, where there was so much specialization. As we read in the Odyssey,[16] 'In medical knowledge, the Egyptian leaves the rest of the world behind'. The blending of magic with reason, of knowledge with faith, and of physician with priest, inevitably associated the care of the sick with the Temple. To the Temple no doubt the medical school was attached; and here sometimes the sick were brought to be laid reverently in the care of the Gods.[17] The Aesculapian temples, of which some 200 were built throughout Greece and Asia Minor in the thousand years that followed upon the first at Trikkala in 1200 B.C.,* had something of the flavour of hospital care. Buddhism, like Christianity later, stimulated humanitarian feelings for the sick and suffering. Under the great emperor Asoka, from about 260 B.C., Buddhist hospitals were established throughout India and Sri Lanka. But the Far Eastern hospital, including institutions then arising in China, resembled the hospice of our own monasteries. Fa-Hsian, the Chinese monk who visited India and Sri Lanka during the years A.D. 399–413, said, 'The poor, the orphans, the lame, in short all the sick of the provinces repair to these houses, where they receive all that is necessary for their wants.'[7]

They were perhaps better described, as in A.D. 629–45, by another Chinese pilgrim to India, Hiuen-Tsiang, as Houses of Benevolence.[7] The Roman valetudinaria, although more truly hospitals for the sick and wounded, were military establishments attached to the camps of the legionaries.

The word hospital has clearly changed its meaning, with the growth of ideas, from a place of refuge to a centre of skilled medical care.[8] In the form of which we think of them today, the Arabian hospital may have been first in the field. Islam built hospitals specially designed for medical treatment from Bokhara to Seville after A.D. 750. As Khairallah[12] has said:

> Every patient who needed hospital care was admitted, with no reference to colour, creed, sex, or social status. . . . Each hospital was divided into two main sections, one for men and one for women. Each section was then subdivided into wards and rooms for internal medicine, diseases of the eye, surgery, and orthopaedics. The medical section was further subdivided into wards and rooms for fevers, wards for cases of diarrhoea, and special wards with barred windows for the care of the mentally afflicted and insane.

* Trikkala in Thessaly, traditionally the birth place of Aesculapius, is the most likely candidate for the first temple hospital; that at Epidaurus, larger and more renowned, followed soon after.

Arabian hospitals were certainly more in keeping with modern ideas than those which began to be founded by Religious Orders in Europe about A.D. 1200, although according to Mumford,[14] the medieval town was by the fifteenth century well supplied with hospital beds at the rate of one to every 2,000 inhabitants. Leprosaria, which began in ancient Rome, to protect the community, were widely used in the Islamic civilization before being adopted by Europe in the Middle Ages.

There were, of course, good reasons why the sick should not have been gathered together for treatment. The art of scientific diagnosis and of surgical and medical treatment generally was lacking. Nursing care was better in the home. For those not in the immediate vicinity of a centre of culture there was the problem of transport. But more important than these reasons was the increased danger. Hospital care provides unusually good opportunities for the spread of infection, to which our language has given poignant testimony. Hospital-fever betokened 'a kind of typhus fever arising in crowded hospitals from the poisonous atmosphere'; and hospital-gangrene, 'a spreading sloughing gangrenous inflammation starting in a wound and arising in crowded hospitals'. The description of the Hôtel-Dieu in Paris by Tenon[20] in 1788 in which he said that *'Quatre et six couchent dans le même lit'*, makes gruesome reading, even more that by Max Nordau,[11] who wrote:

> On the same couch, body against body, a woman groaned in the pangs of labor, a nursing infant writhed in convulsions, a typhus patient burned in the delirium of fever, a consumptive coughed his hollow cough, and a victim of some disease of the skin tore with furious nails his infernally itching integument. . . .

Although hospitals will not always have fallen into such evil practices, they are likely always to have been dangerous. Writing of the much vaunted Islamic hospitals, Elgood[9] says:

> In spite of this apparently elaborate organization the hospitals were not popular. I have nowhere come across in Persian or Arabic writers any eulogy, such as modern patients so often give when they are discharged. On the contrary it was generally considered a very grave misfortune to be taken into hospital and kept there.

As the merchant in the story of Ganem in the Arabian Nights[9] said: 'I will gain Paradise by means of this poor person; for if they take him into hospital they will kill him in one day'. The dangers increased with the growth of population in the Western world when hospitals became more and more overcrowded and the practice of sleeping several in a bed was commonplace. They were aggravated by lack of professional nursing. As late as 1848 in Charing Cross Hospital, London, according to Lord Inman, a benefactor and governor of the hospital, nursing was done by 'watchers' paid 5s a week living out; patients were admitted on one day a week, often to beds just vacated by fever cases, and bed linen was changed when worn out.[4] Thus it is that hospitals, the centres of healing and sources of professional and intellectual aid, as we think of them today, are largely new to man. They were made possible by Pasteur, Lister, and Florence Nightingale, in the middle of the last century. The twentieth century had dawned before the hospital began to occupy the centre of the medical stage.

The growth of the hospital, and its remarkable transformation with the discoveries of the last century, are important to our understanding of world public health. Public Health began in Europe and the New World before the era of asepsis. When Edwin Chadwick (1800–90) started his life work in the 1830s, Florence Nightingale (1820–1910) was only just beginning to think of nursing as a profession, and the work of Louis Pasteur (1822–95) and Joseph Lister (1827–1912) had all to be done. Hospitals continued to ocupy a relatively lowly position in public esteem, as places in which to segregate those who were a danger to public health, or an inconvenience – the sick poor in workhouse infirmaries; the lunatics in asylums; and the infectious in fever hospitals. As places for treating sickness, apart from quarantine or incarceration, hospitals differed little from their predecessors for many centuries. No one then looked to them as more than a limited answer to problems of public health. In her *Notes on Nursing* (1858)[15] Florence Nightingale spoke of the need to teach people how to live. The remedies, she said, for the enormous child mortality are well known 'and among them is certainly not the establishment of a child's hospital'.[15]

The thoughts of the medical profession were then centred upon problems of health and disease throughout the community – how infections spread; what steps to take to prevent illness in industry; the importance of diet, housing, and habits of living. The records of the Epidemiological Society in London in 1850 contain the names of physicians and surgeons of great eminence. T. Spencer Wells (1818–97) read a paper on *Technical Results of Quarantine* a quarter of a century before he became Hunterian Professor of Surgery and Pathology; T. Clifford Allbutt (1836–1925) spoke 'On the Prevention of Disease by Reconstruction of the Dwellings of the Poor' a long time before he became Regius Professor of Physics at Cambridge. The nineteenth-century doctors passed easily from the study of the individual to that of the community. Men with the outlook of John Snow or William Budd, M'Cready, Thackrah, Greenhow, and Patissier were not difficult to find.

The world today is wedded to the hospital. In the developed and underdeveloped countries alike, where there is nationalization and where there is none, with and without social security, hospitals are being built everywhere on a large scale (see page 138). In fifty years the hospital has come to dominate the medical scene. It absorbs the best of the brains of the medical world, the lion's share of time and effort, and, of course, money. Medical students and nurses, who receive nearly the whole of their training within the four walls of a hospital, leave it to practise their professions in the community, imbued with its ideals, but with an inadequate understanding of its true significance. The approach to public health, which the Western world sponsored, and from which it derived such immense advantages, takes second place. The world community itself is hardly aware of the advantages and disadvantages of the change.

The essential needs of public health remain the same. Public health is rooted in the environment; in the way people live, in the social factors of the home and the workshop. For these the hospital, however much relief it may give to the sick and suffering, is only a partial answer. But public health must face the world as it finds it, and be prepared to re-examine it constantly in the light of changing values. The modern hospital constitutes a new problem in public health.

Every country can be said to have two particular needs – interlocked and in many ways inseparable, in some ways favourable and in others antagonistic – one for a healthy community, the other for specialist care in hospital. World health needs a proper balance between them. The amount of hospital provision is a reflection of the success or failure of public health. Every community must spread its resources, so as to achieve the greatest measure of prevention with a proper regard for the calls of human suffering. This is not easy, but it can be accomplished by building up strong public health services and by making the hospital an agent of public health.

The hospital within a strong public health service

The first essential is to shift back the focus of medical care to the community and to lessen the emphasis upon hospitals: to create everywhere sources for community health in terms of the family at home and at work. The dramatic appeal of the hospital both for doctors and laymen alike, which the development of scientific techniques of treatment continually fosters, must be held in check. The Public Health Service in every country must be given first priority to develop measures to keep the community healthy. One of its main objectives is the good home which builds up health and supports in sickness. This can be done in many ways in the widely differing circumstances that the world presents; but little doubt remains that the establishment of *health units*, directed by health officers trained in public health, and equipped with *health centres* for day-to-day work in preventive and curative medicine, has the greatest possibilities for general use.[23] In this way medical and social care are firmly united, and the general medical practitioner is enabled to work with midwives, health visitors, sanitarians, and other social agents. This provides the means for a continuous study of disease and ill-health within the community. In those countries where general practitioners of medicine exist in large numbers, or where health assistants are used, general medical care and public health should operate as one administrative unit (see Chapter 20).

The real focus of interest of public health – a healthy nation – is thus clearly established. Within such a system the hospital is better able to take its place as an essential arm of a total service. The need for hospitals, as with those for infectious disease and to a lesser extent for children, can be reduced by successful public health. Their construction should never be too lavish. Many have said, with some truth, that any nation can fill unlimited beds in mental hospitals. But, if the focus of mental care is shifted back to the community, too many beds may be a positive disadvantage; quite apart from the cost, which must cut heavily into other community programmes. Budgets must not be so weighted with hospital expenditure that social and preventive measures are hampered: hospitals must be weighed carefully in the balance with other forms of community care. Hospital work should not be more highly esteemed or better paid than medical care for the community outside; nor should greater emphasis be laid upon training for specialist work in hospitals.

The superiority of hospital care over home care also needs to be critically examined in all societies – on social, psychological, and financial grounds. Children fare badly[2, 18] and old people likewise[6] when removed from their homes for care in an institution. Schemes of 'home care' such as that for children from St Mary's hospital, London and for the chronic sick from the Montefiore hospital, New York are highly desirable alternatives to hospital. About the mentally ill, the Royal Commission of 1954–7 in England and Wales said:[10]

In relation to almost all forms of medical disorder, there is increasing medical emphasis on forms of treatment and training and social services, which can be given without bringing patients into hospital as in-patients, or which make it possible to discharge them from hospital sooner than was usual in the past.

The treatment of the tuberculous in sanatoria was a brilliant innovation by pioneers of social medicine at the end of the nineteenth century. But today, with the means to diagnose and treat tuberculosis within the community, it is doubtful whether many countries now setting out to overcome the White Scourge would be wise to make more than limited use of them; monies can be better spent on dispensaries and home treatment associated with health centres.

Hospitals are an essential need of all communities in all stages of development; but they have to be seen in the perspective of a sound community based upon good homes. The stay in hospital should be a step in rehabilitation to full life outside – neither unduly prolonged nor unwisely considered. It is not a substitute for a good home, such as the excess of single persons in hospital on Census night in the UK suggests to be the case.[1]

The hospital as an agent of public health

Secondly, the hospital must be an agent of public health. As the first report of the expert committee on the rôle of hospitals in community health protection said:[25]

The hospital is an integral part of a social and medical organization, the function of which is to provide for the population complete health care, both curative and preventive, and whose out-patient services reach out to the family in its home environment; the hospital is also a centre for the training of health workers and for bio-social research.

It may help sometimes to day dream. Few hospitals have this outlook and many are unlikely to develop it. We must indeed realize that the interests of the hospital are sometimes in conflict with those of public health. The hospital is not unique in seeking to seal itself off from the community affairs: most institutions have the same urge. The combination of hospital with health centre, recommended by Bridgman in his *Rural Hospital*,[3] may be one of the means to overcome this difficulty; but this expedient can fail where the interest and appeal of curative medicine come to dominate the scene. The responsibility must be with the public health organization, either working with headquarters in the hospital, or distinct from it, to draw out the hospital gently but firmly into a wider sphere. 'The hospital should organize itself to serve the community in all aspects of health care and can contribute much to improve the community health';[25] 'The general hospital ... should not limit its functions to the restorative sphere, but should ... organize itself to serve preventive, educational, and research ends as well.'[25] In short, the hospital should be an integral part of society, and not, as so often and so long, a monastic institution separated from the world around by high walls of brick and prejudice.

What this means in more particular terms must depend upon the social organization of each country. It may be that the hospital will be the centre of preventive work through a system of peripheral health centres; that it will be the leading spirit in a scheme 'to link together all aspects of the healing art and to prevent disease';[25] that much of the vital work of public health in case finding, health teaching, and special examinations will be organized as part of central out-patient departments with satellites throughout the area; that the hospital will be the centre of home care schemes and other extramural activities. This is already becoming the case in many parts of the world. On the other hand, many countries may not wish to centre too many activities for the promotion of health upon institutions primarily for the care of sick people. For them the health centre will perform many of the functions of out-patient departments, retaining a close link with the family, home, and factory, and obtaining specialist advice from the hospital. Such details are for local decision.

But all hospitals everywhere must be *socially orientated*.[5] The ideal is to use the hospital to the best advantage socially as well as medically. Every patient in hospital should be regarded as a social problem for himself and for the community. Hospitals should also be dynamic, seeking to establish themselves as centres of rehabilitation; as places to which the sick can enter for diagnosis and treatment and from which they will return home. Retention for long periods, as has happened for mental disorders, mental deficiency, and the chronic sick, can often be avoided, where the hospital is working in partnership with the health unit. Since the hospital reflects an important aspect of the picture of disease in the community, it must be both a centre of statistics and a source of information on infections on which it can provide a running commentary; quite apart from the spread of infections within the hospital itself, which occurs despite the success of medicine and nursing. Of every 1,000 children admitted to hospital, in terms of the survey by Watkins and Lewis-Faning,[21] 71 were given a new disease, and four or five killed. Paul[18] has said that 'it is more dangerous to admit a very young child to hospital than to allow him to play on an arterial road'.

Hospitals collect together many who are in need of teaching; and they provide admirably the milieu for health activities. Every advantage should be taken of this in the out-patient departments and in the wards. Every hospital should also have a centre of social work with specially trained staff for interviewing patients and relatives and for obtaining background reports. Such a dynamic approach, in these and other ways, more than any other measure, will help to bring the hospital into closer touch with the community.

Such a development could best be achieved as WHO recommends,[25] by arranging for every general hospital or group of general and special hospitals, to have a department of social and preventive medicine directed by the medical officer of health of the local health unit, thus reinforcing the specialist clinical team by a 'social physician'.[5] Such an arangement which is gaining ground in Europe, and particularly in Britain, will be aided by the creation of the 'community physician' on the staff of the new area boards (see p. 121). In this, as in other advances in public health, the prestige of the hospital is so high today that it can afford to lead the way in breaking down the barriers which may exist between itself and other services.

12. Food

The world's menu

Man in his most primitive form will have known that his health and strength depended upon having enough to eat. Throughout his development, in and out of civilizations, food gathering has been one of his chief preoccupations. But the influences at work, for good or ill, have been many and varied. Man's diet has been the expression, as it were, of their inter-action; population growth, agricultural development, the existence of local hazards or advantages, the bending of nature to man's will by artificial or natural selection, scientific advancement, the introduction of new dangers by harmful practices or social customs, these and other considerations have taken part in an endless and dynamic struggle.

With so many variables to determine the menu, the diet of the human being has been subject to kaleidoscopic changes. Throughout history some people have fed well while others have fared badly. The skill in husbandry, for which the Roman and Greeks were famous, gave abundance. The millions who lived around the Mediterranean seaboard lived in dietetic luxury. So too the English countryman of 1740 fed well.[6] The renaissance of agricultural learning had reached Britain from the Continent; the potato, after a century of neglect, was being grown in large quantities; garden vegetables had spread beyond the estates of the wealthy; livestock abounded; and the grain was whole and nourishing. The result was a full diet of dairy produce, meat, potatoes, vegetables, and oatmeal or wheaten bread.

But these periods of good feeding, as so many others at different times and places throughout the world's history, have been followed by scarcity. Inefficient strip farming, with its low production and poor cattle rearing, followed the break-up of the Roman Empire. The new townsmen and women of industrial England exchanged the diet of the countryman for a roller-processed wheat adulterated with alum, a disgraceful episode to which Tobias Smollett (1721–71) refers when he makes his character, Matthew Bramble, say:

> The bread I eat in London is a deleterious paste mixed up with chalk, alum and bone ashes, insipid to taste, and destructive to constitution.

Many similar contrasts can be found in the world today, for example the wholesome diet of whole wheat, milk, meat, and cheese of the hill tribes of India is strikingly different from the diet of polished rice of the lowland peasant.[13, 14] Moreover, food has always been a social ingredient, unequally distributed in quantity and quality; good living has been for the rich, bare subsistence for the labouring poor; the manchet loaf for the Lord of the Manor and cibarus, the bran loaf, for 'all servants, slaves and the inferior type of people to feed on.[10] Therefore the social class gradient is one of the main considerations of public health.[5] Poverty results from the interaction of income with basic essentials, of which food is the most important. The poverty line which Rowntree described in 1899,[16] mainly based on food, has always existed. But the distinction between primary poverty; where there is too little money to buy food, and secondary poverty, where the household budget has been improperly spent, is steadily getting less. The household budget should permit of other expenditure than that upon 'minimum necessaries', if we believe that the full life and the fair diet should be inseparables.

Family life exerts its own biological forces which cannot be easily countered. Expenditure upon food per head within a static budget gets less as the number of children increases. The tighter the budget, the worse the quality; the fewer the calories, the more carbohydrate, less protein and protective elements. Calorie needs are satisfied by cheaper carbohydrates to the exclusion of more nourishing foods. Bread will supply 2,500 calories at one fifth the cost of milk, even in countries where milk abounds, and at about one twentieth the cost of eggs.* Thus, as the family grows in size the diet deteriorates and its balance is upset.[2]

Nations are like families in this respect. All over the world where there is little money and few calories, the food consists mainly of cereals, alone or with sugar, the cheapest satisfiers of hunger; thus, in India cereals and sugar provide 1,500 calories out of a total of 2,000. New Zealand and Denmark, with high average food consumption (about 3,300), have a low cereal intake of approximately 900 calories with high milk and meat consumption. Java, with a daily average per head of less than 2,000 calories, has a wholly un-balanced diet with animal protein as low as 4 grams.[2] To feed the people according to their biological needs calls out the best in every nation – in education, statecraft, and social organization. But of all influences at work upon the diet, man's multiplication has been the most potent. Food, until recently, has provided an automatic check upon the numbers living in any region; causes of decline have been, as in the animal kingdom, 'density-dependent', since overcrowding promotes contagion, and the under-nourished are an easy prey to infection and hardship[8] (see also Chapter 3). To this simple law of mass action, another force has been added – understanding. The Malthusian spectre dogs man like a shadow, but we can keep one step ahead with the aid of science. Skill in husbandry, and public health, are the way forward to a new balance with food.

Man himself has often made things worse. The plague of rickets came to Northern Europe, already deprived of sunshine, with the smoke clouds of the coal-burning domestic chimneys and foundries; and to Asia Minor, where the sun pours from cloudless skies, with the over-clothing of infants, which religious custom demanded. The use of chemicals to whiten bread – alum in the last century, agene yesterday, sulphur dioxide today – and the polishing

---

* In Britain in 1952, 2,500 calories cost 7½d in the form of bread, 3/1½d as milk, 8/- as vegetables and 16/6 as eggs.[2]

of rice, to satisfy social demands, have all robbed man's staple diet of much of the vitamin B complex, and of other essential nutrients. The introduction of small power-driven mills rapidly increased the consumption of highly milled rice in areas where previously rice could only be hand-milled.[3] The excessive use of refined 'sugars' may well also add to the man-made hazards.

The soil upon which man depends for his very existence has been lost to him by carelessness and ignorance. In his haste to cultivate it he has often heedlessly removed the trees, bushes, and grasses which sustain it. Dried by the winds, it has blown away in the dust clouds; soaked by the rain, it has been carried to the valley bottoms. The barren sub-soil, denuded of its lush covering, has been added to the deserts. Soil erosion is one of man's greatest enemies, for the earth's surface is limited. The 3,500 million acres now in use might be doubled by the inclusion of deserts and marginal lands. Every acre added to the present land in cultivation is important, but the overriding need is for scientific farming everywhere. Great areas of the world yield only 6 to 7 cwt of wheat per acre in comparison with 20 cwt or even 50 cwt in Europe and the New World. It has been said that India could use twenty times as much fertilizer and increase its yields in ten years by 30 per cent. Milk and meat may be similarly increased by breeding and the elimination of cattle disease.

Harnessing the soil

Since man began a settled life, his diet has depended on his ability to harness the soil. Some regions of the world will have been naturally more productive than others; but, this apart, food production has called forth many skills – irrigation, terracing, drainage, fertilization, instrument making. The cultivation of grain in areas cleared by fire began agricultural experiments. Chemical fertilizers, first produced in abundance in the middle of the nineteenth century, are but the latest method of soil enrichment, which dates back to early times, guano in Peru, powdered pumice in the Gilbert Islands, human excreta in China, Mexico, and elsewhere. Much has depended on mechanical aids, advancing with a spurt here, lagging a few centuries there, but always tending to improve the yield per acre and the acres tilled. Expansion and development, as in the breaking and cultivating of the black land of the Middle West of America, have been the greatest challenge.

Every generation has contributed agricultural implements. The scythe replaced the sickle; the modern plough is the direct descendant of the digging stick, still in use in primitive societies. Threshing with the hand-flail, or by driving animals on a treading floor, and winnowing by hand, were ingenious innovations for earlier civilizations – destined to spread throughout the world. Thus, the nineteenth century, which ushered in the age of mechanical farming, was building on a long past. Newbold's cast-iron plough (1797), Bailey's mower with the circular blade (c. 1820), and the early threshers (1825), were adaptations of old ideas. Forty years of trial and error were needed before the binding of sheaves could be done by machinery: the Appleby Knotter

(1878) probably influenced man's diet more than any improvement since the introduction of the horse. The modern grain separator which sails over Canada, the Middle West of America, and the Ukraine, threshing, cleaning, weighing, and bagging, is a combined effort of all men, at least from the Stone Age to the present day, in search of a decent diet.

Foods of particular value to man, the results of natural selection which have made their appearance in different parts of the world, have been carried by traders and adventurers to distant parts. Oranges and lemons, which cling to the warmth, have been cultivated for export to less favoured regions, northern territories, whose native fruits, apples, pears, plums, and even the cherry which the Roman legions transported, are deficient in vitamin C. Rice has been unwilling to leave the tropical zone, but other cereals, wheat, oats, rye, millet, dura, have slowly spread to cover a large part of the earth's surface. The potato and tomato, which appeared in South America, have each been transported to far distant places at different times in history. The wheat grain, Red Fife, specially suited to the southern prairies of Canada, and later its offspring Marquis, Yeoman, and Holdfast, which thrive also in the shorter summers of farther north, have helped to increase the area in Canada under wheat cultivation from 2·7 million acres in 1891 to 27 million acres within half a century.[17] Enormous yields are now claimed for the new wheat *Maris Huntsman*.

Extensive cultivation of *Solanum tuberosum*, the humble potato which the Spanish discoverers of America brought back to Europe, dispelled the dreadful scourge of scurvy and may well have been a stimulus to set on foot the industrial and agricultural revolutions. But the struggle has been one in which nature has often lent an unwilling hand, or none at all. In countries where maize has been the staple diet, there has been pellagra from lack of nicotinic acid; in others the alkaloids of the senecca plant act as liver poison. Everywhere seasonal shortages, floods, and pests have brought malnutrition and even famine. The land food gathering has always been a struggle against the hostility of physical and ecological powers, to be fought by ingenuity and knowledge. And since the health of the whole human family now is involved, it has become a problem for world health.

More recently, artificial selection has been added. No doubt it has been in operation, for both plants and animals, with periods of rapid advance and others of stagnation, as long as civilization. Robert Bakewell (1725–95) in the early eighteenth century inaugurated a century of intensive selection which produced breeds of cattle, pigs, and sheep yielding twice or three times. These have populated the New World. But he built on what had gone before. Roman livestock may well have been fattened and kept through the winter, an art which was lost to Europe for a thousand years. The art of growing the turnip and clovers and the common garden vegetables, so necessary to beast and man, was re-discovered in Europe in the early eighteenth century. Plant genetics is now helping to breed stronger wheats resistant to disease, and with better quality protein; and is giving us drought-resisting grasses which can make grazing lands out of marginal wastes.

Our ignorance of causes has been largely dispelled. The spirit of James Lind, who on 20 May 1747 took '12 patients in the scurvy on board the *Salisbury* at sea'[12] has lived on. Takaki, Eijkman, Barlow, and others, have added clinical observations about the relationship of food to health. The chemistry and biochemistry of food have been laid bare. In 1906, rats subjected to a purified diet told us perhaps the greatest truth of all, that 'In diseases such as rickets and scurvy we have had for long years knowledge of a dietetic factor, but the real errors in the diet are to this day obscure. They are certainly of a kind which comprises *minimal qualitative factors*'.[9] Since that time, the accessory food factors have one by one been hunted down – the 'real errors' have become known. To the importance of food as a source of calories and nitrogen, we now add several substances needed in minute amounts. But always there are new horizons – scurvy, beri-beri, rickets, keratomalacia, and pellagra are milestones. Today's problems are equally momentous, millions with kwashiorkor in tropical countries,[11] atheroma in the ageing peoples of the Old and New Worlds (see Chapter 3).

Food and world health

No uniform plan can ever be devised to meet the needs of all countries; but all should make the feeding of the people with a balanced diet their ideal. The needs of growth, protein, calcium, vitamins A and D, and the B group, give rise to much the same problems everywhere. Calcium and vitamin D are universally limited in their distribution in nature and the vitamin B group is always needed in greater amounts as the carbohydrate increases in the diet. Protein is everywhere so expensive, when the national or family budget is near the poverty line, that it is difficult to obtain in sufficient amounts.

Public health cannot work in the dark; it depends on accurate knowledge of what is required for a realistic food policy, i.e., upon a knowledge of the existing state of the diet.[2] This entails the use of the dietary survey, to discover what people eat and how diet is related to custom, prejudice, ignorance, money, or cooking. Of the four types of dietary survey, statistical studies of national resources, and the study of groups, families, or individuals, each can be used in different circumstances by questionnaire, log book, or weighing techniques. Surveys such as those by Edward Smith (see p. 269) and John Boyd Orr[15] have played a vital rôle in the building up of an understanding of nutritional needs in individual countries.*

The results of successive sample surveys of food consumption and expenditure (see p. 263) have made it possible to study family needs at various income levels and the effects of social policies upon them.

In the UK, a national food survey has been conducted (in 1972 by means of a three stage stratified random sample) annually since 1940. Housewives are asked to keep a record for one week of all food purchased for the family, and of all food from garden and allotments and otherwise obtained without actual cash payment. Visits of investigators are preceded by introductory

* Surveys are discussed in detail in Chapters 25, 26 and 27.

letters to explain the use of the log book for recording weight and cost of food. During the week of the survey two visits are made; food stocks are weighed immediately before and after each visit. The results in Table 12.1 for 1950 and 1972, in relation to family size show that the decline in diet with increasing family size was less marked in 1950 than in 1936/7[2] and that the advantage had generally been maintained in 1972:[5]

Table 12.1 Results of national food survey for 1950 and 1972.

Nutrients	Childless households		Families with more than 3 children	
	1950	1972*	1950	1972*
Energy value (cals)	2,804	2,460	2,168	2,030
Protein (g)	91	64·9	65	59·7
Animal protein (g)	47	38·2	30	33·2
Fat (g)	118	93	86	85
Calcium (mg)	1,212	1,010	959	850
Iron (mg)	15·9	13·9	11·3	11·3
Vitamin A	3,949 I.U.	1,460 μg	3,201 I.U.	980 μg
Vitamin B (mg)	1·17	1·30	1·33	1·10
Riboflavin (mg)	2·17	1·84	1·43	1·55
Nicotinic acid (mg)	15·4	17·9	10·4	13·6
Vitamin C (mg)	102	60	61	40
Vitamin D	167 I.U.	2·76 μg	201 I.U.	2·53 μg

* In 1972, households compared contained 2 adults, and housewives under 35 years of age.

There had been a levelling out in the lower social classes of expenditure, particularly of eggs, butter, fresh meat, and vegetables – a clear result of national food policies.[5] Every country can study with advantage its own social pattern – how people feed and what they need.

When the national larder is examined for protective foods, milk, unpolished rice, whole wheat, fruit, and vegetables, many nations find a disturbing imbalance. Sugar, whose shortcomings are plain, occupies too large a place. The pressures to mutilate the staple grain of the country are always strong, although the loss of the vitamin B group together with the essential amino acid lysine and much valuable iron, and even possibly of essential fatty acids, is harmful. Milk, the main source of calcium, and containing valuable protein and other nutrients, is hardly obtainable throughout most of the underdeveloped countries. A low milk production in any country usually means that the children are undernourished, and that the process of gestation is endangered. In 1956 UNICEF provided skimmed milk to some 50 countries involving 2,700,000 children.[18]

Since then important developments have taken place in the preparation of milk substitutes which, if properly exploited, will go far to remedy the grave evils of protein starvation particularly among the young. C.S.M. (cornflour 70 per cent, defatted soya flour 25 per cent, and skimmed milk powder 5 per cent) is now widely used by UNICEF: 124 million lb were shipped in 1973 to Bangladesh and the Sahel. Plants to manufacture 'superamine' (wheat flour, chick peas, lentil powder, milk, sugar, pre-mixed minerals and vitamins) have been established with UNICEF assistance in Algeria, Egypt, Iran, Morocco,

Tunisia and Turkey.[20] The Institute of Nutrition of Central America and Panama manufactures 'incaparina', a powder consisting of finely ground corn (29 per cent), soya bean (29 per cent), cotton seed (38 per cent), Torula yeast (3 per cent) and chalk (1 per cent), which can be given easily as an 'atole' or hot drink or incorporated in soup and puddings. Many other milk substitutes are now being manufactured in different parts of the world, with the additional advantage of making the developing world more independent of outside aid.[19, 21]

In 1971, the general assembly of the UN recommended that a protein advisory group be set up with membership from its specialized agencies. The five sponsoring members of PAG (FAO, WHO, UNICEF, IBRD, UNIDO)* at the 21st meeting discussed global maldistribution of protein.[20]

The manufacture of protein by unicellular organisms (yeast, microbes, amoebae) is now advanced; this makes use of a mixture of petroleum or paraffin (for energy) and nitrogen compounds (urea, ammonia) with added minerals. So also is the manufacture of Lysine, an essential aminoacid which can raise the nutritive value of cereals, rice and cornflour, from 50 per cent to 75 per cent now far advanced. The artificial production of protein and lysine together may well revolutionize the world protein situation, dependent of course on three still unexplored factors – cost, toxicity and acceptability.

Feeding according to biological needs has more to offer to the world than almost any other form of public health. Special feeding for vulnerable groups is likely to be needed everywhere: milk distributed through schools, child health centres, or hospitals; vitamin preparations for pregnant women; meals, and high protein concentrates, for children. School meals are of particular value, since they ensure that children get the full benefit of national expenditure. The subsidizing of essential foodstuffs, priority distribution, and fortification of foods with essential nutrients, such as margarine with vitamin D, rice with nicotinic acid, or salt with iodine, are valuable steps. The ill effects of vitamin A deficiency (corneal scarring and blindness) in S. and S.E. Asia are being countered by the distribution of vitamin A in capsules.[20] Farming developments can, with advantage, be closely related to nutritional status and to the findings of dietary surveys.

Yet an even more fundamental solution is needed – teaching the family to make the best use of local foods, which local experiments have shown to be fruitful.[18] All measures designed to feed people properly will succeed only if closely integrated with public health teaching – fully alive and sympathetic to the customs and beliefs which determine the pattern of life in the household (see Chapter 6). Nutritional advance, like so much else in public health, is not solely a question of techniques.[4] How strong are the forces with which public health has to contend was seen in the persistence in Coonoor, South India, of age-old customs of feeding infants, long after the establishment of health centres.[3] In the past workers tried, by repeated blows of didactic teaching, to hammer through the haze of tradition, taboo, and magic; more recently, we came to realize that beliefs about food are part of the whole fabric of the

* International Bank for Reconstruction and Development (IBRD).
  United Nations Industrial Development Organization (UNIDO).

people and cannot be changed in isolation.[3] The most effective channel of nutritional teaching, if given by well-trained doctors and nurses, is the maternal and child health centre.

The great advances in knowledge have not so far solved man's difficulties, for the problem of human nutrition is economic and social as well as bio-chemical. The saddest of all happenings to an ill-fed world is the destruction of surplus crops when swollen markets have caused a slump. Economy has often turned a blind eye to the world's suffering. And for many countries, higher nutritional standards cannot be achieved without an improvement in trade. When people live at a low subsistence level, hunger is a driving force to be satisfied irrespective of protective foods – kwashiorkor with, rarely but tragically, cancrum oris, keratomalacia, and many other nutritional disasters, must follow (see Chapter 3). Economic development often provides the only means to break the vicious circle of poverty, hunger, malnutrition, ill-health, and physical inefficiency. Europe needs to import food, and has the money to do so; but so on balance must the Far East, and it has not. The Western Hemisphere and Oceania need to continue their exports of food if the world diet is not to decline still further; but already surpluses decline and exporters (e.g. the USSR and China) have become importers of food.

Every nation must put its own house in order.

The spectacular rise in food production in North America over the past few decades was not the result of good luck. On the contrary, in a world with a growing population and a growing multiplicity and complexity of wants, the advantage lies with nations possessing a large territory under unified economic control, where land and other resources are ample in relation to population, and where modern techniques can be developed and applied without hindrance. In many of the less developed regions, land and other potential resources are available in abundance, but unified control has been largely absent and modern techniques have not penetrated the masses. In other parts of the world, as in Europe, some national units have become too small for full advantage to be taken of modern forms of industrial organization and technique. Persisting trade and other barriers have resulted in diminishing returns to a point at which economic standards can scarcely be maintained. Second World Food Survey, Rome, 1952.

If present technical knowledge can be spread, potential food production is extremely large. The use of organic and inorganic fertilizers, control of pests and disease, better seed and appropriate methods of cultivation, together with the large possibilities of extending irrigation and double-cropping, provide the means of increasing crop and fodder yields. Better and scientific feeding, timely use of forage crops, control of animal disease, and an efficient breeding program can likewise increase yields of livestock. Without any expansion of the cultivated area the production of crops could well be doubled. For livestock products the prospects are even better, although yields as high as those in some developed countries are not likely to be obtained until the scarcity of feeding stuffs has been overcome. Third World Food Survey, Rome, 1963.

These encouraging words did not take sufficiently into account the rapid expansion of population and the increasing disparity which affluence in the developed world would produce. In the 15 years since the first edition of this book, the total world population has increased from 2,600 to 3,800 millions and the diet of Western Europe, in its protein content, has approximated to that of North America (150 g daily). Moreover, the increases in food production which FAO considered to be necessary in 1963 (see p. 21) have not been met and the likelihood of a 174 per cent increase by the year 2000 seems remote in the extreme. Despite all that can be said about the possibilities of increasing food production all is jeopardized by our inability 'to make rational use of nature's bounty' (FAO 1963).[7] International acceptance and vigorous pursuit of family limitation by all or most countries of the world will be needed to prevent further disastrous decline in nutritional standards.

The nutritional problems of the world also call for concerted *international* action to expand the crop area, to raise yields, to improve livestock, and to reduce waste. Few nations can now hope to solve their problems alone and unaided. The pooling of resources, technical knowledge, and experience through WHO and FAO has already given rise to great improvements. But international collaboration is needed on a wider scale if the great obstacles to development are to be overcome and the orderly marketing of foodstuffs at reasonable prices is to be ensured. A World Food Board is needed to stabilize prices, to establish a world food reserve, to provide funds for the disposal of surplus, and to organize international credits. Countries, like human beings, must help each other. Tentative steps to this end have been taken. As the director of FAO said in 1963; 'The World Food Programme launched jointly by the UN and FAO on an experimental basis is a welcome indication of our awareness of this task'. The FAO conference in 1973 recommended international reserves of food for emergencies; and the conference in 1974 that 15 per cent of the world's annual grain should be held in reserve for nations most in need.[20] With the passage of time, sheer necessity will drive nations to work together for a fairer distribution of the earth's bounty.

13. Industrialization

In terms of public health, and possibly of other evaluations, industrialization implies radical alterations in society, with far-reaching effects for every member of it. Industrialization is new, in this sense, but industry is not. If industry is large-scale manufacture, it was in operation in the mines of Rome and Greece and in the mills of Antioch and Tyre. Pottery has likewise been manufactured on a large scale for ages. The five towns of Staffordshire (England) – Burslem, Tunstall, Hanley, Stoke, and Longton – were loading immense quantities of pottery on to pack-horses, for transport along muddy lanes to far-off ports, for two centuries before industrialization began.

The manufacture of cotton goods flourished throughout the East from earliest times. For centuries this was the chief source of India's wealth, owing its reputation to the exquisite skill and delicate touch of the Hindu. India clothed much of Southern Asia. The cotton industry was introduced to Spain by the Moors in the tenth century, by the twelfth century exports of cotton from Genoa were brisk, in the fifteenth century fabrics were being produced in Flanders and, after the arrival of religious refugees from Antwerp in the late sixteenth century (1585), in England. For two centuries the cotton industry flourished in England without the phenomenon of industrialization having developed. Kay's flying shuttle (1733) and Hargreaves' spinning jenny (1770) made no essential change. It was not until Arkwright's roller spinning process was patented (1769, 1775) that industrialization in the cotton industry began.[2]

Industrialization cannot easily be described in terms of one factor. It displays a number of different characteristics, dependent to some extent upon where and when it has taken place. The most ubiquitous of these is *transformation of a peasant society* into a community dependent upon the factory. A peasant society works in crafts and local manufactures, mainly in its own homes and generally in its own time. It exists on locally-made goods and locally-grown food. For the sale of its wares, peasant and townsman deal directly in local markets and pedlars and travelling dealers take the place of shopkeepers.

A peasant society is knit firmly together by long-established practice and belief. Thus authority tends to be concentrated in one member of the family; in Europe it was generally patriarchal. In most parts the ties with the land – the essential feature – are strong. The hard life with few luxuries is the lot of nearly all, especially in countries, as in Europe, where the climate can be severe. Man and beast may share the same dwellings. So too the forces of nature, food, famine, and pestilence, impose their will upon everyone, while foremost there are customs from which it is not easy to depart and which restrict activities and curtail initiative[5, 6] (see also p. 47).

The peasant has a sense of security which flows from his attachment to land and family and from the customs which contain his daily life within a narrow compass. Yet paradoxically on his translation to an industrial society he becomes bound in other ways, for he loses the right to use his own initiative and to exercise choice in the way he does his daily tasks. Impersonal discipline now replaces the authority of a relative or friend. Time often has a new value, imposing fresh strains upon those who have lived in societies where people work as necessity calls and who can enjoy to stand or sit for long periods in contemplation. It has been said that from a craftsman in his own right he becomes a cog in a machine. Nevertheless he must often have escaped from the restrictions of authority within his own family by acquiring an independent source of income; and the industrial society into which he enters, if without ties of kinship, may restrict his movements less. He may also eventually, as his horizons widen, be less a prey to superstitious beliefs and be freed from anxiety about the forces of nature.

The factory where men and women are collected together for work is an almost universal concomitant of industrialization. While cotton goods were made in the home, even after the introduction of the flying shuttle and the spinning jenny, the age-old tradition of a family occupation, with family and village responsibilities, continued. But the roller spinning frame, worked by water power, took cotton into the factory, and began industrialization. Although physically factories may vary from mines, or brick ovens, to an establishment with large shops for assembling motor cars, yet all are alike in introducing new features into the community life. The mass of persons taking part have no property in the land, the capital, or the instruments; they work away from home; they are paid by wage; and they must tend machinery. The factory, although not universally, relies upon machinery driven by mechanized power. It is true that Staffordshire pottery-making became industrialized with the throwers' wheel as the main machine, identical in mechanical principle with that used by the ancient Egyptians, and without, at least immediately, any mechanical propulsion; but this is an isolated instance.[2]

The factory involves society in *migration*. Often whole communities have left a settled country life to live, at a distance, in towns. Or the men may travel away from home to work, spending perhaps the whole day, or, as in Africa and elsewhere, being absent for weeks and months. But men have left home in fishing communities, for days or months, for many ages past. Men have left the Balkans, and other countries, to earn money, for their families, possibly even fortunes, in distant lands, where standards are higher and opportunities greater. From far and wide they come to pedal a samlaw in Bangkok, Jakarta, or Rangoon, and, if they survive, return to their villages after months or years to live in relative opulence. Yet migration of peasants to towns is one of the hallmarks of industrialization; and even where it it transitory it either represents a transition phase, or it may mean industrialization elsewhere.

The factory also tends *to take the women from the family*. They leave the spinning and weaving in the home, the keeping of livestock, the laundering on the slab by the village fountain, or on the rocks by the stream, for something like the life of a man ordered by the same rules, and subject to the same hazards.

The factory introduces *the money economy*, if this is not already present; and the use of money can help to break down traditional practices and family relationships, especially in those societies where wealth has lain in herds of cattle under the head of the family, or extended family, to whose authority all have bowed.

Yet the factory is not a new invention. Men and women have long been collected together in mills and mines. The distinguishing feature of the factory in an industrialized nation is chiefly the extent of its development, so that the community becomes dominated by it, and life centres around it. The establishment of only a few factories in a peasant society may mean the beginning of the irreversible process of industrialization.

'Industrialization' implies that *occupations become more sharply defined.* In the old pottery industry, master potters each had a single oven with six men and four boys. They undertook the whole range of operations. Journeymen potters were accustomed to pass from one kind of labour to another, just as impulse or convenience demanded.[2] When industrialization began – as oven was added to oven and the brick factory replaced the master potters' family concern – the work was divided into many distinct categories; throwers, turners, oven men, flat pressers, hollow ware pressers, dippers, etc. Subsidiary and complementary trades, crate makers, colour makers, lathe makers, grew up around it. Moreover, *occupations tend to change* as processes alter with new inventions. Thus, the use of coal instead of charcoal in the production of pig iron changed the character of work for many thousands in newly industrialized iron districts. The master hammersmith disappeared almost overnight, and in his place, puddlers, rollers, and other new classes appeared. Not only 'change', but the possibility of it, and to some extent its inevitability, provide one of the most significant contrasts of an industrialized society with the age-old life of the village, hallowed by long tradition. Any change in technological processes in turn affects the whole life of the community.

Industrialization is also distinguished by its emphasis upon *production for the masses* – designed to meet the needs of mankind as a whole, and not, as was generally the case in earlier centuries, dependent upon the making of luxury goods for the few. This has been described, not very accurately, as satisfying the needs of the poor, so that in 1831 it could be said that two centuries before, not one in a thousand wore stockings, whereas by then not one in a thousand was without. Industrialization thrives upon the width of market which only the inclusion of everyone, rich and poor, can produce. And in its turn it revolutionizes the life of the members of society by making goods which affect almost everything in life from diet and travel to hospitals and television. It is based upon commerce with other nations, and it encourages its further growth.

Finally, industrialization determines a *different economy,* which in turn reflects upon the structure of society. It can only take place when large resources of capital exist, and it promotes a process of further accumulation. This again is not new – Roman and Venetian industries depended upon capital – except in the extent to which it became the driving force in society. The industrial revolution gave to capital a much wider control over the lives of men. Capital, whether from the State or private sources, provides the motive force which drives the whole industrial machine.

The influence of industrialization on public health

Industrialization came first to the world chiefly in England during the later years of the eighteenth century. It created an upheaval, social, environmental, and cultural, and gave rise to changes which had not been previously encountered. This first episode coincided with the great inventions and discoveries which began to make man more quickly the master rather than the slave of his environment. But it found the world unprepared to meet the evils to which it could give rise, although able to benefit from its advantages. The factory system was called the English System, but it travelled fast to some other countries, particularly Belgium, and more slowly to others such as Germany. In all these it reproduced much the same phenomena. Fielden referred to American factories in 1833 in his *Curse of the Factory System*.[2]

This is not the place to examine in detail the reasons why this phenomenon, which affected the world's health and welfare so extensively, should have begun mainly in England. The usual catalogue of circumstances can be paraded, but they are of little relevance except so far as they help us to understand how much industrialization depends for its effects upon the social background of the country in which it occurs. Before the remarkable series of inventions upon which it was based began, England had a government favourable to commerce; it had internal free trade and a prosperous and growing textile industry; it was already an exporting nation with large commercial connexions; it had a banking system and had evolved joint-stock companies; its common law gave a measure of individual freedom; its aristocracy had the tradition of engaging in trade; nature had given it coal, abundant and near to the ports, and a climate suitable for spinning cotton; world events had placed it on a great water route between Europe and America; and the Elizabethan adventurers, seeking outlets for commerce, had taken its ships and trading companies to Eastern markets.

Everything was favourable to industrialization. There was no special barrier, as in Rome or Greece, to prevent the use of inventions on a large scale – no high-minded Roman to tear up as dangerous a proposal to mechanize a traditional process, and no Greek Hero to see in the steam engine the means only to pump libations for the temples. It was as natural for the disciples of Newton to think of industry as it was for those of Archimedes to turn against it, for inventors were free to experiment, with the near certainty that the results of their genius would be put to productive purposes. Thus it was essentially the political, economic, and social background of England which determined the course of events. So it is today.

Industrialization in the eighteenth and nineteenth centuries led immediately to ugliness, squalor, and insanitary dwellings, to exploitation of the wage earners, to high mortality and spreading infections, to a loosening of family ties and morals, and to employment of children in conditions that the twentieth century hardly likes to recall. These circumstances arose because the state of society favoured them. Exploitation of the worker was part of the same set of values which allowed the traffic in slaves in which the new industrialized societies were engaged. The wealth of industry then played little part in achieving harmony with the physical environment because money became an end in itself; so that towns of the first industrial period, without plan or beauty, were symbols of the age, just as were the cathedrals of medieval Europe, or the amphitheatres of Rome.

Everywhere throughout the world it is the structure of society and its culture with which we must be concerned in garnering the fruits of industrialization and in mitigating its evils. In the country which gave it birth this was soon to be seen in the variations which occurred in different areas. In Manchester, where there was already a strong social framework, and powerful voices for reform and the remedy of abuses, the impact was modified and mollified – whereas in South Wales, with thousands of immigrants and without the restraints of tradition, experience of government, or common history, conditions resembled those in a gold rush. So the effects in Japan will differ from those in America or Africa.[9]

The developed nations, now that they have for the most part overcome infections, find themselves beset with a multitude of social problems. Some appear to be due to a loosening of family ties, others to a sense of uncertainty from loss of faith in divine purpose, still others to increasing difficulties of human relationships. Much illness, as seen by the general practitioner or in the outpatient departments of hospitals, appears to be psychosomatic, or as part of an escape mechanism, or of a stress phenomenon. Mental illness is more obvious, if not necessarily more frequent, and the extent of departures from mental health is thought by many to be widening. Both adults and children have behaviour difficulties (see p. 23). In different ways underdeveloped and developing countries are involved in the same process. Separation from wife and home, for example, is the cause of spreading venereal disease in many African communities. Promiscuity, alcoholism, and syphilis accompanied the break-up of the African family.[3] Cash crops and a wage economy, which upset subsistence farming and introduce processed foods, can be blamed for nutritional disease. Destitution and poverty may be the lot of the displaced industrial worker who no longer has his place in the family and his attachment to the land.

That these social ills arise directly or indirectly from industrialization can hardly be doubted.[8, 12] Many are clearly connected, particularly those associated with a break-up of the family (see Chapter 7) and those that result from changed social conditions. In an industrial society, for example, the mentally handicapped, the aged, and epileptics become problems in social medicine, when in a simpler society they may not.[11] The increased complications of life, and the diminished resources of the family, weight the balance against them; as the old become problems, irrespective of infirmity, when the traditional jobs of the countryside and the fireside chair in the family house are no longer available. Epileptics and the mentally subnormal can be accommodated in industry only when careful social systems are devised to meet their needs.

Mental illness is more obvious in the developed world, but this does not necessarily mean that it could not be found equally, if not more, in less developed countries. Yet, if anxiety results from conflict, and this in turn arises out of the need to exercise choice, or from difficulties in personal relationships, here may be found some part of the cause of the psychoneuroses and the psychosomatic diseases, such as the peptic ulcers, which recently have appeared to excess in industrialized societies.[4]

The manner in which this course of events is set in operation is far from clear. There is hardly likely to be less conflict in the personal relationships within the factory than in a peasant family, living, as already described, on the land. Among the many cultures of the world there are probably few where conflicts within the family circle do not occur. The dominant personality in the extended family, whether father or mother-in-law, or, in different circumstances, both, may be as much a cause of anxiety as the unsympathetic foreman. Daughters-in-law everywhere may display hysterical phenomena, although they will not always complain of them. The indictment of industry for causing greater frustration in highly repetitive and specialized jobs, and for denying the individual the satisfaction of creative work, may also be exaggerated. Life outside the factory may well compensate for monotony within; moreover, thoughts can wander, and social concourse provides its own interest. Industry, however, in giving rise to perplexing choices and loss of security, to which the peasant in performing traditional roles is not subjected, may well be a factor in the production of our social misfits and of the psychosomatic disorders which prevail. But it is not the only, nor even the major cause. The syndrome of conflict is more likely to be related to many things than to any one particular aspect of industrialization.

To some extent the industrialized world has made a rod for its own back. When it calls for punctuality, reliability, and regularity in its workers, absenteeism, hardly recognizable in a peasant society, becomes a social illness. Yet in many parts of the world workers tend to cease work for no other reason than that they do not have a sufficiently strong incentive to earn money, or the urge to buy manufactured goods. Peasants, as in Turkey and elsewhere, generally prefer agricultural work to the factory, so that a transfer to industrial life sometimes takes place only under the compulsion of economic necessity. In the more industrialized societies the sickness certificate may cover up the same phenomenon. We should ask ourselves whether perhaps absenteeism, in seeking to avoid the shackles of the factory and in preferring the simple life, is not a sign of a healthy outlook rather than of social disorder. They have '. . . cut the invisible wires of steel that pull them back and forth, to work . . . hooked fishes of the factory world' (D. H. Lawrence).

Industrialization is not reversible.[10] It must eventually cover the world. For millions living at or near starvation level it appears to be the only answer to a multitude of health problems. It seems unlikely that industrialization, any more than education or public health, can be artificially limited to modify its impact upon societies of different types.[9] But if the process itself has to be given a free rein, there is much that can be done to forestall the disorders.

Where the integrity of families is involved they may be transplanted to the neighbourhood of the factory, or alternatively, where appropriate, industry itself may seek the peasant in, or near to, his own village. Workers can be fitted in to the right job. The working mother and her young children can be given special consideration. Industry can be given a new structure so that workers feel themselves to be part of it;[4] and it can associate itself actively with the life of the worker and of the society of which it forms part. Health departments can widen their outlook and seek to promote the health of society, as well as of its individual members.[1] The family can be made the basis of any health service; and particularly in the underdeveloped world, where the infrastructure of health outlined in Chapter 20 can base much of its work on *home visiting*.

Towns can be built as true centres of the 'good life'. Security can be given to the worker and his family, no less than that which he enjoyed in his peasant culture. The formula must vary in every society, and in many different circumstances. But, as it is hoped previous chapters have shown, the effects of industrialization on the many different aspects of the life of any community – town living, food production, culture, population, occupation, family life, medical care – can be guided to the benefit of both individuals and society. It is for the twentieth century to show that none of the unhappy sequels of industrialization is inevitable, and that, with due consideration, its advantages can outweigh its disadvantages.

Part Four: The Development of National Systems of Public Health

14. The European Movement

Early attempts

Public health – the application of scientific and medical knowledge to the protection and improvement of the health of the group – calls for organization, a conscious effort by authority. Some form or organization for public health has existed in most societies from the earliest times, but always, until recently, limited by the lack of technical knowledge and often hampered by an inadequate appreciation of the value of health, or by a lack of social understanding. The State doctors of Egypt and Rome, the leprosaria of the Middle Ages, the quarantine procedure of Venice, the sanitary inspectors of Cordoba and other Arabian cities, the regulation of brothels in many societies from the Golden Age of Greece onwards, all these are illustrations, though limited in scope; as also are the councils of health in Paris and other European cities, the central council of health in England (advocated by Richard Mead in his *Treatise on the Plague* (1720)[34] and coming into existence nearly a century later (1805)[11]), and the local boards of health in Baltimore (1793)[47] and Manchester (1795).[12]

In the form we think of it today Public Health is new. The highest measure of health for all, not only the privileged few, has never until recently been a national objective. Smillie, writing about North America before 1790, says that during the entire colonial period, 'We find little evidence that the authorities realized that they have a direct and continuing responsibility for the health of the people. Certainly there was an almost complete lack of community organization for health services.'[47]

And so might it have been written for the rest of the world at any stage and in any land from the dawn of history. Some or all of the many ingredients which go to the making of public health have always been lacking. When, in the days of the ancients, health was highly valued for itself, and when the social organization existed through which protective measures could be applied, the social conscience was weak. Significantly, Galen persuaded himself, when physician to the School of Gladiators in Pergamos (A.D. 157), that there was, as he said, 'a certain art of hygiene', but he wrote his book on 'Hygiene' entirely for a privileged aristocracy.[22] When later, at least in the Western world, every man began to be accounted as of value, the health of the body was no longer so highly prized, and disease was often a grace to purify the soul. The cult of individual hygiene flourished through many centuries without giving rise to services for the protection of the community health. The advice on mothercraft which Galen made the basis of his first volume on hygiene might have led to the foundation of a maternity and child welfare service throughout the Roman

Empire, as logically as that which followed the teaching of Florence Nightingale and the practice of Pierre Budin and William Ballantyne, in the twentieth century.[11,12] The healthgiving thermae of Roman cities, where baths and gymnasia went hand-in-hand with social activities, might have produced the health centre, if Roman minds had had the social outlook of Andrija Stampar of Yugoslavia. Why did our preoccupation with diet, long recognized as one of the main hygiene agents, have no application as a public health measure? Why did seafaring men need to await the graduation of James Lind and his appointment in 1749 to HMS *Salisbury*, before they were given a service to maintain their health?

> Behind us lie
> The Thousand and the Thousand and the Thousand Years
> Vexed and terrible and still we use
> The cures which never cure.
>
> *Fry*

'For the life of many men', said Galen, 'is involved in the business of their occupation, and it is inevitable that they should be harmed by what they do and that it should be impossible to change it.[22] Galen might have argued the case for rather than against an occupational health service, as logically as did Patissier in 1822 (see Chapter 9). So much has depended upon the development of ideas: about the sanctity of human life, about the rights and privileges of all men, and about community organization and the propriety of action by government in matters which concern the individual. Even more has depended upon additions to human knowledge which have encouraged us to think that something effective can be done.

Public health has, even then, often had to await the enlightened self-interest of those who are capable of getting things done; so that it has been practised when it seemed to lead not only to 'pastures new', but to pastures pleasant. Thus the rich in England played a more active part in sanitary reform once they were convinced that the diseases of squalor might endanger their own lives, as well as those of the poor. Likewise factory legislation followed an appreciation by the employer of the economic value of improved health in the worker.

Public health begins in Europe

The eighteenth century had almost passed before public health in the modern sense had begun to develop. It had many points of departure, reflecting the varying ideologies of the peoples among whom the pioneer thinkers lived; and what we see today throughout the world still shows much of the early patterns. It was natural for Johann Peter Frank (1745–1821) to write about social medicine as a police measure, for this viewpoint was an expression of the autocracy under which he and his forefathers for many centuries had lived. Frank's *System einer vollständigen medizinischen Polizey* grew naturally from *Cameralism*, as enlightened rulers conceived the idea of people as the natural wealth of their country.[44] Frank's exposition of social medicine was far ahead of his time; any general concern, for example, for hygiene in the schoolroom awaited the passage of well over a century. But we find little in his teaching to satisfy present-day concern for 'participation by the people', for 'an appeal to the individual', for 'local government', or for 'doing things with people in tune with their culture'.

The new birth of public health in England, to which the industrial revolution gave rise, was very different, again reflecting the prevailing philosophy of local government and distrust of autocratic rule, however benevolent. Edwin Chadwick (1800–90) is justly famed for hammering relentlessly home his conviction that health depended upon sanitation. Chadwick's circulation of vital fluids, from pure water to purified sewage, protected water courses, pipes, drains and sewers intact and inviolate, return after purification to the soil – has been as momentous for man's progress as Harvey's discovery of the circulation of the blood.[12] If Chadwick were alive today he would find nine-tenths of the world still suffering the torments of intestinal infections from which Europe and the New World, in following his teachings, have escaped. Nevertheless Chadwick's claim to our undying respect might rest even more firmly upon his less considered teachings: the use of local government in public health administration, and also of the medical officer of health as a specialist adviser, both of which gave rise to far-reaching effects.[12] The people began to participate in their own health protection by franchise from among themselves for voluntary service on local Boards of Health; and by supplying the means to finance the services needed to remedy sanitary evils out of their own pockets. Doctors, locally appointed, advised the boards in the discharge of functions placed upon them by Parliament. Their appointment soon became compulsory and their tenure of office protected. Their duties outlined in detail in a circular issued by Chadwick's General Board of Health dated 12th February 1851,* required an annual presentation of data of sickness and mortality in terms of 'the several streets, squares, courts, lanes, yards and alleys'; this began in earnest the nationwide epidemiological studies, based upon statistics which William Farr's registration data now made possible (see Chapter 21).

This is the English scene – with its attention focused unromantically upon sanitation – which was Chadwick's gift to the world.*

Throughout Europe, North America, and the British Dominions the general plan of organization followed, not of course consciously, one or other of these two prototypes, although Edwin Chadwick is recalled to mind now only as the domineering policeman and the name of Johann Frank, benevolently academic, has been virtually lost to the world. France, Spain, Austria, Germany, Italy, Belgium, and the Scandinavian countries all developed their public health along paternalistic lines. To this, no doubt, the French Revolution added an appreciable impetus. No sort of uniformity existed, and each European country grew apart from its fellows in a hundred different ways; but in the background can be seen the web of centralization, the reliance upon the State official. Perhaps France is now the greatest example with its public health services based on the *département* under the supreme authority of the Préfet, *'fonctionnaire nommé par l'Etat'*, and with a medical director on the staff of the central organization.[18]

* See Brockington, C. F. (1965) *Public Health in the Nineteenth Century*. Edinburgh: Livingstone for a full account of this development.

Speaking in 1954 of the failure of the *Conseil Départemental d'Hygiène* established in 1902 to advise the Préfet, Pequignot[40] says significantly that since the method of dealing with questions of techniques in preventive work is essentially by means of national circulars, 'it is difficult to imagine a policy of official services different in the Savoy and in the Morbihan'. In England it would have been difficult to imagine them the same.

The paternalistic countries also tended to develop Frank's ideology of social medicine, with emphasis upon hospitals and medical care. The French prefects received their first national circular about hospitals in 1840.[41] Most if not all the European countries began to build State hospitals at an early date. As early as 1931 Newsholme's report spoke of 'an admirable system of municipal and county hospitals throughout every part of Denmark'.[37] Both Denmark and Sweden, he said, had 'a hospital system supported out of the taxes, which removed hospital treatment for all needing it from the category of problems still to be solved'. With Germany as the pioneer, European countries also tended early to insure, voluntarily or compulsorily, for care in sickness by the medical practitioner. Denmark succeeded in the seemingly impossible task of obtaining virtually complete cover on a voluntary basis. Perhaps we can see in this also a reflection of Frank's concern for poverty as a cause of disease, which he put so eloquently in his oration as Dean of the Medical School in Austrian Lombardy (1790).[20]

In contrast Chadwick's emphasis on disease as a cause of poverty – 'the pecuniary cost of noxious agencies'[43] as he said – led to sanitary measures. England came much later (1911) to adopt health insurance. The USA, confidently expected by all political parties to be about to adopt some form of national health, was still in 1974 without complete cover.*

Thus while Europe gathered its administrative forces at the centre and attacked the problem of how to get the sick treated, England and the New World got down to sanitation with the responsibility firmly place upon the shoulders of the local citizens. Chadwick rubbed their noses brutally in the dirt.

The American scene

The influence of England on America, although with long-delayed action, was striking.[3] The Shattuck report (1850), if it had had a greater appeal to the emotions, might have been written by Chadwick.[33] Shattuck followed the English report in most of its main recommendations, including that for full-time medical officers of health specially trained and qualified in public health and independent of private practice. 'Statistical investigations', he said, much as did Chadwick, 'are our best friend and severest critic.'[33] As a result English and American public health have had their roots in biostatistics.

At the American Sanitary Convention of 1859 the finger was pointed across the Atlantic to Chadwick and the 'noble Government of England', noble for what it was doing to promote health and preserve life.[54] In 1876 the first President of the Massachusetts State Board of Health said that England, which 'had

---

* Personal communication from Dr Myron Wegman, Ann Arbor.

far outstripped any country in the world in the direction of State Medicine', exerted by far the greatest influence upon America. 'When the time came for the American cities to pass sanitary ordinances', he said, 'they did so in the tradition of English Common Law.'[26]

The development of the public health movement follows so closely the English pattern that Welch's classical dictum that the Panama Canal and the public health nurse have been America's two great contributions to public health, could, with modification, have been coined for England. Both countries also used voluntary effort for much of the pioneer work. Hanlon writes: [26]

> While the official, governmental, or public health agencies were still in the process of development, a complementary and supplementary force appeared in the form of the voluntary non-official health agency . . . spurred by public interest, desire for private philanthropy, and sometimes by impatience or dissatisfaction with governmental programmes, over 25,000 such agencies were established during the ensuing half century (after 1892).

The same could be written of England. English and American Public Health have both in the course of development favoured local government with considerable autonomy. In 1961, Wyatt said in his study of intergovernmental relations in the USA: [60]

> The role of national government is confined primarily to providing plans, financial aid, advice, and supervision; and in varying degrees this is true of state governments as well, although they provide also most of the legislation and sanctions for public health. In most communities and many rural areas the direct public health functions are performed mainly by local officials, though with the assistance, support, and supervision of state agencies; and it is the hope of most public health authorities that this system of primary local responsibility will be extended to cover the entire country.

Yet, both, as the second half of the twentieth century progressed, have tended to centralize and to limit local autonomy in health matters. In the USA, the establishment of 'regional planning councils (1966), together with 'regional medical programs', and in Britain the creation of regional hospital boards (1948) and regional and health authorities (1974) have sharply diminished the influence of local authorities in health matters.

Variations in development within the European movement

The countries that pioneered public health were remarkable rather for their differences than their similarities. The control at the centre assumed many forms and no two were alike. The public health of Denmark, which has been in advance of the world, has functioned without a Ministry of Health, nor even a separate health department within an existing ministry. The Sundhedssty-relsen, 'the chief supervisor of public health and nursing', is a separate institution which must be consulted by the various departments of the central administration whenever matters requiring expert professional knowledge are to be decided.[19] Some countries with less corporate spirit might easily fail to develop under such a loose rein.

Where a central government department of health exists there is no known instance of its embracing all health matters, and the extent to which functions are spread over other ministries has varied. In the USA, the Children's Bureau, created by congress in 1912, was until recently an independent unit directed 'to investigate and report upon all matters pertaining to welfare of children and child life'. In Uruguay and in Brazil, the administration of care of mothers and children is still undertaken by distinct national organizations. And in many parts of the world voluntary agencies for maternal and child health have developed independently, an aspect which is fast disappearing, particularly in developed countries. In Spain, two central bodies (health and social security), in parallel and with much overlap, are still engaged in providing hospitals and organizing medical care.[13]

At the periphery there has been likewise every variation. The development of Local Public Health units has been, to all appearances, quite haphazard. In England they began to be formed in 1831; the country was covered completely in 1872–5.[12] In the USA they began in 1793; but despite the Shattuck Report (1850), the concept of a well-organized health department, supervised by a whole-time Medical Officer of Health, was not widely applied, in the USA, until the 1920s.[45] Three-quarters of a century lapsed after the first Board of Health in Baltimore in 1793 and the foundation of that of Michigan in 1873.

The power wielded by local councils and their officers was also developed along different lines. The relative autonomy of cities and counties in the USA, subject to supervision and final authority of their state governments,[26] has to be seen in contrast with the relative subservience of the council of a French *département*. An English city or county council, or a Swedish county, lay somewhere between. The Swedish autonomy at the periphery, as in Denmark, has been limited by the central appointment of governors, prefects, or chairmen, and, of course, of the medical adviser.

The system of local units for health administration in Holland, which relies on what might be called voluntary local authorities and is unique,[1] illustrates well the great variety in organization which can exist. Holland has a chief medical officer responsible to the Minister of Social Affairs with twelve departments, all but one headed by doctors. In each province there is one Medical Inspector of Health, who is responsible, without executive authority, for what happens in public health in his province. Public health practice, as it concerns maternity and child welfare, tuberculosis, child guidance, mental health, and many forms of child care, is conducted by voluntary agencies – the Green, Yellow, and Orange Cross societies. These are organized on a village, province, and state basis. Since most of their funds are derived from the government, the medical officer advises their central departments, and the provincial medical officers exert their influence locally. The doctors at each level are thus able to guide the service, in much the same way as under the grant system in England or the United States.

The extent of the power to be wielded by the medical officer of health has been strikingly different, both as between different countries and often within the same country. The health commissioner in an American city governed on the managerial system, making and executing his own laws, but generally liable to removal by political whim, will have enjoyed a very different daily round of life from that of a nominated official of the State on the continent of Europe.

The British medical officer of health, whose duty it was to discover everything in his area prejudicial to the health of the people, virtually independent of control from the centre and yet the servant of a locally elected council with its own chairman, stood again in a category of his own. Symbolic of the whole variegated picture of public health practice throughout the pioneer countries were those large areas of the USA in which, at the time when Emerson was writing (1945),[15, 16] no health department existed.

The pattern of administration has been further complicated by individualistic trends in devising new fields of action. 'Hitherto, most countries have evolved measures for reaching their hygiene objectives only as each pressing need has emerged.'[37] Not even Frank's omnibus of social medicine, the work of a lifetime, could stamp a blueprint which all would follow. This is understandable, when human needs and circumstances vary so greatly and are so constantly changing. Public health has to be paid for, and the money chests are opened reluctantly. Yet the differences in approach and rate of advancement are difficult to explain, except in terms of the whole philosophy and system of values of a people. Scientific knowledge has been at everyone's disposal. Yet Denmark began a system of gratuitous treatment of venereal disease for all patients, irrespective of social and financial status, in 1790, 126 years before Britain (1916). In Switzerland gratuitous treatment began as late as 1931, and then for the indigent only; so that 'the struggle against venereal disease was described in 1935 as in a relatively early stage of development'.[37] France made vaccination against smallpox obligatory 105 years after Jenner's discovery, and nearly a century after Germany. Sweden pioneered vital statistics. As early as 1758, Sweden had an official statistical commission charged with the tabulation of details received from the clergy. She now has the longest continuous series of vital statistics of marriage, births, and deaths in existence. Sweden likewise began the notification of sickness much in advance of other countries. In Holland and Scandinavia the midwife reached professional status in the early part of the century; disasters in pregnancy in these countries had fallen to a low level shortly after the end of World War I, to the envy of others less fortunate. In contrast the United States of America has not found it necessary to develop the midwife. Examples could be multiplied many times.

Few things, indeed, are so striking as variations in development of public health. While England concentrated on sanitation, at least from the time of Chadwick's Public Health Act (1848), France hardly approached the subject before the Law of 1902, which established at one sweep all that painstaking trial and error and empirical action had achieved across the Channel in the preceding half-century. As late as 1954, Pequignot said that France's sanitary services although in advance of underdeveloped countries, lagged behind those of 'les nations plus modernes', such as England and the United States.[42] Equally striking has been the unevenness of the advance towards the acceptance of medicine as a social science, and of medical and hospital care as an essential agent in public health. While Scandinavian doctors accepted a co-operative rôle from the nineteenth century onwards, the professions in England, the USA, and France have fought rearguard actions to avoid what they considered to be an infringement of their liberties.

Cameralism v. local autonomy

Much has been said about the advantages and disadvantages of the two main European systems of public health administration. Newsholme, speaking particularly of France (1931), said that the system implied 'a shackling of local enterprise, and an influence tending to keep at a very low ebb the training of local patriotism'.[37] Perhaps the lag in French sanitary services, to which Pequignot referred, might have been due to this, since local autonomy in a matter so rooted in local habits and customs, will be of particular significance. Particularly disheartening was the need to refer to higher authority on small matters of expenditure. 'If a public lavatory is needed, this may involve an addition to the budget and the central power must approve.'[2] Yet it would seem that the Clochemerles of France, as elsewhere, have escaped from this dilemma by one expedient or another. In Denmark and Sweden the solidarity of national culture, above all the acceptance by the medical profession of social and preventive medicine and its participation in a social service, has done much to remedy the inadequacies of bureaucracy.

On the other hand, local government in public health, which relied in both the United Kingdom and the United States of America on local initiative, has not been able to escape the defects of its virtues. Some might say that what was gained on the swings, in participation by the people and by local initiative, was lost on the roundabouts in a muddle of inefficient units. In practice, neat parcels of administrative territory, the legacy of paternalism on the European continent, had many advantages as a basic framework of public health, in comparison with the haphazard areas of local government in the United Kingdom, or in the United States of America.

Thus, for example, the Minnesota State Board of Health, which consists of 15 members 'nine of whom shall be broadly representative of licensed health professionals and six of whom shall be public members as defined for the purposes of the Act', appointed by the governor with the advice and consent of the senate, has all the powers for the promotion of health of the people of Minnesota which the lawyers could devise.[60]

The state board of health acting through its secretary shall have general authority as the state's official health agency and shall be responsible for the development and maintenance of an organized system of programs and services for protecting, maintaining, and improving the health of the citizens. This authority shall include but not be limited to the following:

a. Conduct studies and investigations, collect and analyse health and vital data, and identify and describe health problems;

b. Plan, facilitate, coordinate, provide, and support the organization of services for the prevention and control of illness and disease and the limitation of disabilities resulting therefrom;

c. Establish and enforce health standards for the protection and the promotion of the public's health such as quality of health services, reporting of disease, regulation of health facilities, environmental health hazards and manpower;

d. Affect the quality of public health and general health care services by providing consultation and technical training for health professionals and paraprofessionals;

e. Promote personal health by conducting general health education programs and disseminating health information;

f. Coordinate and integrate local, state and federal programs and services affecting the public's health;

g. Continually assess and evaluate the effectiveness and efficiency of health service systems and public health programming efforts in the state; and

h. Advise the governor and legislature on matters relating to the public's health.

(Minnesota Statutes 144.05)*

In addition to these considerable general powers, other statutes exist to regulate the reporting of vital statistics; to order the discontinuance of dangerous pollution of drinking waters; to hold hearings and issue orders concerning 'offensive trades'; to inspect and license hotels, restaurants, resorts, and small boats; to examine, license, and administer the special laws relating to the licensing of plumbers, embalmers, and funeral directors; to provide instruction for the protection of maternity and infancy; to administer state narcotic laws; and to inspect and license hospitals, rest homes, maternity homes, and homes providing care for the aged. To complement its functions, the Board may issue regulations of permanent application having the force of law. It elects its own secretary, who may or may not be a member of the Board, but who is the executive officer of the Board – the state health officer, a medical man (by job description, not statute).[60]

The disadvantages of local government have arisen, not only in the USA and the UK, but almost universally, from its inability to adjust to the changing character of Public Health, as new techniques and ideas develop. Admirable at first to deal with down to earth problems of environmental hygiene, the areas of local administration are quickly too small, and, even more important, too disparate, to build on the larger schemes of social medicine, as it seeks answers to the problems of the vulnerable classes and is involved in surveys and other esoteric matters. In Minnesota, for example, no less than 1,831 towns, 97 cities, and 87 counties were required to appoint Local Boards, and 649 villages had the right, if they wished to do so. The stage, so admirably set for dynamic public health, took on the appearance of a chessboard for a slow and protracted contest, as each of the towns, counties, cities, and even villages placed a piece. Obstruction, apathy, and vested interests can be doughty opponents of local interest and sympathy; the enthusiastic advance of the Central Departments can be lost in a stalemate.[60]

The inability of small local units to practise public health on modern lines was probably one of the reasons why the USA remained so long without a complete health cover. Less than half the Minnesota towns, according to Emerson's Survey, had appointed a medical officer of health by 1945.[15]

Since all towns, most villages, some cities, and even many counties have considerably smaller populations that can economically support public health programmes . . . it is not surprising that the law has not been enforced for towns.[60]

Many answers to this difficulty have been devised. Minnesota, and other American state departments, developed 'state health districts', which temporarily at least replaced local boards.[60] To bridge the gap elsewhere, the state

* Personal communication, 1974. Professor John Westerman, School of Public Health, Minnesota, USA; revised terms of reference.

duty of supervision and advice was widely interpreted to help the growth of local initiative and to provide essential services in the meantime; state inspectors of food and hygiene worked all over the state – often, especially in the smaller communities, without making any official contact locally, lay or professional. Since 1966, the regional councils mentioned earlier, have further increased the power of the state and diminished those of the local boards.

The influence of federalism

The inadequacies of local government may have been exaggerated in the USA by federalism. Federalism has had so marked an effect upon public health development that the analogy between two such widely different countries as Switzerland and the USA, where state autonomy preceded a federal constitution, strikes even the casual observer.[37] Where the care of the public health is primarily the responsibility of each individual state, there can be little uniformity. The 22 almost completely self-governing cantons of Switzerland and the 50 sovereign United States present infinite variations both in enactments and in methods of public health administration.

Newsholme's study led him to indict federalism rather than local government for the slow development of 'public health administration in both USA and Switzerland'.[37] Public Health in both countries, he said, 'would advance more rapidly if these were organized on a minimum order of uniformity, with full freedom to experiment and extend beyond the stage of minimum equality of establishment'.[37]

This may have been true in the early thirties. But more recently grants-in-aid, introduced by the inspiration of Surgeon-General Parran, have been responsible in America, as for long in England, for vigorous development in public health programmes – despite, at least in the USA, strong resistance from the local bodies that they have been designed to help. The US Public Health Service and earlier the US Children's Bureau, charged by Congress with the administration of the majority of the federal grants-in-aid for public health purposes have been constantly called upon to convince their beneficiaries that their freedom of action would not be unduly limited. The development of uniform services within a federal system has been well illustrated by the National Office of Vital Statistics, first established in the US Bureau of Census in 1950 to encourage the States to develop a uniform system of registration and tabulation of vital data. By this means the national collection of vital statistics covered all states by 1953.

Colonial systems

The influence of the European movement spread to colonial lands, to peoples who, for the most part, had no understanding of, and little sympathy with, the philosophies upon which it had been founded. Africa and many parts of the East, including some countries to be described later for their independent efforts, thus received a first innoculation with the doctrine of public health, with services developed on the pattern of the parent country. Public health in these regions has inevitably been a watered-down version of the original, particularly in the British system in which the Colonial Office tended to take up a paternalistic rôle. The forces which Frank and Chadwick had released, reinforced and canalized by the great men of many nations – William Farr and John Simon, Lemuel Shattuck and Stephen Smith, Parent-Duchatelet, to mention but a few – met the resistance of people with entirely different philosophies of health and little scientific understanding. Europe had to learn how much public health depends upon a willing co-operation of the people; and this in turn upon standards of living rising with technological development.

No adequate description can be given of services provided in so many different ways and under such varied circumstances; but it may be possible to see in the practice of public health in India and Sri Lanka something of what has been happening everywhere. In both these countries, as elsewhere, the burden of sickness, and the absence of social services, proved to be an overriding consideration.

India

The Bhore report (1946) said of India, comparing it with European countries: [27]

In India the rate of progress in health administration has been much slower . . . reference may be made to one aspect of health administration in which India differs from other countries. In the latter, the provision of medical relief for the community has largely developed in the past through the efforts of voluntary agencies and through the growth of an independent medical profession. In India, on the other hand, medical relief was accepted by the State as its responsibility from the beginning. Indeed, it received much more attention than the development of those preventive health measures which may collectively be termed 'public health activities'.

When the Commissions of Public Health in Madras and Bengal (1864) put forward far-reaching recommendations, which included the employment of trained public health staffs in towns and districts, these came to nothing. Sanitary commissioners were appointed to the provinces. But 'each provincial sanitary commissioner had only one assistant to work with him and, apart from this lack of adequate trained staff, the main emphasis continued to be laid, during the period, on the development of medical relief. Medical administration did not give preventive medicine its place.'[27] The reason appeared to be the vast numbers of India's sick, 'so obviously demanding attention that it was to the practice of curative medicine that by far the majority of doctors of the State health service turned'.[27]

This same appeal of the sick must have happened in all underdeveloped countries. It still happens today. But it is difficult to find in this the whole answer. The difficulties of excessive sickness applied earlier, if in a lesser degree, in the homelands too. It is true that the development of hospitals, even if only as places of refuge or isolation (see p. 93), had reached, in Europe, a point where minimum needs were satisfied. The average conditions, too, in the new industrial areas, if shocking to European eyes, were in advance of those in India. Great differences existed in the cultural and social background. There were doctors of a sort in England, and none in India. All these considerations were formidable obstacles, but constituted no absolute barrier, to the application of the

Chadwick philosophy. Some part, at least, of the genius of England's pioneers in public health should have been India's. Nowhere in the world can peoples have existed more in need, in desperate need, of Chadwick's sanitary science. And yet the country which gave birth to this idea could not give it to India. England, that had set aside medical care and hospitals as of secondary importance to the hygiene of the environment, exalted them in India to an exclusive and privileged position. The driving force of self-interest, which so greatly influenced the development of public health in home territories (see p. 118), was no doubt largely lacking in administrators overseas.

The development of public health in any real sense began in India only in 1921, after the Government of India Act (1919) had transferred health administration to the provinces. This late entry of India into the field of public health action, whatever the causes, can be compared with that of the United States of America. As history has shown so often, public health, illogically, is not accepted as an immediate need by developing societies; the fight for existence in both new and old environments can be all-absorbing. Disease and death then become no more than incidents in a life of toil. When life is cheap, the motif of self-interest is slow to develop and the vicious circle of disease and poverty continues unbroken.

In the years following World War I, public health in India, under the new directors of public health, began to develop, particularly in certain provinces. But in many parts the subservience of preventive to curative medicine continued to exercise a baneful influence. Preventive health duties formed part of the responsibility of the civil surgeon in each district. 'The duties of the latter in connexion with medical administration as well as his professional work in the district headquarters hospital and his private practice generally take up so much time that the public health functions which he is required to perform remain largely undischarged.'[27]

The drive to clean up the insanitary environment which kept England intensely occupied for the latter half of the nineteenth and the first quarter of the twentieth century – legislating for health in a hundred or more enactments, developing local government within a slowly extending 'franchise', and training medical men and medical auxiliaries in public health techniques – for long passed India by.

Nevertheless, England's public health practice could be seen represented in a hundred ways in the Indian institutions – in maternity and child welfare, midwives, health visitors, sanitary inspectors, school health, factory health – even if imperfectly developed. India may have waited a half century or so, but in the end local government began to administer 'general sanitation, control of infectious disease, regulation of housing construction, control of purity of food and water supplies, abatement of nuisance, and registration of vital statistics. Speaking generally, all local bodies were given power to appoint and control their own establishments, including the health staff'.[27] India reproduced the English and American mistake of having areas which were too small for effective public health work, so that the Bhore report recommended the abolition of many and their replacement by district health boards. Characteristically, the security of tenure of the medical officer of health was reproduced by a statutory requirement that the provincial government must give prior sanction to his appointment and dismissal.

The English obsession with local government – its autonomy, its integrity, its dynamism – may well have been her greatest gift to India's public health. Her belief in sanitation, as the first requirement of any public health system, is a close second, for it would be wrong to conclude from the obvious preoccupation with curative medicine that the sanitary ideal was wholly ignored. At the time of the Bhore report the vast majority of areas in India did not have the benefit of safe water supplies; in a total population of 350 millions the number living in areas normally served by sewers 'was probably only seven millions'.[27] Yet Chadwick's enzyme was at work. It is more remarkable that there were seven million under the protection of an adequate sanitary system than that 343 million were without. With time, and particularly with nationhood free, the whole will be leavened.

Sri Lanka

Public health practice varied in every colonial territory. In Sri Lanka, so near to India, the introduction of an organization designed to protect public health was similarly delayed, for reasons which could not differ greatly from those in India or in any other colonial territory. A sanitary department, with full-time medical officers of health in large districts, was not established until 1913.[46] After this time progress in many ways was greater, so that Sri Lanka illustrates what must have happened in many other colonial territories, the advantages of enlightened local leadership. In 1926 the first of a series of health units, covering 40–80,000 population, was established. The development was modelled on America, not, as might have been thought, on the British pattern. Health units have been the basis of continuous public health action in Sri Lanka in surveys, statistics, health education, maternal and child health, school health, sanitation, and control of disease, for 30 years. The favourable state of the island today and the ease and readiness with which it has adopted modern public health services after World War II, is not a little due to this fortunate development.[35]

Japan

The colonial dependencies, apart, the public health movement, despite its practical advantages, hardly spread beyond the immediate spheres of influence of the Western European countries in which it was born. The East, Middle, Near, and Far, except where colonial services operated, lived up to its sobriquet and continued unchanging. To this generalization there is one obvious exception – Japan. Late in the nineteenth century Japan came under the influence of Germany; as a result of this she adopted something, if not all, of the public health practice of the paternalistic school. She established public health almost literally as a police system and as part of the local police service, with such peripheral health administration as could be imposed upon an exceptionally complicated social background having its roots in antiquity.

The 46 prefectural police departments took their orders from the State; and the medical officer of health – sturdily independent and outspoken in his criticisms of sanitary evils, who featured so strongly in the British and American scenes, was absent. As in Germany, health insurance was a prominent feature, and, unlike Britain, sanitary science, including housing, remained largely neglected. But Johann Frank's paternalistic public health, as seen in Japan, was never more than a general reflection of the European scene. The emphasis on hospitals and medical care was absent, possibly because Japanese culture included an exceptional ability to withstand hardship and was affected in its attitude to human survival by many influences, including a rapidly expanding population.

Local health departments on the European pattern began in Japan only in 1938. By 1956, no doubt encouraged by American advisers who saw the possibilities of decentralization which these offered, 783 public health units had been developed throughout the provinces, undertaking health education, vital statistics, improvement of nutrition and food hygiene, environmental sanitation, public health nursing, maternal and child health, dental hygiene, laboratory tests, and the prevention of tuberculosis, venereal disease, and other communicable diseases.[30] American influence is to be seen chiefly in the reorganization of the Ministry of Health and Welfare and the creation of a prefectural health department apart from the police. The 'health officer' became an important, if badly paid, servant of Japan's public health.

The success of Japanese health practice, despite many inadequacies, has been considerable. Her achievements in recent years for example, the sickness surveys which she shares with Canada, Denmark, Britain, and America give promise of rapid progress. In the background are to be seen, a little incongruously perhaps, the shadowy figures of Frank and Chadwick. As with Sri Lanka and India and many other countries to which the European movement spread, even if only as the faint outer ripples of an ever-widening circle, Japan benefited from philosophies alien to her culture and development.

The final patchwork

These are but pen sketches. A richer and deeper picture might be painted if the canvas were available and the time opportune. In machinery and in content, public health – the basic institution created and maintained by society to preserve the life and health of the people – is, in Europe and the New World, a many-splendoured garment. The philosophy of public health has been given many interpretations; and the human being, subjected broadly to the same occupational, ecological, nutritional, psychological, and other hazards, has nowhere been given any uniform protection. The visitor from another planet might well ask upon what general plan the developed countries had used their new technological and social weapons in the interests of Public Health. Nevertheless, although the practice of public health is, and is likely to remain, so varied, there has been a growing together. Each nation has incorporated new ideas to meet the needs of its developing society at varying dates and times; but the final patchwork which each country presents, i.e. sanitary science, control of communicable diseases, protection of vulnerable classes, biostatistics and surveys, health education, mental health, welfare of the aged and child care, industrial hygiene etc., is not now dissimilar.

Recent developments in comprehensive medical care have tended to hasten the development of a common pattern. Most of the countries which began their public health in the nineteenth-century movement are once again in the throes of revolutionary thinking towards the new goal of social medicine, which involves public health in curative medicine and vice versa. The concept of good public health now demands a full medical service, at home and in hospital, available to every citizen irrespective of ability to pay. Britain, Australia, New Zealand, Canada are engaged, more deeply even than the Scandinavian countries where such developments were pioneered, in operating schemes of medical care, financed by the State or by insurance, according to taste. These have resulted in increasing emphasis on the hospital, a phenomenon which every country in one form or another has experienced. The future in Europe and the New World may well become a fight to prevent the hospital from taking control.

15. Newcomers to Public Health after World War I

After the First World War there were three particular newcomers to the public health scene – Yugoslavia, Turkey, and the USSR. They are to be included together in this account because each set out – in very different ways – on the same track to technological development, seeking to achieve in a few years that state at which Europe and the New World had arrived after perhaps 200 years of evolutionary change. Yugoslavia, Turkey, and the USSR sought to pull themselves up, as it has been said, by their own shoe-strings. It would not be true to say that these countries had previously been unaffected by outside influences, or that they had done nothing in the field of public health. In Turkey, where the Ottoman Empire had left the care of public health largely to religious and other voluntary organizations,[51] perhaps least had been done. The USSR certainly had the Zemstvo, a form of local government body, with salaried doctors, who were responsible for both curative and preventive medicine in their districts. Large parts of Yugoslavia had taken part in Austrian public health developments. But in fact, despite everything that had gone before, these three countries in 1920 presented the typical picture of the underdeveloped world; high infant and child mortality, low expectation of life, widespread infectious and nutritional diseases, almost complete lack of sanitary science, with practially no measures to combat widespread evils. In the post-war movement for development, public health was regarded in each case as a first consideration. Each country wiped the slate of past endeavour clean, and drew out afresh a plan for public health practice. The public health of these countries in consequence differs in many fundamentals from the European pattern which we have already considered. The fact that these bold enterprises have now been in operation for more than half a century gives them greater fascination.

Many, as Newsholme has said,[37] must 'envy Yugoslavia in having begun its work without the impedimenta which undue multiplication of units and administration implies'; and indeed the USSR and Turkey too. Nevertheless, other countries have had the same advantages without seizing them. The USSR and Yugoslavia resembled India in this, as well as in the extent of disease, and in the many different races and civilizations, diverse in character and development, of which they were composed. It is significant that the recommendations of the Bhore Committee in 1946 would produce a service in India very similar to those of the USSR and Yugoslavia. The USSR and Yugoslav services, like the writings of Bernard Shaw, seemed more revolutionary and esoteric when first produced than they do today. The principles on which they were based, complete integration of curative and preventive medicine, medicine as a social service, the predominance of preventive medicine, health centres as the basis of operation, and community participation, taken together, shocked Europe, as did *Pygmalion,* after the First World War; yet they went little beyond the statements made in the various White Papers which preceded the National Health Service in Britain (1948). Many have been advocated, and some operated, for some years in different parts of Europe.

The health centre, combining medical care with preventive work, which is perhaps the most distinctive feature of the USSR[8, 17] as to a lesser extent in Yugoslavia[6] and Turkey,[5] was recommended, independently, by the Dawson Committee (1920) in England.[25] After the government White Paper of 1944, which reflected the views of a succession of planning committees, it was incorporated in the National Health Service Act (1946). Similarly in South Africa the National Health Service Commission (1944) recommended a service based upon health centres, each serving about 25,000 people.[21] The South African scheme was to be a family health service, as already demonstrated in their pioneer health centre at Pholela. But in England and South Africa these ideas came to nothing. Medicine perhaps was not sufficiently a social service, or maybe, as in South Africa, the pull of curative medicine towards the hospital was too strong.[21] The European Conference on Rural Hygiene convened by the League of Nations Health Organization (1931), in which 23 countries participated, recommended health centres wherever 'a modern public health organization is to be created in new territory' (see p. 184). Health centres were recommended by the World Health Organization Expert Committees on Public Health Administration (1952–54),[55] and during the Technical Discussions of the World Health Assembly, 1954.[56] The key to the Bhore report recommendations for India was the primary health centre with two medical officers, four public health nurses, four midwives, four trained dais, two sanitary inspectors, and two health assistants.

The union of curative and preventive medicine has been a long-cherished ambition of most health planners. First advocated *officially* in the report of the Dawson Committee (UK) in 1920 (see p. 184), it has appeared in many subsequent reports and writings in different parts of the world. 'Once the essential environmental and infectious disease services have been completed, health will not further progress to a satisfactory level until preventive and curative medicine are brought under a single co-ordinated administration which includes the general practitioner....' (Grant.)[24] 'The co-ordinated application of curative and preventive measures can alone help to secure an adequate control over the incidence of disease' (Bhore).[27] Many have also believed that preventive medicine should come first in planning[24] (see p. 183). In the mid-twentieth century there is little that is remarkable in the principles on which the USSR and Yugoslavia have operated their public health services, except that they were put into practice so long ago.

The first outstanding feature of the USSR was the policlinic, perhaps better called a health centre, of which some 30,000 were established in industry, and, separately for children and adults, outside in the community. The health centre differs from a dispensary in having social and preventive functions; it combines preventive and curative work for a surrounding area. The USSR health centre employs three types of doctors : general practitioners who cover a defined sector; 'specialists' who work in the centre in various branches of medicine, and; public health experts. The centre does most of the work which in Europe and America would be channelled in hospital outpatient departments; so that the hospital lies, as it were, in the background, as a second line of defence, leaving to the health centre the bulk of the work of maintaining health and caring for the sick. Preventive examinations are conducted not only of schoolchildren, mothers, and infants, as in the Western world, but also of adults, particularly in industry, using a team of specialists – a process known as dispensarization. Factory health, school health, maternal and child health, other special branches of public health work, are based upon the centres. The training of doctors has been designed to use medicine as a social service. More time is spent than in the Old World on training students in the principles of public health. Furthermore, students can separate into three streams, so that the final product is adapted for general medicine, for sanitary and hygiene work, or for paediatrics. Also in the sixth year, until 1955, students specialized in one or other of the branches of medicine, in order to be able to occupy special posts in health centres – after a period as general practitioners.[7, 48]

The second feature is the use of soviets in public health work. Such local committees of citizens exist in streets, blocks of flats, and other units. In Stalingrad in 1956 there were said[8] to be 400 and 70,000 in the whole of the USSR :

These undertake social welfare work under the direction of a committee of the Stalingrad Council, with a prominent member as chairman. They are responsible for sanitary matters, for taking steps to see that those in need of care get it; for work in connexion with problem families and marital disharmony; for following-up schoolchildren (in collaboration with parents' committees) and much else.[36]

Each Republic has a central health administration, under a director of public health, which directs and controls the whole of the health services, including medical education and research. But the control of all the republics from Moscow tends to produce a uniform pattern, somewhat on the French plan.

Health services in the USSR, clearly unique, may be an expression of political thought; but they bear in many ways the imprint of a powerful but unknown mind. They are of a piece; designed to an end – the protection of the health of the Soviet citizen from birth to death. Health centres, medical education, and soviets, fit together, as one logical whole.

In contrast, in Yugoslavia the presiding genius is well known – Andrija Stampar, the first head of the hygiene section of the Ministry of Health in the newly-formed Kingdom of the Serbs, Croats, and Slovenes. The history of the new Yugoslavia was chequered; one regime followed another in bewildering succession. But through all this period, little affected by changes in political systems, the imprint of Stampar on the health services stands out. Most striking was the creation, in each of the nine provinces, of a *central hygiene institute*, which combined administration and research. By this means, the administration of all forms of public health work, epidemiology, industrial medicine, bacteriology and parasitology, food hygiene, maternity and child welfare, nutrition, etc., has been kept in touch with scientific investigation. In 1931 Newsholme[37] found this combination to be eminently satisfactory, with little risk that the administration would become 'stereotyped and rigid', so long as it was linked with the scientific investigation of current problems. The passage of nearly half a century has borne out the truth of this prediction.

The Institute of Hygiene, in the Yugoslav form, has, no doubt, a lasting message for all countries. Stampar also started a section on social medicine in the new School of Public Health at Zagreb. At this very early date public health teaching included 'the study of the biologic and anthropological peculiarities of the people in general and of the different groups'.[37] As in the USSR, but without the peculiarities in medical training, health centres were established as the focal points of combined preventive and medical care of the community. Both the USSR and Yugoslavia, in their different ways, subordinated medicine more obviously to the needs of the community, requiring that it 'be a social service working with the people'. The wisdom of enlightened autocracy has imposed upon the people what 'local participation' and initiative, as a deliberate democratic choice, has found difficulty in doing.

Turkey differed only in its social pattern from its two near neighbours. It had the same familiar background of poverty, excessive disease, and scarcity of trained personnel, a handful of doctors and few nurses or medical auxiliaries, which is familiar to a large part of the underdeveloped world. The death rates from all or most infectious diseases were high, although their true magnitude was, and still is, unknown from lack of valid statistics. The Republican Government in 1920 established the first real health service that the Turkish people had seen, and in between the two World Wars, Turkey made great progress in health. The successes lay largely in those spheres where centrally run schemes could operate successfully, as in the control of malaria, venereal disease, and trachoma. The tradition of local autonomy and participation, and the will to subordinate curative to preventive medicine, were absent.[29] The Ministry of Health and Social Assistance controlled the organization, operating through directors of health as their representatives in the provinces. The Governor of the province was head of a provincial public health board composed of officials. Corresponding district boards existed.[50] The service was thus almost completely bureaucratic, without the saving grace of the soviets. As has been said, after 1920 'a campaign almost on military lines was organized to attack the problem of disease'.[51] But the rate of increase of doctors, nurses, and other health personnel was slow and the training of doctors particularly lacked the preventive bias which the USSR and Yugoslavia, each in its own way, introduced. The spectacular appeal of curative medicine was too great, and critics[29] early reported an exaggerated and disproportionate hospital plan. When so much preventable disease was directly attributable to low standards of hygiene – trachoma, typhoid fever, worm infestations, gastroenteritis – the first need was for basic sanitation. The spirit of William Duncan, the first medical officer of health in England, one of the pioneers of the Chadwick era, would be a notable addition to the fight against disease in many Turkish towns. As Lightbody said in 1951[29] in his critical analysis of Turkish services:

As fast as sanitary inspectors can be properly trained, their energies should be applied to the abatement of nuisances, public education on the value of clean surroundings, the protection and improvement of water supplies, better methods of sewage and refuse disposal, and inspection of housing and food. Urban communities should be provided with water purification plants, or at least emergency chlorination plants. Regular inspection and frequent bacteriological analysis should be made of all major supplies of water . . . inspection of supplies from source to consumer . . . greater attention to the effective enforcement of regulations regarding septic tanks and cesspools and to the controlled collection and dumping of refuse, is vital in towns and hardly less important in villages . . . etc.

But this unglamorous and unspectacular ideal had to await the development of an effective infrastructure of health. The first step in this direction was taken in 1950, when the country began to establish health centres, incorporating a rural hospital on the Bridgman plan[4]; by 1955, 181 such centres were operating in rural areas. This plan had limited success because the doctor in charge had no special training in preventive medicine and no time to devote to the work. In 1967, the nationalization act began free medical care in the eastern territories, following broadly the pattern of western Europe.[5] Health centres (ocaks) of standard pattern for 8,000 persons, and sub-centres staffed by midwives for 2,500 persons, were set up. The general practitioners, with a team of paramedical workers were to combine curative and preventive medicine in family health care, as originally advocated by Dawson.[25] Nationalization, extending westward province by province, had by the early 70's covered about one third of the country. The programme encountered grave difficulties in lack of staff, insufficient training, and inability to integrate earlier schemes designed to deal with individual diseases. There was in fact virtually no infrastructure of health, so that, as was said, 'it resembled a house built on sand'.[5] These basic difficulties will resolve as the training of staff gathers impetus. Turkey has in recent years made astonishing progress in establishing colleges for training most types of paramedical workers, and the teaching of social and preventive medicine at Hacettepe medical school in Ankara equals that to be found anywhere.

In each of these three underdeveloped countries, the drive towards public health has produced great improvement; but for various reasons the USSR has outstripped her neighbours. Here the health picture, if statistics were available, would almost certainly be seen to have been transformed into that of a developed country.

16. Newcomers to Public Health after World War II

The whole world encompassed

At the end of the Second World War a further movement towards public health began in sovereign states, new and old; of these the most notable were Indonesia, Burma, Thailand, the South American States, China, India, and Pakistan. This period was remarkable for the influence of the World Health Organization, described later (Chapter 17), and of other specialized agencies of the United Nations. The rapidity with which less favoured nations now began to 'develop', under the influence of international aid, was remarkable. As was said of Thailand in 1958:

> Thailand has developed fast, through the work of international organizations and with direct aid. Many nations have poured in money – the USA., 100 million dollars since 1950. There are 325 projects in operation, from a $10 million scheme for providing hydro-electric power to the $30,000 education scheme for the teaching of English in Thai schools. WHO, UNICEF and UNESCO give aid, sending staff for training overseas and developing public health schemes parallel with, and sometimes overlapping, those of direct aid.
>
> Thus the nation is carried along on the crest of a wave of international aid. There are projects for abolishing malaria and yaws; villages are being persuaded to have privies; public health nurses go into the homes; and education becomes general. Hospitals, clinics, and all that goes to make scientific medicine, is growing rapidly. There is squalor, ignorance, and superstition; babies die; eastern diseases abound. But it is only now a question of time before Thailand becomes a developed land (1958).[9]

Of this late awakening, urgent and impulsive, much less can be said in concrete terms for a variety of reasons, including lack of statistics and, as in the case of China, lack of published information. Of China, amounting to perhaps a quarter of the globe's population, nothing official has yet been made known and we must rely on travellers tales.[32] These tell of accelerated progress much on the lines of the USSR as seen in the last chapter.

The general range of health problems which faced these countries exceeded those of the USSR, Turkey, and Yugoslavia in the 1920s, and even those of Europe in the early nineteenth century (see Chapters 3 and 4). Communicable and nutritional diseases abounded. Intestinal infections and worms of many kinds were almost universal. Special diseases, such as yaws, leprosy, or filariasis, prevailed over wide areas. Widespread lack of sanitation caused untold illness. In nearly every part of these vast regions, childbirth remained in the hands of village handywomen, with deplorable consequences. Thus, in Indonesia a woman died in childbirth every quarter of an hour, and a baby every minute.[49] In Thailand, motamnys were still attending five out of six deliveries in 1958, although over a thousand midwives had been trained, mainly for work in the jungle, since the Second World War.[9] Doctors, nurses, sanitarians, and other auxiliaries hardly existed. Indonesia in 1956 had one doctor only to 55,000 people.[31] The social framework, upon which health services depend for their support, had in most cases hardly begun to develop. The means to meet the burden of sickness and suffering were as limited as its needs were great; while the absence of a scientific background, and the existence of deeply rooted customs and beliefs, introduced difficulties which Europe at least has experienced relatively little (see Chapter 6).

Despite all such evidence of preventable disease, the spectacular appeal of curative medicine now hynotized the developing world. The hospital, increasingly the scene of drama in Europe and North America under the influence of advancing technology, seemed to the uninformed to answer all imaginable problems of health. The lessons of European medicine after the renaissance of learning, if ever marked or sufficiently digested, were forgotten. The building of hospitals generally exceeded the rate at which trained personnel, particularly nurses, could be provided; and the shortage of nursing staff, exacerbated by the reluctance of women to take up this profession in so many parts of the world, added greatly to the hazards – much as had been the case in medieval Europe. The building programme moreover consumed a large fraction of available funds and thus encroached on the monies available for developing public health in the field.

Yet public health did now begin in special and often limited forms. In countries where social development was insufficiently advanced to permit of an effective local organization, administration tended, although not universally, to be centralized. This was almost inevitable where the services consisted for the most part of special schemes to meet particular problems. In South America, despite the USA pattern of federal, state, and local services, with emphasis upon local control, the main responsibilities were, and still are, federal. The paternalistic pattern of the Continent of Europe, which came to South America via Spain and Portugal, was allowed conveniently to outweigh the American influence. The federal government of Brazil concerned itself with the solution of public health problems on a nation-wide scale with local services operated essentially as executive agencies at the national level.[39] Thus there were national services for malaria, leprosy, yellow fever, mental diseases, cancer, plague, and tuberculosis. The Federal Government also operated the Port Health Service, the Bio-Statistical Service, the National Drug Control Service, the National Health Education Service, and eight federal health commissions, the activities of each being limited to a group of states. Such services were in addition to the supervision exercised by the central health department over all activities from nursing and sanitary engineering to hospitals.

Yet large parts of South America were still without any health services, and where these existed they were largely deficient in essentials – in Brazil there were municipal services, but these did not employ full-time health personnel.[39] The effects of this lack of development in areas with so much preventable disease were far-reaching. In Bolivia, where systematic vaccination began in 1953, 'although vaccine of good quality and sufficient quantity is prepared, it was not yet possible to eradicate smallpox because of the lack of an adequate organization to carry out the vaccination campaign on a national scale'.[39] So it was in many places. Special schemes of various kinds helped to fill the gaps: in eight South American countries the reporting of communicable disease was done by 'reporting areas', which covered from one-fifth to four-fifths of the total areas of the countries. Public health had begun, but it was as yet 'a thing of shreds and tatters'. The support of the citizens was little more than a faint stirring of interest; and the professional staff, who could put public health into practice, teach the people, and awaken their interest, was yet to come. In all that was happening expediency seemed to control events; there was a grave lack of National Health Planning (see pp. 186–188).

In this new setting, many countries began to organize a permanent framework in which to develop the sanitary ideal. Health centres were early adopted, and, in varying degree, developed as fast as the training of staff permitted. Burma, using health assistants with 21 months training, had 300 in operation by 1957 and 903 in 1973/4 (with 251 sub-centres). India implemented the Bhore report[27] in this as well as other respects;[28] in the state of Bengal there were 106 health centres by 1950 and 286 by 1972 (with 1,291 sub-centres). Chile divided her territory into health zones, which by 1958 contained 163 health centres. Leimena suggested five health centres in each of 12 new model areas in Indonesia,[31] each to have one public health nurse (co-ordinator), one midwife, one mantri for protective work, one hygiene educator, five assistant midwives, four assistant nurses, 10 village hygienists, and five home visitors. The social centres of Egypt[53] and the development projects in India[52] incorporated the health centre in a wider approach to community development. The surprising thing about the underdeveloped world was not that so much remained to be done, but rather the immense strides that were made in so short a time.

Experimental health centres and special schemes under central control point the way, but they give no final answer to public health, to which there are few short cuts. Long-term projects cannot be completed overnight. There remains the much more difficult step to take. In order to develop long-term public health, applying medical and scientific knowledge to the prevention and cure of all disease and to maintain services in face of difficulties, it is necessary to devise a *general public health infrastructure* to cover the whole country, soundly based at the local level. For the development of such a 'permanent framework', we must look back to the European movement and its lessons (Chapter 14), and forward to the particular needs of the less developed world (Chapter 20); but first we should examine the contribution made by international health organizations.

Part Five: International Public Health

17. From Quarantine* to World Health

The quarantine period

The origins of international collaboration in public health, as in those of national public health, are to be found in the fear of epidemic spread. The possibility of contagion was recognized by many even during the centuries when diseases were little differentiated; when fevers were attributed to exhalation from the ground, or to putrefying odours, or to the state of the atmosphere; when millions believed that sickness was a punishment from the gods. The Court left sixteenth century London so soon as the Bills of Mortality gave warning; Boccaccio's young aristocrats fled to the country from plague-stricken Florence[21]; in times of pest people in Constantinople hurried along the side-walks fearing the touch of another.[19] The people of the little village of Eyam in Derbyshire, England, to which the plague was brought in 1665 in a box of old clothes, isolated themselves and died, nearly to a man, in putting this belief into practice.[21] There have been examples of the 'cordon sanitaire' from A.D. 630, when armed guards were placed on the roads leading from Provence to Cahors, to A.D. 1720, when Marseilles was ringed with sentries. The movements of armies, of traders, and of pilgrims along the golden road to Samarkand, and by other land routes, and of ships along the Black Sea, the Mediterranean Sea, and the Persian Gulf have been known to carry disease from the East to Europe for upwards of a thousand years. Europe has reciprocated. Traders and adventurers from the West have carried infections, as well as colonies and commerce, to most hemispheres.

Each nation thought only of itself. The obvious practical answer was quarantine – a remedy which was operated at least from the fourteenth century, when Venice first set up a sanitary council of three noblemen (1348).[21] The first lazaretto was established in the following century (1423). After 1585, when Britain first attempted quarantine, every European country, and most seaports, adopted its own regulations.

The value of quarantine, in days when modes of transmission were unknown, can never have been great. Rats infected with plague, and infested with the fleas which carry infection to man, will often have run along the ships' hawsers to the dockside; passengers in the lazarettos with few symptoms, but heavily infected with the vibrio of cholera, will have gone ashore to contaminate water supplies and food. But the appearances of protection were not wanting, since epidemic

---

* Quarantine, a period of 40 days, originally the time during which a ship arriving in port and suspected of being infected with a 'malignant infectious disease' was obliged to forbear all intercourse with the shore; later came to signify the place where vessels are stationed and also the practice of isolating or being isolated.

spread depends on many variables and is almost unpredictable. In 1720 when plague spread from Africa to Marseilles it failed to cross the English Channel; who was to say that this was not due to the quarantining of all ships which Richard Mead, physician to St Thomas' Hospital, London, had again recommended in his *Treatise on the Plague* (1720)?[24] Much of public health has had its beginnings in equally empirical action.

It would be pleasant to record that international collaboration in public health began with the need to discuss the eradication of smallpox, following the publication of Jenner's discovery in 1798 of the preventive qualities of vaccination with cowpox; or, indeed, at any time during the previous century when inoculation from arm to arm had been in vogue. It might equally have had its origins in a determination to abolish scurvy from the world, following James Lind's demonstration of the virtues of fresh oranges and lemons on board HMS *Salisbury* in 1747.[23] Smallpox and scurvy shortened life and brought untold misery to millions. They were the first two diseases for which scientific proof of prevention was obtained; their elimination had immense possibilities for human happiness; they were an admirable subject for concerted international action. Much too was known about the means to combat malaria, which even in 1857 may have been the cause of a million deaths yearly; enough at least to have made international discussion valuable.[28]

At the beginning of the twentieth century there were extensive anti-malarial drainage projects in many places, as widely separated as New York and Sierra Leone, Brazil and Hong Kong. Soon after 1820, the alkaloid quinine replaced cinchona bark, used in prophylaxis at least since the mid-eighteenth century, when two English naval surgeons, Bryson and Lind, made use of infusions and tinctures for this purpose.[28] But the time was not ripe for international public health in this sense. Perhaps there was so much sickness in the world that a little more or less made no difference.

It was the subject of quarantine which brought nations together in the first international meeting in 1851. From the outset quarantine had had great inconveniences, particularly to sea-going nations. When rigorously imposed it could be brutal: defaulting sailors were treated as felons and might suffer death. Ships had not infrequently been burned as Mead had advocated, or they might be marooned, like the *Matteo Bruzzo* in 1884, unable to land for four months on either side of the Atlantic.[13, 29] At its least the continual waste of time for passengers and crew alike was profoundly irritating. More generally, on payment of adequate consideration, it was honoured in the breach. But whether applied or misapplied, the damage to trade was considerable. And so it came about that this mundane consideration of how to protect trade, and not humane feeling about how to prevent disease, was the main item on the first international public health agenda.

International conferences 1851–1909

Quarantine, and the orgins of infection, provided the main topic not only for the 1851 health congress in Paris, but also for the nine further international meetings – Paris 1859, Constantinpole 1866, Vienna 1874, Washington 1881, Rome 1885, Venice 1892, Dresden 1893, Paris 1894, and Vienna 1897 – which took place before the turn of the century.[21] Interest was heightened after 1869 when the Suez Canal was opened.

Nothing came out of these meetings, except the fact of having met. The two diseases that could be prevented were not discussed. Other diseases were discussed at length without any of the scientific evidence which alone could have made such deliberations of value. That fleas carried plague was not certainly known until 1905;* the role of the mosquito in yellow fever not before 1900–02 and that of the louse in typhus fever not before 1909. Even the diseases themselves were confused. At the 1851 congress many of the delegates confused plague with typhus. Typhus fever had in any event been distinguished from typhoid fever by William Jenner only two years previously (1849). The main topic of all these discussions was the nature of infection, with the contagionists ranged against the miasmatists. As the nineteenth century passed scientific epidemiology was born; but slowly. John Snow† had given the first scientific proof of the transmission of cholera by faecal contamination of water supplies in his Soho study (1854), first suggested in a 'slender pamphlet' in 1849.[33] Now that the world is drowned in words, it does good to contemplate so much benefit to mankind from so few. The work of Pasteur (1822–95) had its culmination in preventive inoculation against hydrophobia in 1885.

The discovery of the tubercle bacillus in 1882, and two years later the vibrio of cholera and the bacilli of diphtheria and typhoid, literally ushered in a new era. The specific organisms of many of the great problems of public health were discovered at short intervals with almost bewildering speed up to the turn of the century: pneumonia (1886), brucellosis and cerebo-spinal fever (1887), the fungus of actinomycosis (1891), the bacillus of plague (1894), dysentery (1898); the spirochaete of syphilis waited until 1905. None of this work seemed immediately to affect discussions at the international level. As in most meetings, international, national, or local, there was special pleading. The British delegation in 1851, influenced no doubt by considerations of trade, denied that cholera was contagious; epidemic constitutions, as Sydenham had postulated, or perhaps the odours, they said, of putrefying matter, as the Greeks had thought, was the cause of outbreaks of pestilence. Yet, the medical member of this same British delegation, Dr John Sutherland, had his office in the General Board of Health at Gwdyr House, Whitehall, in Westminster, only 850 yards from Soho, north of Piccadilly, where John Snow had made his revolutionary observations on the transmission of cholera. But it is always hard for administrations to accept new teachings. The fact that it took up to fifty years for the medical colleagues of John Snow to accept and act upon his teaching may be a pointer

---

* The transmission of plague by fleas was first suggested by Ogata in 1897, Simond (1898), and Gautier and Raybaud (1903), but the flea theory was specifically developed by W. G. Liston (1905).

† *On the Mode of Communication of Cholera*, 1849. In the second edition (1855) John Snow said, 'The first edition of this work, which was published in August 1849, was only a slender pamphlet.'[33]

for those who find action upon modern epidemiological discoveries too slow to follow.

The nineteenth century in Europe was also remarkable for a series of international statistical conferences devoted to the development of a uniform classification of causes of death. From earliest times much of the difficulty in producing worthwhile statistics of mortality had been seen to be rooted in lack of scientific accuracy in disease classification. William Farr in his first annual report to the Registrar General in Britain (1839) had said:

> The advantages of a uniform statistical nomenclature, however imperfect, are so obvious that it is surprising no attention has been paid to its enforcement in bills of mortality.

The first international statistical conference was held in 1853 at Brussels, when William Farr and Marc d'Espine were instructed to prepare *une nomenclature uniforme*. The general arrangement of this early list, based upon anatomical sites, has survived to this present time. Further congresses were held in Paris 1855, 1864, London 1870, Paris 1874, 1880, 1886. The Bertillon classification followed the Vienna congress of 1891, to be further adjusted in Chicago (1893) and Christiana (Oslo) in 1899. The first international congress on statistics, for the revision of the international classification of causes of death, was held in Paris in 1900, at which delegates from 26 countries attended. The advance to uniformity in respect of causes of death had been considerable, with far reaching results for public health. But during all this time there had been no common classification for both death and disease, from which so obviously the greatest benefit could come. Farr early recognized this need and put forward a suggestion 'to extend the same system of nomenclature to disease which, though not fatal, caused disability in the population. . . .' Florence Nightingale submitted a statement to the London congress in 1870 in which she urged hospitals to adopt Farr's classification, so that 'the laws which regulate disease action would be better known.'[25] 'Up to the present time', she said, 'the statistics of hospitals have been kept in no uniform plan'. She continued:

> Every hospital has followed its own nomenclature and classification of diseases, and there has been no reduction on any uniform model of the vast amount of observations which have been made in these establishments. So far as relates either to medical or sanitary science, these observations in their present state bear exactly the same relation as an indefinite number of astronomical observations made without concert, and reduced to no common standard, would bear to the progress of astronomy. The material exists, but it is inaccessible.

No action was taken and, as classification became more sophisticated, the achievement of this ideal became more difficult. International congresses occurred roughly every ten years (1909, 1920, 1929, 1938), but the fusion of codes of mortality and morbidity had to await the birth of WHO after the second World War.

L'Office Internationale d'Hygiene Publique

The idea of a permanent international organization for health gradually emerged. It was first suggested in the fourth international health congress of 1874 and finally accepted in the eleventh at Paris, 1903. The year previously a Pan-American Sanitary Bureau (1902) had been formed with headquarters at Washington. L'Office Internationale d'Hygiène Publique, popularly known as the Paris Office, came into being in 1909[21] with the following terms of reference:

> To collect and bring to the knowledge of the participating states the facts and documents of a general character which relate to public health and especially as regards infectious diseases, notably cholera, plague, and yellow fever, as well as the measures to combat these diseases.

The Paris Office, directed by a committee consisting of one technical representative of each participating state, had a small permanent whole-time staff, consisting of a director, a secretary-general, two or three technical assistants, a librarian, and an accountant.

It was concerned mainly with quarantinable diseases – to gather information, to revise conventions, and to arbitrate on differences. Speaking generally, international public health during the first 75 years of international collaboration up to the end of the First World War was restricted to epidemic intelligence, and this in a limited form; mainly how to stop the major diseases from spreading to the developed countries. The possibility of fighting disease on a broad front everywhere had hardly yet been considered. The concern for health as a state of mental, physical, and social well-being, and the right of every man, was even more remote.

But it would be an injustice to the Paris Office to omit to mention the genesis of a wider view. The office began to widen out the range of subjects for international regulation. Most notably, it obtained agreement by fourteen countries for certain measures against the spread of venereal diseases along the shipping routes. A campaign was then begun that is not yet brought to a successful conclusion. It also began the standardization of sera and the control of the drug traffic. Within its own committees, it began to discuss other public health problems – ranging from anthrax in shaving brushes to the organization of hospitals. These may be regarded as the forerunners of the 'expert committees' of WHO, which have done so much to spread an understanding of the scientific approach to public health.

The health organization of the League of Nations

In 1923, the Geneva Office, the health organization of the League of Nations, was created, and this functioned until the Second World War, alongside the Paris Office. It had the following terms of reference under the Covenant of the League of Nations, article 23(f), to 'endeavour to take steps in matters of international concern for the prevention and control of disease.'

Within this wider framework, international public health began to advance. The Geneva Office produced a system of epidemic intelligence of greater efficiency, with a peripheral centre at Singapore (1925). Thus it recognized that the great epidemic diseases, which are occasional trespassers in Europe and the New World, are a perpetual menace to the vast regions of the East from Vladivostok to Australia and from Mombasa to Hawaii. In its weekly epidemiological record it covered not only the five 'convention' diseases – plague, cholera, yellow fever, smallpox, and typhus – but also many others, such as poliomyelitis, enteric fever, scarlet fever, and dysentery.

The Geneva Office also carried on the work of international standardization and the control of the drug traffic begun by the Paris Office. It gave particular attention to codes of vital statistics.

Much the most effective part of its work was, however, done by means of *expert committees,* then called technical commissions, of which, in the field of international public health, it must be considered as the inventor. International committees of experts met in Geneva and elsewhere to consider malaria, cancer, nutrition, housing, health centres, syphilis, tuberculosis, rheumatism, heart diseases, the teaching of medicine, and other subjects. Many of these had far-reaching results. The commission on nutrition (1936), for example, laid down a standard minimum diet which made it possible to examine, by means of dietary surveys, the state of nutrition throughout the world.[22]

Of equal importance was the *International Conference* which the Geneva Office also developed. A European Conference (1931),[12] and a Far-Eastern Conference (1937),[16] produced well-documented statements about public health needs in underdeveloped countries. These remain as classics to this day. African conferences were held at Cape Town (1932) and Johannesburg (1935). The Geneva Office began the system of organizing tours and exchanges for study abroad.

No doubt to many, including those who framed the terms of reference for the Geneva Office, it was a disappointment that more practical steps were not taken to help with public health in the field. Unfortunately the total maximum budget of £78,500 was too slender for such ventures. Practical assistance was, in fact, given in combating epidemics of typhus fever with which the war had ended in Poland, the USSR, Rumania, and Greece; and aid was also given in establishing permanent health services in Greece and China. Courses of instruction in malaria control were organized in S.E. Asia. But, after this, money and staff were not forthcoming. The work of 'practical aid' in the field had to await another war and the creation of an international organization with a more generous budget. Until then such efforts remained with voluntary agencies, among which the Rockefeller Foundation is outstanding; this was the first to demonstrate the practicability of mass campaigns against hook worm in 52 countries throughout the tropics before the First World War, and against yellow fever a few years later in Central and South America and Africa.

World War II greatly interfered with the work of the Paris and Geneva Offices. To all intents they came to an end. In 1944 UNRRA (United Nations Relief and Rehabilitation Administration) was created to help the devastated world; and for somewhat over two years it acted as an international health organization. It had a staff of 1,134 persons, including nationals from thirty-five countries, and it spent over £58 million. But it was no more than a stopgap in the interval before a new world-wide organization could be erected.

18. The World Health Organization

The interim commission 1946-8

The Charter of the United Nations, signed at San Francisco in 1945, inserted the word 'health' on the proposal of the delegate from Brazil. The delegations of Brazil and China then recommended that a general conference be convened within the next few months for the purpose of establishing an international health organization. As it was minuted:

They intend to consult further with the representatives of other Delegations with a view to the early convening of such a General Conference to which each of the Governments here represented will be invited to send representatives.

They recommend that, in the preparation of a plan for the international health organization, full consideration should be given to the relationship of such an organization and methods of associating it with other institutions, national as well as international, which already exist or which may hereafter be established in the field of health.

We recommend that the proposed international health organization be brought into relationship with the Economic and Social Council.

Although the Governments of Brazil and China followed up the Declaration by suggesting that a Conference be held before the end of 1945, the resolution relating to this proposal was adopted by the Economic and Social Council only on 15 February 1946. In accordance with the terms of para. 3 of the Resolution, the Economic and Social Council established the Technical Preparatory Committee and directed that it should meet in Paris not later than 15 March 1946 to prepare a draft annotated agenda and proposals for the consideration of the Conference, to be held not later than 20 June 1946.[26] The technical preparatory committee sat under the chairmanship of Dr René Sand. The international conference of fifty-one nations, which was held in New York, adopted the draft constitution drawn up by the preparatory committee with few changes of substance. It also established an interim commission of eighteen states to bridge the gap until the constitution of a world health organization could be ratified. This was not brought about until 7 April 1948, when the necessary 26 states had formally assented. The interim commission, first under the chairmanship of a Russian, Dr Krothov,* and then of a Yugoslav, Professor Stampar, remained in being for over two years.

These two years of delay were not wasted. The Interim Commission dealt successfully with great emergencies, such as the Egyptian cholera outbreak, and with the day-to-day international health work which it inherited from the Paris office and the League office. But more than this, it had two years in which to plan; two years in which to use the exceptional genius of Andrija Stampar, who twenty years before had started his Institutes of Hygiene and health centres in

* Dr Krothov remained in office only two days.

the new Yugoslavia, with social medicine incorporated in the work of the Zagreb School of Public Health. Much that has followed may be due to this happy chance.

Constitution of WHO

The first World Health Assembly, which met at Geneva in June and July of 1948, was attended by 52 out of 54 eligible states, only Afghanistan and Jordan being absent. The new body, which began work in September 1948, absorbed, in addition to UNRRA, both the Paris and Geneva Offices. WHO thus became the sole international health organization, excepting the Pan-American Sanitary Bureau, which continued independently, but worked in close association with it and became, in 1949, the regional office for the Americas. A severe and unexpected blow, after the favourable opening address of the delegate from the USSR, Dr N. A. Vinogradov, was the virtual withdrawal in 1949 of the USSR and, during the next eighteen months, one by one, of all the other eight Cominform countries, from active participation in the work of the organization. The reasons given were inefficiency and poor administrative machinery. Since the charter contains no provision for any resignation, these states continued on the roster of WHO membership, but were designated as 'inactive'. In 1956 the USSR again expressed a wish to take an active part in the work of WHO and in 1957, with some of the other countries of Eastern Europe, she returned to full participation. In 1974, the membership was 140 full members, including the recent addition of China, with three associates; it covers a wider area of the globe than the UN itself, with very few states (including N. Vietnam) outside the organization.

The World Health Organization operates as one of the organizations active in the economic and social sphere known as specialized agencies of the United Nations.[32] By a specialized agency is meant one which conducts a programme of importance to the United Nations, in a special field of competence, under the general review of the General Assembly and the Economic and Social Council, but with important scope of autonomy in matters of membership, programme, personnel, and finances.[1] It has an office in New York to maintain liaison with the United Nations and other agencies. The headquarters is located in Geneva, where the Assembly, the parliament of the organization, usually meets. Between the annual meetings of the Assembly the work of the organization is directed by an executive board acting as a cabinet. This is non-political, and consists of 24 persons, designated by 24 nations elected for the purpose by the Assembly. Eight members retire and are replaced each year. The Director-General of the organization has a whole-time staff of about 5,000 persons,* recruited in rough proportions from the constituent nations. These are divided in approximately equal parts between the Geneva headquarters, regional offices, and field work. The staff is predominantly medical. The work of the Geneva

* The total staff in November 1973 was 5,003, including 35 in the International Agency for Research in Cancer. In June 1957, it was 1,413 (including 262 doctors, 171 nurses, 44 sanitarians and 158 other medical and para-medical staff).

headquarters is administered through fifteen divisions: Legal; Coordination; Internal Audit; Malaria and other parasitic diseases; Communicable Diseases; Environmental Health; Health Statistics; Strengthening of Health Services; Family Health; Non-communicable Disease; Health Manpower Development; Prophylactic and Therapeutic Substances; Personnel and General Services; Budget and Finance; Public Information. There are separate offices for Mental Health; Publications and Translations; Science and Technology; and Library and Health Literature.

The World Health Organization is independent; and its decisions, unlike those of the health organization of the League of Nations, do not need to be endorsed by a higher body. Its constitution is wide enough to permit it to undertake any health work within the limits of its budget. The ceiling of expenditure, first fixed at 5 million dollars, was raised to 13·5 million dollars (1958), to 53 million dollars (1967), and in May 1974 the 27th World Health Assembly adopted an effective working budget of 115,240,000 dollars. Payment by member states is based on the United Nations scale. In 1975, the USA was assessed to pay about 26 per cent, the USSR 13 per cent, the Federal Republic of Germany and Japan 7 per cent and France, UK and China 5 to 6 per cent.

WHO also benefits substantially from the UN Development Programme, which aims to help low-income countries to create conditions in which capital investment is both feasible and effective. UNDP, created in 1956 by the General Assembly of UN, is a consolidation of earlier machinery for economic aid, namely, *technical assistance* and the *special development fund*. It functions under the Economic and Social Council, with its policy controlled by a 37 member governing council, through 82 field offices. Technical assistance provided WHO with 9 million dollars in 1957, 10·25 million in 1966 and 23 million in 1973. The technical assistance component of WHO's total expenditure has declined; for field projects it was 52 per cent in 1957 and 16 per cent in 1973. Money from a *Voluntary Fund for Health Promotion* established in 1960 provided 11 million dollars in 1973 to be used in activities over and above the regular budget; this gives flexibility, as illustrated by the community water supply programme, which spent about a million dollars in 1959 to meet urgent requests for it in various parts of the world. International health projects also benefit from equipment and supplies made available by UNICEF estimated to be worth 37 million dollars in 1975 (see p. 161). Each national government bears a large share of the cost of health projects which it undertakes with international assistance; expenditure by governments in 1967 amounted to 353,586,190 dollars.

Terms of reference

The World Health Organization has grown out of the past. But its terms of reference are much wider.

The first article in the Charter of the World Health Organization gives as its objective, 'The attainment by all peoples of the highest possible level of health'. This, says the introduction in a clarion call, is to be regarded as 'one of the fundamental rights of every human being, without distinction of race, religion, political belief, economic or social condition'. 'All governments', it adds, 'have a responsibility for the health of their peoples which can be fulfilled only by the provision of adequate health and social measures'.

The Charter is thus remarkable for its breadth of vision. The aim is health: 'a state of complete physical, mental, and social well-being and not merely the absence of disease or infirmity'. This implies public health on the highest plane – to promote health, to prevent disease, and to rehabilitate suffering. Public health in the nineteenth-century sense of overcoming infectious agents of deadly diseases is to be widened to encompass practical social medicine. The twentieth-century public health is concerned with social factors before, during, and after the onset of illness – all disease, degenerative as well as infectious, mental, and physical. It is keenly interested in handicaps and other biological infirmities, which cannot be avoided; it believes in education about what we know and do not know in health matters; and it wants accurate records of morbidity and mortality and allied social phenomena. The specific inclusion in the Constitution of responsibility in the fields of mental hygiene, nutrition, and medical care, are illustrations of this modern concept of public health.

The scope of activities laid down for WHO by its Constitution goes far beyond the work done by previous organizations.[10] The following nine powers, among 28 major provisions, give an idea of its scope:

1. To assist governments, upon request, in strengthening health services

2. To promote improved standards of teaching and training in the health, medical, and related professions

3. To provide information, counsel, and assistance in the field of health

4. To promote, in co-operation with other specialized agencies when necessary, the improvement of nutrition, housing, sanitation, recreation, economic and working conditions, and other aspects of environmental hygiene

5. To promote co-operation among scientific and professional groups which contribute to the advancement of health

6. To promote maternal and child health and welfare and to foster the ability to live harmoniously in a changing total environment

7. To foster activities in the field of mental health, especially those affecting the harmony of human relations

8. To promote and co-ordinate research in the field of health

9. To study and report, in co-operation with other specialized agencies where necessary, on administrative and social techniques affecting public health and maternal care from preventive and curative points of view, including hospital services and social security.

The constitution of the World Health Organization takes in the whole of mankind. In this respect also the Organization differs from any of its predecessors by its worldwide character, by the absence of discrimination between races, and, perhaps most of all, by the shift of emphasis towards underdeveloped countries. WHO in fact takes up the challenge which the remarkable variations in the health picture throughout the world throws down (see Chapter 4).

The developed world consists of countries which have, for the most part, a century or more of industrialization behind them; they have overcome the major infectious diseases; infant and child mortality have fallen to a small fraction of the losses of last century. Life has lengthened out so that half the people live now beyond seventy years of age, four out of five dying of degenerative disease, mainly of the circulatory system. In contrast, as we have seen, the under-developed world still dies young; it has a high infant and child mortality; it suffers immense loss of life, and still greater illness from many infectious diseases. Degenerative disease, which people do not live long enough to experience, is much less common. What one part of the world gained, should not be impossible for another.

Yet, although WHO may lean towards the underdeveloped countries, it has a responsibility also to those countries where public health began. The problems of degenerative disease, of mental illness, of the viruses and of social disorders are, in their way and at a different level, as pressing as those in less favoured regions. There is, in any case, no firm line to be drawn between the two types of country and many degrees of development exist. Some problems, such as overpopulation with grave implications for the human race, transcend all boundaries.

Regional offices

The extreme variety of problems throughout the world, the immediate urgency of need in the underdeveloped countries, and the fact that local international organization already to some extent existed, made regionalization inevitable. Thus regional organizations were the subject of special provisions in the Constitution, including the following:

(1) The Health Assembly is required to define the geographical areas in which it is considered desirable to establish a regional organization. (2) With the consent of the majority of member states situated within each such area, the Health Assembly may establish a regional organiza-tion to meet the special needs of such area. (3) Each regional organization is an integral part of the world organization. (4) The regional organization consists of a regional committee and a regional office. (5) Regional committees are composed of representatives of member states in the region.

This left much to be decided as to the measure of autonomy which the regional offices should have. Some areas favoured regional services without immediately implementing the provisions of the Constitution, on the argument that nobody is expected to produce a family before the age of maturity. The existence and pressure of the Pan-American Sanitary Bureau, already operating effectively in many fields, including malaria eradication, helped to determine the course of events. In the result, WHO is alone among the specialized agencies to have adopted a policy of full regionalization.

The six regional offices, under the direction of regional committees composed of member states and associates, came into operation at different times. The first to be approved by the Executive Board was that for South-East Asia (New Delhi) in 1948; in 1949 there followed the Eastern Mediterranean (Alexandria), and the Americas (Washington) by agreement with the Pan-American Sanitary Organization to use the existing Pan-American Sanitary Bureau; finally in

1951 the Western Pacific (Manila) and Africa (Geneva); in 1952 Europe (Geneva). The irregular timing depended on many factors. Agreements of the countries involved took time; New Zealand and Australia, for example, for long opposed the Western Pacific office. The location of the regional office was not easily determined. Africa and Europe, first located in Geneva, moved respectively to Brazzaville (1952) and Copenhagen (1957).

Further decentralization with a measure of autonomy has been carried out by the Regional Office for the Americas. The American continent has been zoned with subsidiary headquarters at Washington, Mexico City, Guatemala City, Lima, Rio de Janeiro, Buenos Aires.

The regional committees have wide powers, including that of formulating policies and of calling conferences. They co-operate with other regional groups having common interests; they may nominate the Regional Director for appointment by the Executive Board. The regional offices have considerable autonomy. They are responsible for drawing up, in collaboration with governments and within the allotted budget, a plan of international assistance for health projects. After approval and allotment of funds by the Assembly, the regional office is again responsible for the conduct of the work. Regional offices have shown individuality in their development. They differ perforce, in their mode of operation from the headquarters at Geneva, largely because the responsibilities of the regional offices are those of assisting governments directly upon request.

There is little doubt that regionalization, so liberally interpreted, has been one of the factors which has contributed most to success – particularly in securing worldwide co-operation. As the Director-General said in 1950, the increased decentralization which this permitted,

has brought the Organization into close touch with the most immediate needs of the member countries, and has enabled WHO to begin to assist each country in taking the next appropriate step towards developing its health services within the limits of its economic, social, and cultural circumstances.[10]

The World Health Organization at work

The work of the World Health Organization can be divided for the sake of convenience into two parts:
1. Central technical responsibilities
   a. Epidemiological services
   b. International standardization
   c. The dissemination of knowledge
   d. Applied research
2. Services to Governments
   a. Expert guidance on specific topics
   b. Practical aid with short-term objectives
   c. Practical aid with long-term objectives.

1. *Central technical responsibilities and activities*

In the matter of central technical services the Organization has followed in the footsteps of its predecessors. When it began in 1948, sanitary conventions had existed for a century. For nearly half this period there had been an international bureau of epidemic intelligence, and also agreements about common standards for biological products and vital records. With a larger budget and the goodwill of nearly the whole world, the approach has naturally been more vigorous and the scope greater. What was previously done on a limited scale could now be applied generally.

a. *Epidemiological services*

The first fruits of world-wide collaboration were seen in the control of epidemics. The muddle of sanitary conventions, of which no less than thirteen existed, was replaced by a new code adopted by the Assembly in 1951, designed to protect countries, without irksome interference with travel and freight. The new regulations differed fundamentally from what had gone before: the system of bills of health, for example, was abolished. The adoption of these new regulations was made easier by the new powers vested in the World Health Assembly. In particular, it is empowered to discuss and adopt international health regulations to which member states become parties *without positive act.* Previous international conventions took years to ratify. Procrastination now favours unanimity where before it hindered. Of a possible 89 countries only 25 submitted limited reservations.* The International Sanitary Regulations came into operation in October 1952.[2] † Concurrently, the new centre of epidemic intelligence at Geneva gradually extended its range of interest to infectious diseases of all kinds and in all countries.

Fear of invasion by quarantinable diseases – cholera, plague, typhus, smallpox, and yellow fever – and the effects upon international traffic, are no longer necessarily among the chief preoccupations of health administrators. The endemic foci of these diseases quickly dwindled; and the frequency and extent of their occasional excursions diminished.[13] Modern epidemiology and public health have become effective safeguards, where before little, if any, existed.

Nevertheless, although the risks have been so much reduced, there is increased need for vigilance in a world in which carriers of disease can spread with the speed of an aeroplane. 'A typhus louse or a plague flea, brushed off the rags of a beggar in an Eastern bazaar can be in Tokyo or Oslo, New York, Moscow, London or Sydney, within a few hours'[8] – although it is not certain what harm they would do so far from their native habitat. A worldwide radio network, based on Geneva, came into use in 1948. Today, a daily bulletin of epidemic news, broadcast on nine wavelengths, can be picked up by sea ports, airports, ships at sea, and public health authorities everywhere. Regional stations of epidemiological intelligence exist for the Americas (Washington) and for the Eastern Mediterranean (Alexandria).

In addition to introducing uniformity in national action at frontiers, WHO has furthered epidemiological work, by sponsoring and co-ordinating research

* A state which submits a reservation that is rejected is excluded from the operation of the regulation unless it withdraws its reservation. In 1967, 162 states and territories have accepted the International Sanitary Regulations without reservations and 28 with reservations found admissible by the World Health Assembly.

† Within six months, 126 countries had accepted the International Health Regulations which came into force on 1 January 1974.

into communicable diseases, and by technical assistance to nations for combating the diseases themselves (see later).

The problems of infectious diseases, to which so many research workers and administrators all over the world have paid attention for many years, have lent themselves admirably to discussion in expert committees. Experts have considered and issued reports upon tuberculosis, malaria, treponematosis, poliomyelitis, onchocerciasis, rheumatic diseases, hepatitis, yellow fever, plague, cholera, smallpox, typhus and other rickettsial diseases, bilharziasis, trachoma, leprosy, rabies, brucellosis, influenza, the zoonoses (jointly with FAO), enteric infections, helminthiases, gonococcal infections, trypanosomiasis, filariasis,[2] schistosomiasis and viral diseases.

Epidemic intelligence – giving information about pestilential diseases, quarantine restrictions imposed or withdrawn, and details of current epidemics of, for example, influenza or poliomyelitis – is issued weekly; an epidemiological and vital statistics record is published monthly.

'Improved health facilities and the application of modern prophylaxis', says the WHO *Chronicle*, have 'greatly changed the health situation of the Mecca pilgrims and of the inhabitants of the region, where, between 1831 and 1912, forty different epidemics of plague, dysentery, typhoid and cholera were recorded during the pilgrimage seasons.' My own memories of a pilgrim voyage in 1927 are vivid.* Steaming slowly from Jeddah in the Red Sea through the Indian Ocean with 1,200 Malays, mostly sick and ailing, on the return voyage to their own lands, we had to stop daily to bury our dead. The 1973 pilgrimage, in contrast, was declared free from infection.

b. *International standardization*

The Organization has pursued, like its predecessors (see Chapter 23), the endless quest for statistical perfection in the analysis of causes of disease and death. The first revision of the international list under the auspices of WHO (the 6th of the series in this century) fused the codes of mortality and morbidity (see p. 227). The international death certificate which followed has given the opportunity to make mortality statistics valid and comparable everywhere. The national committees of vital and health statistics have been seeking to build up organizations adapted to the needs of their own countries. Statistical centres have been established in London, Paris, Caracas and Moscow, for advice (see p. 228).

Perhaps the most remarkable achievement in standardization has been the publication of the *Pharmacopoeia Internationalis* (1st vol. 1950, 2nd vol. 1955; 2nd edn. 1967, supplement 1971). This has been a longfelt want, since every nation had its own specifications, making international comparison of drugs difficult. The great variety of new drugs, many of great potency, which poured out from laboratories all over the world every year, added to the need for a common reference work. Little more needs to be said about standardization of biological substances, except that WHO has continued the work. Nine new standards, for example, appeared in 1954, including one for Schick toxin as a

* *Guy's Hospital Gazette*, January 1928.

test for susceptibility to diphtheria; cholera vaccine was standardized in 1958 and rabies in 1973.

c. *The dissemination of knowledge*

If existing knowledge of how to promote health and prevent diseases were to be generally applied, nine-tenths of the present volume of illness in the world would shortly disappear. The world does not lack knowledge, but rather the wisdom to apply it. But this criticism of man's good intentions overlooks the difficulties in communication, the conflict of voices, the variations in local conditions, and a dozen other barriers to a common understanding. In seeking to promote a common scientific understanding WHO may be doing more, with the least pretension, than in many other fields. What is needed is a clearing house of medical and scientific information; a machine for weighing and sifting the experience of different countries; the means to make the common accepted results available to all, governments, public, and workers in the field; and these WHO provides.

In this the *international committee of experts,* pioneered by the Geneva Office, economical to run* and infinitely elastic, has been admirably adapted to this wider purpose. During the past 25 years, committees have produced reports on some 50 different subjects, most, if not all, of those set down for prior study. In 1953, for example, committees studied and reported on the following: alcohol, biological standardization, drug addiction, environmental sanitation, health education, international pharmacopoeia, malaria, onchocerciasis, poliomyelitis, public health administration, rabies, rheumatic diseases, vaccination against tuberculosis, treponematosis, yellow fever, and protein malnutrition in infants and young children. A joint committee with UNESCO studied the mentally subnormal child. In 1974, 2,724 scientists were available to serve on expert committees in an honorary capacity as members of 44 panels maintained for consultation on a permanent basis.

Seminars, international conferences, working parties, study groups, study tours, and research symposia, which serve the same purpose, have also been widely used. The *research symposium* on epilepsy, which (October 1955) sat for a week in London, illustrates both the method and its adaptation to the widening scope of public health. It consisted of ten doctors from different parts of the world, who had spent substantial periods of their lives working with epileptics. The approach to epilepsy was as to a great social problem and what could public health do about it. In September 1953, 22 nations sent delegates to a European conference on public health training at Göteborg, Sweden. In 1955, with the object of improving the techniques of education in nutrition, which is one essential in the campaign against kwashiorkor, a joint FAO/WHO seminar was held in the Philippines. The research symposium held in Rome (October 1953) discussed the need for research into the insect vectors of disease, with the bogey of 'resistance' lending a note of urgency to the recommendations for research, before too late, into insect physiology and biochem-

---

* Expert committees and conferences together cost 238,000 dollars in 1966 representing 0·55 per cent of the regular budget.

F*

istry. *International conferences* played an important role in malaria eradication, not only in helping to synchronize plans, but also to thrash out the realities of an extremely complicated problem.

Second to none as a means to spread understanding are the *fellowships* granted to doctors and other workers in the health field for travel and study abroad; in 25 years (1948–1973) five thousand were awarded. In furtherance of antimalarial work alone, 2,774 fellowships have been given to medical graduates, entomologists, and engineers. One of the principal stipulations is that governments benefiting must guarantee a permanent post to the 'fellow' on his return. The wise use of fellowships has continually sent new life pulsating through the world's body politic, bringing enthusiasm and keenness to banish apathy with new ideas. The same can be said for many thousands of professional men and women consultants and experts, otherwise confined within their own narrow horizons, who have been given the opportunity to learn from the experience of other lands; and for the delegates from member nations who meet together in Geneva, Alexandria, Brazzaville, Washington, New Delhi, Manila and Copenhagen, to return fortified in spirit and enlarged in understanding to their own countries; and for the many research workers and others who meet on expert committees or on visits to different countries, to exchange experience and knowledge.

To all these means to further international understanding of scientific matters must be added the publications of the organization: the *Weekly Epidemiological Record*; the *WHO Chronicle*; the *Bulletin*, and the *Epidemiological and Vital Statistics Report,* issued monthly; and annual compilations *World Health Statistics Annual*; the *International Digest of Health Legislation*; and (1974) 55 *Public Health Papers*, 60 *Monographs*, 549 *Technical Reports* and 3 *Offset Publications*.

d. *Applied research*

But before knowledge can be pooled it has to be gained. One step back from the Expert Committee, the Study Group, and the Conference is the laboratory.

The experience gained by WHO during its first 25 years has continually shown how much success in public health depends upon a better understanding of specific problems and of the particular local conditions under which the work has to be done. More and more, therefore, the work of WHO involves *research* which arises out of work in the field. A practical venture in public health meets with difficulties; these are examined for suitable ways to find a solution; and a suitable laboratory or organization is then encouraged to undertake the necessary research. Thus, WHO sponsors research, but itself conducts little; it seeks problems, defines them, stimulates others to solve them, and co-ordinates the plan of operation. Where, as in research into epidemiological problems of infectious diseases, several laboratories in different countries agree to work on the subject, they do so according to a protocol drawn up with them by the technical section of the headquarters at Geneva. In 1974, there were 255 international or regional reference centres and 208 collaborating institutions involved in such research.

Where the control of spread of infection depends upon survey work or upon classification and comparison of pathogens isolated all over the world, WHO sponsors special international centres. In 1973, there was a network of 35 WHO international and regional reference centres for virus diseases (influenza 2, other respiratory viruses 7, entero-viruses 7, arboviruses 10, smallpox 4, trachoma 2, mycoplasms 2, rickettsiae 1) and a further 20 collaborating laboratories. A WHO brucellosis centre in Moscow, with 12 reference centres in other parts of the world, makes possible the world-wide survey of human and animal infections with brucella. Similarly, there are centres for shigella in London and Atlanta (Georgia), salmonella in Paris and escherichia in Copenhagen.

The search for new knowledge is often the only means to further success in public health work; the means to overcome or circumvent resistance in insect carriers of disease; the development of a dry smallpox vaccine stable at 45°C which will keep for two years in hot countries; the prophylaxis of rabies by serum and vaccination; the methods of spread of yellow fever in the jungle regions of Africa and South America; the means to destroy the snails in the waterways of Egypt and elsewhere, which carry bilharzia and help to produce widespread debility; the nature and prevention of kwashiorkor, the protein deficiency disease, which under 20 different names occurs in children throughout vast regions of the world; the health problems of the use of nuclear energy; these and so many other matters form the basis of research.

An early success for international research involving successive research ventures and trials in different parts of the world was in the field of deficiency diseases – goitre.[7] The first step was taken in 1949, when the subject was discussed by the first Nutrition Expert Committee. Consultants visited countries in Europe, Asia, and South America to examine the difficulties of supplying iodine to deficient populations. England, the USA, and the countries of South America collaborated in research to overcome first the difficulty of iodizing crude salt, then in determining the suitability of sodium iodate, and finally in conducting field trials. In 1954, five years after the subject had first been raised at an international level, two consultants – a chemical engineer and a doctor, with extensive experience of goitre – visited 16 countries of Latin America to advise the government on appropriate measures. The means to control goitre are now within every country's reach.

The work of stimulating and co-ordinating research, now a relatively small part of the total activity of the Organization, assumes increasing importance, as, year by year, the countries of the world perfect their basic public health services and look increasingly for help in overcoming particular difficulties. In perhaps ten or fifteen years it may have become the major rôle.

Nevertheless many hold the view that fields of research, closely related to the work of WHO and best performed by an international agency, did exist; such were, or seemed to be, problems of *computation,* e.g. in nomenclature, filing, adapting computer languages to biology, studying epidemiological models, monitoring drugs and pollution agents, storage of literature; of *biometry,* e.g. somatic and genetic effects of the wide range of toxic agents which increasingly pollute man's environment; or of *epidemiology,* e.g. cancer, psychological illness, drugs and world phenomena generally. A proposal in 1964 to found a $43 million centre with computer laboratory and a technical staff of 700 was finally shelved by the 18th Assembly in 1965. It was agreed that international monies could best be spent on action already clearly supported by existing knowledge, or alternatively that all new knowledge could be adequately sought by national research centres. The problem will surely be raised again and may well on another occasion be determined in favour.

In the meanwhile WHO has begun to develop its own research, for example in cardiovascular disease; it has established a division of research in epidemiology and communicable disease; and it has established a computer unit which appears to be extending its range of work. Seminars, advisory committees, working groups, conferences and symposia have been held (London 1968, Washington 1970, Bratislava 1970, Geneva 1971, 1972, and Luxembourg 1972) to discuss 'medical computing'.

The 19th Assembly (1966) agreed to create 'an international agency for research in cancer', now supported (1974) by ten countries.* The agency has its headquarters at Lyon in France and operates in 5 administrative divisions (epidemiology and biostatistics; Environmental, biological and chemical carcinogenesis; and research, training and liaison); it has an effective staff of 129 (26 scientists and 48 technicians). This is concentrating on 'the relationship of environment to human cancer', e.g. global distribution, migrant populations, industrialization, identification of aetiological factors in liver and gastro-intestinal cancer. It maintains a close working relationship with WHO's cancer control unit.

2. Services to governments

WHO follows in the footsteps of the Rockefeller Foundation in giving services to governments, service as distinct from advice; but in this it is distinguished clearly by the vastly greater range and extent of the work undertaken.

Aid in the field can be in one of two forms – either (a) as expert guidance or (b) and (c) as practical projects.

a. Expert guidance

Expert guidance is the least spectacular method of giving practical aid, since it is mainly concerned with administration and organization. In 1953 the Burmese government asked for advice in re-organizing the Central Health Department; Bogatá (Colombia) and Panama sought advice about local public health services; and Turkey about the development of a sound system of health statistics. In 1963, Jordan, well advanced in its services for two million people, asked for advice on the best means to direct them. WHO consultants, assisted, willy nilly, by a team of business consultants under bilateral aid, suggested means to strengthen the central and regional administration. In 1966, a team of three consultants (Egypt, USA, UK) advised Kuwait on its proposal to establish a medical school. In 1968, a medical consultant spent 3 months in the eastern Mediterranean region evaluating auxiliary training in Libya, Somalia, Ethiopia

* Australia, Belgium, Federal Germany, France, Italy, Japan, Netherlands, USSR, UK, USA.

and Saudi Arabia.[4] The range of advice is wide and varied. In any objective analysis of WHO this aspect must rank high; it is economical and it deals with fundamentals. So much that is being done in public health throughout the world fails for lack of sound advice and effective administration. How great, therefore, an advance it is that high-level advice, unstinting, unprejudiced and without strings, should now be available to governments everywhere.

An important development of expert guidance has been in the field of National Planning. Most countries have experienced the frustrations of developing services over the whole field of work without the guide lines of a national plan (see p. 186). When the range of possibilities is so great and the resources necessarily limited; when there are conflicting claims as for hospital care on the one hand and a health infrastructure on the other; when the priorities of disease prevention have not been adequately established nor has the full pattern of staffing in all parts of the service been clearly outlined – in such circumstances confusion is inevitable; waste and frustration follow. After 1951 a series of expert committees studied the problem of national planning and their reports laid down the basic principles.[37] This led in turn to Regional Seminars and meetings (as at Manila 1964 and Addis Ababa 1965) and to expert guidance on national planning from the Centre and from Regional offices to individual countries, e.g. Gabon, Mali, Niger, Sierra Leone. Liberia, Somalia, Libya and various SA states. This is an approach to National Health which must eventually encompass the whole world.

Practical projects

Practical projects to help in the establishment of public health services are undertaken in collaboration with other specialized agencies of the United Nations, notably with FAO, UNESCO, ILO and UNICEF.* UNICEF collaborates in a wide range of projects which directly or indirectly affect children; in schemes specifically aimed to benefit maternal and child health; in campaigns against individual diseases, such as yaws and leprosy; and in projects for water supplies, environmental hygiene, training staff, and construction of training schools and hostels for students. In 1973, UNICEF spent 8·5 million dollars assisting water schemes in 68 countries. It collaborated in a scheme to aid the Indian National Institute of Health Administration to make a study of district health administration; and, between 1970–74, it helped to provide refresher courses in Beirut for 162 doctors from 15 countries in the Eastern Mediterranean region in child health, school health and family planning. For some years it was one of the mainstays of malaria eradication, furnishing insecticides, spraying equipment and transport, between 1949–53, covering 71·8 per cent of the cost.†

Much help for WHO schemes also comes from the United Nation's Development Fund (Technical Assistance). Such joint schemes do something, at least in

* Food and Agriculture Organization of the United Nations (FAO). United Nations Educational, Scientific and Cultural Organization (UNESCO). International Labour Organization (ILO). United Nations Children's Fund (UNICEF).

† UNICEF has virtually terminated assistance to malarial campaigns in favour of more fruitful forms of international aid; but it still provides antimalarial drugs to enable health services, particularly in Africa, to lessen the impact of malaria in heavily infected communities.

the health field, to channel the rising flood of international aid now pouring into less developed countries. In all projects the expenditure from international funds is at least equalled by national contributions. For much of the work in the field, the Organization uses a permanent staff, but where problems call for special knowledge there is an effective and elastic system of temporary consultants.

Practical projects can have either immediate or long-term objectives, i.e., they can seek to eradicate disease by a blitz or mass campaign, or, alternatively, they can use methods which rely on the establishment of permanent services or on the furtherance of education and social change.

b. *Practical aid with short term objectives*

Technique. Mass campaigns are outstandingly the most spectacular innovation. These can be defined as: *Short-term temporary schemes for the control or eradication of a single disease, generally directed by a 'special epidemiologist'.* They operate on military lines with control from a central point, irrespective of local government boundaries and generally independent of the country's permanent health service. They are concerned chiefly with primary prevention and, when made use of, secondary prevention is limited to the treatment of infectious conditions. The campaign is conducted in three phases: attack; consolidation; and maintenance. Prior to the attack the area must be surveyed, a plan developed, and staff recruited and trained; with consolidation comes the problem of integration into the general public health service. Maintenance (see later) is a function of general public health.[20, 34, 38, 39]

Mass campaigns have the following advantages:

1. They can be conducted as *military campaigns.* The forces of liberation, so to speak, move into the occupied country, operating a well-planned campaign, destroying ruthlessly the bacterial enemy, its vector, or its power to attack the human host.

2. They provide their own *discipline.* This is 'built-in' by imported supervisory staff which trains and controls an army of workers.

3. They can succeed largely *without the active participation* or partnership of the people of the country in which they operate. Thus they can in large measure be imposed upon the people, or at least be applied effectively in the absence of sympathy, understanding and co-operation (but difficulties do arise from human resistance, see later).

4. They require *little or no pre-existing health infrastructure* for the attack phase; although (see later) they cannot be brought to a successful conclusion in its absence.

5. They make use largely of *auxiliaries,* who need no lengthy education and can be trained in-service with relative ease for simple repetitive techniques.

6. They ensure a high level of *technical achievement* based upon controlled trials and continuous supervision.

7. They *reduce prevalence rapidly* and thus give immediate economic and other benefits, including a striking demonstration of the benefits of modern scientific medicine.

8. They can be directed over a wide area simultaneously with a minimum of highly trained 'special epidemiologists'.

9. They lend themselves admirably to international planning and aid.

Mass campaigns depend for their success on man's ability to find an inexpensive means, chemical, biological or immunological, with which to sever the chain of causation of disease in one relatively simple operation, or at most in a limited series of such operations repeated at intervals. The weapon selected to interrupt the epidemiological process may be employed directly against an organism or its vector, or indirectly in raising the resistance of the human host. Diseases selected for such treatment – malaria, leprosy, filariasis, tuberculosis, yaws, typhus, smallpox – are all due to organisms of the bacterial, viral or protozoal world; in those due to causes other than bacteria the chain of causation cannot be severed with the ease, simplicity and finality needed to make the cost of a mass campaign worthwhile.

By 1974, many hundreds of mass campaigns had been conducted throughout the underdeveloped world, generally with remarkable success. As early as 1954, WHO was helping to control tuberculosis in 28 countries; by 1974 nearly three-quarters of a billion persons had been tuberculin tested and over a quarter of a billion vaccinated against tuberculosis. Filariasis has been treated with diethyl-carbamazine, with, e.g., in the Western Pacific region, a reduction in carriers of micro-filaria from 19·6 to 1·63 (1973). Endemic typhus has been eliminated in Afghanistan (345,000 persons, 19,275 homes, 2·5 million pieces of clothing, 1,294 horsedrawn tongas, and 29 public baths were dusted with DDT).

Malaria is the outstanding example of this type of activity. It was the subject of the first expert committee which met in Geneva in 1947; first on the list, not only for the ravages which it made, but also because DDT and other insecticides, with prolonged residual activity, had been made available for killing adult mosquitoes. The spraying of the surfaces on which insects, gorged with blood, are likely to rest, is a weapon of remarkable potency. At some time during the ten days required for the development of infective sporozoites, most mosquitoes will have received a lethal dose. When reinfection is thus prevented, the two main malarial infections of man, even if untreated, are quick to disappear; with few exceptions, falciparum parasites do not last longer than a year and vivax two years. If the mosquito population is held in check and transmission prevented for three years there can be no more malaria parasites either in the human, or the mosquito, host.

Yaws, and allied treponemal conditions, have been attacked by means of penicillin, involving the examination and treatment of some quarter billion people. In Thailand during 1950–4 seventeen teams each consisting of a medical officer and four auxiliary workers, local people trained for two months in the epidemiology of yaws, visited the scattered villages and townships of the jungle in teams, like a judge on circuit, examining everyone and giving a single injection of PAM (penicillin G with aluminium stearate) to all sufferers.[3] Throughout Asia, where Yaws had been a scourge for centuries, the disease has been reduced to low levels at which it could be contained by a well developed public health service.

Smallpox eradication eventually provided comparatively the greatest success story and one which would surely have delighted the heart of Jenner had he been here to witness it. In 1967, some 20 years after WHO came into existence, when eradication began, smallpox prevailed in 30 countries; by 1974, the countries with endemic smallpox had been reduced to four (Pakistan, Bangladesh, India and Ethiopia) with every prospect of eradication becoming complete by 1975.

The success of smallpox eradication carries two important lessons. First it demonstrated the weakness of the health centre as a preventive agent, since in most of the countries, where smallpox continued to be endemic, health centres had been in operation for some years. Inundated with sick people and staffed by doctors trained in traditional clinical medicine they had been ill-equipped to take Jenner's vaccine into the villages and homes of the people. Second, it showed how, by grafting on the mass campaign to the existing health centres, a new and dynamic outlook could be brought about. The scheme was operated by experts, medical and lay, at district and group levels (see p. 189) with teams of auxiliaries working from the health centres. Much of the success also depended on an overhaul of the techniques in use for vaccination and for the preparation and checking of the vaccine itself.

The mass campaign has generally been considered a time limited operation, presumably because of the cost in money and effort in maintaining an independent service. It now seems certain that by linking mass campaigns with the health centres in the manner demonstrated by the smallpox campaign, the time element becomes of less significance. From this it also follows that the mass technique, applied in this way, can be adapted to the prevention of diseases, as, e.g., the common infections of childhood, for which immunization has to be continued indefinitely.

The Limitations of mass campaigns. The early expectations of worldwide total eradication of various diseases by means of a mass campaign, operating independently of a permanent infrastructure, proved to be unduly optimistic, mainly because the relative ease and simplicity of the attack phase tended to conceal a number of hidden difficulties.

Residual infections. The chief disability of the mass campaign lies in the fact that it can never, or rarely, reach finality.[20, 38, 39] In trachoma, yaws, malaria, filariasis, and even smallpox, pockets of infection remain, even when the level of endemicity is reduced to near vanishing point. Among the few exceptions to this rule appears to be typhus fever. Yaws provides clear evidence of this dilemma; for eradication involves more than penicillin. It brings into question the whole mode of life and system of values of the people involved:

In the province of Rotburi, 50 miles from Bangkok, jeeps bumped along mud tracks to Nongkog, where 1½ years after the original injections, the yaws team was engaged in follow-up. The school, on stilts with open sides, where the examinations were performed, with the monk's *sala* and their shrine, occupied a clearing in the woods. One hundred and eighty-four persons recorded in the original census were examined in two days. Yaws in its florid state no longer existed; smiling faces replaced misery and suffering. Yet latent and active cases remained. In a social disease of this character, meticulous supervision, early detection and treatment of cases and prolonged health education provide the only real safeguard against a wholesale return. Who is to shoulder this task when international support is withdrawn?

The monks, colourful, persuasive, all-pervading, are unlikely to become effective health educators. The enduring solution of the problem of yaws, as of most other diseases and public health problems, is threefold, (1) organization of public health in local units, (2) professionally trained staff, and (3) the development of social understanding. Can this be done?[3]

It follows that in the absence of a permanent public health infrastructure the mass campaign has to continue in operation. Under these circumstances, as Alvarado has said,[40] in the case of malaria *a ruinous "sine die" prolongation of the consolidation phase would be required until the adequate infrastructure is created*.

All can be lost without a permanent infrastructure of health. Yaws and other endemic non-venereal treponematoses are found mainly in rural areas of underdeveloped or developing countries where social advancement is slowest. It is in these parts of the world where most difficulties arise in creating a health infrastructure.

Special problems of malaria. In the case of malaria, eradication was further complicated by the existence of very high levels of endemicity, particularly in Africa and New Guinea; by the tendency of the insecticide to be absorbed on mud walls, thus losing its efficacy; by the inaccessibility and mobility of nomadic tribes, capable of bringing infection to areas supposedly free; and, most important of all, by the development of resistance to insecticides in the vectors of the disease. Resistance is also found to occur in the malaria parasite itself, both to the drug used in treatment, and to house spraying, an everlasting inconvenience to humans.

Resistance of insects, parasites and humans. The spectre of new strains resistant to the poison (physiological resistance), or of mosquitoes that have learned to avoid sprayed surfaces, where they would be exposed to lethal doses (behavioural resistance), has appeared to complicate an already difficult situation.

Physiological resistance signifies 'the development of an ability, in a strain of insects, to tolerate doses of toxicants, which would prove lethal to the majority of individuals in a normal population of the same species'.* Resistance to one member usually means resistance to others in the same insecticide group, so that the local anopheline population becomes immune to several of the chlorinated hydrocarbons together.[28] For this reason, resistance to both BHC and dieldrin is not regarded as double resistance. The number of resistant anopheline species rose from 14 in 1959 to 32 in 1965 and to 40 in 1973;[27] 38 had developed resistance to dieldrin, 19 being principal vectors of malaria. Resistance to carbamates has been observed in El Salvador, Guatemala, Honduras and Nicaragua; and to organophosphates in Yugoslavia.

In 1958, there were only two species resistant to two insecticides – A. subpictus, in Java to dieldrin, and in India to DDT, and A. sacharovi, in Greece, to both. The situation today is more grave. Double resistance, i.e., to both DDT and to the benzine compounds (BHC and dieldrin) is now widespread

* Discriminating doses are generally as follows: 0·4 per cent dieldrin for one hour kills all susceptibles with the exception of A. sacharovi (which requires 0·8 per cent); 4 per cent dieldrin kills the heterozygous members; 4 per cent DDT for one hour kills all susceptibles WHO/mal/73/803).

and yearly appears in more places throughout the malarial world. The phenomenon is often associated with the use of insecticides for agriculture.* Triple resistance (DDT, dieldrin and propoxur, a carbamate) has appeared in A. albimanus in El Salvador, Guatemala, Honduras and Nicaragua.

Resistance of the malaria parasite itself to chemical treatment may well prove to be a more sinister development; plasmodium falciparum (in SE Asia and in Brazil) has shown resistance to chloroquin.[41] Resistance to collaboration in humans themselves and their governments, which develops once the memories of the disease begin to fade and the inconveniences of periodic spraying become magnified, is spreading, not surprisingly when we recall the unwillingness of Europeans to be immunized against smallpox and diphtheria, now for them forgotten maladies. All these obstacles increase the risks of reinfection, as well as the dangers of the disease itself; and they clearly militate against the final eradication of the disease.[38]

Nevertheless man keeps one ahead in the conflict with the vectors of the malaria parasite. The spread of resistance to DDT singly, and to DDT, and dieldrin jointly, appears to be slowing down.[27] The range and extent of insecticides available for use against mosquitoes extends, with every likelihood of continuing to do so. When resistance has appeared, chemicals can still reduce transmission to a level at which surveillance, with radical medication of sufferers in the reservoir of infection, can finally wipe out the disease. Progress has been made towards the ultimate preparation of an immunizing agent which might replace all other techniques for the eradication of the disease.[42, 43]

The bitter truth. The first malaria conference was held at Kampala, Uganda, in 1950, to discuss control south of the Sahara, where even at that early date, the characteristics of a 'stable' infection (see p. 167) were seen to present well nigh insuperable difficulties for eradication. Many local experts held the view that eradication should not be attempted where, owing to high endemicity, adults were immune following childhood infections. It has to be admitted that this opinion discouraging as it might be, came very near to the truth. Nevertheless, the conference reached the unanimous opinion that *whatever the original degree of endemicity, malaria should be controlled by modern methods as soon as possible* . . .[28] The second conference at Bangkok (1953) was attended by fifty persons from twenty different Asian countries, representing 590,000,000 people living in malarial territories. This conference recognized the dangers of lack of co-ordination in a campaign which appeared at that time to be a race against time; it recommended *the merging of controls wherever the malarial territories are found, irrespective of national boundaries.* The third conference in Baguio, Philippines (1954), concerned with malaria in the Western Pacific and South-East Asia, first introduced the note of urgency: the need to *hasten control in order to keep ahead of resistance* to the insecticides, already well advanced. With the encouragment of the successes of the Pan-American Sanitary

---

* The major vector species showing double resistance are *A. albimanus* (Middle America); *A. stephensi* (Asia); *A. pharoensis* (Central and Lower Nile Basin); *A. gambiae* (Blue Nile Province, Sudan); *A. aconitus* (Java).

Bureau in malaria eradication techniques, the eighth World Health Assembly decided to aim at worldwide eradication within ten years.

Unreal as this decision has subsequently proved to be, indeed it seemed to be so to many at the time, it took several more international conferences to issue warnings before the Assembly bowed to the realities of the world malaria plight. The conference in New Delhi (3rd Asian, 1959) called for *careful planning*; that in Manila (4th Asian 1962) pilloried the *absence of a health infrastructure*, without which consolidation and maintenance were impractical, (see p. 196); the 2nd African (1955) in Lagos stressed the difficulties of eradication in areas with *high intensity of transmission*; the 4th (1962) at Yaoundé spoke frankly of *slow progress and disappointing results*. All very necessary and sobering. Objective conferences slowly led to 'a thorough evaluation and assessment' (1967 and 1968) and to a revised strategy adopted by the World Health Assembly (1969), which, in effect, accepted that in malaria control 'due to complex ecological conditions, a time-limited programme was not likely to succeed'.[42]

Malaria has continued, despite worldwide campaigns, as a major source of illness and continues to menace large areas of the globe occupied by 1,900 millions of people. In these territories, where 306 millions are still in the attack phase, 286 millions in consolidation and 787 millions in maintenance, there is a constant risk of spread.[27] Many outbreaks occur yearly in areas of consolidation and maintenance, as, e.g. in 1969 in Turkey, both East and West, when vigilance is relaxed.[5] The area of involvement, like a vast inland sea evaporating in the sun, slowly contracts, leaving countries like Greece and Portugal on its fringes suddenly and miraculously free. This is not the rapid and dramatic progress to complete eradication once thought possible. In Africa, where malaria is said to be 'stable' i.e. with transmission optimal, vectors highly effective, and the reservoir of human infection from which they draw full to the brim, eradication will probably not be achieved until well into next century, (see also p. 16).

Eradication of malaria throughout the world, now seen as a longer, more difficult and costly exercise than at first thought to be the case, should no longer be looked upon as a race against time. Urgency exists, because areas that have eradicated it are under increased risk, often with tragic consequences, from those that have not. But the disease will yield to steady pressure over years, ultimately to reach insignificant proportions. This will involve more than the mass campaign. There must also be a return to the well tried naturalistic and mechanical methods of reducing mosquito life; drainage, alternating irrigation, oiling surfaces and the use of gambusia, the larva eating fish. Permanent engineering works in some regions can do more than anything else. The greatest importance must be attached to the development of adequate infrastructures through which malaria campaigns can be channelled. The world map of malaria will slowly contract as countries on the fringe of the most endemic regions are freed; and finally, if it does not disappear, it will be held in check by an effective worldwide infrastructure of general public health.

The need for a permanent health infrastructure. All mass campaigns to eliminate endemic disease depend ultimately for success upon a sound public health system. The greater the success the more evident this truth becomes; for new found health now stands endangered by the lack of services whose true significance was never previously properly understood. For some years now the infrastructure has been found wanting and mass campaigns have perforce continued beyond the consolidation and maintenance phases. The teams of specialized auxiliaries are required to do work well within the capacity of a general purpose visitor (see Chapter 20), e.g., in the surveillance of malaria to do house-to-house visiting, enquiring for fever, taking blood for slides, arranging for examinations and giving mass medication; a large scale military machine maintained for this purpose resembles a sledge hammer knocking in a tintack. There's the rub. It is this consideration, rather than the bogies of resistance in its many forms, which gives most cause for concern. The true position is only now being fully appreciated when failure to promote long term public health infrastructures is seen to be at the root of present difficulties in terminating mass campaigns and integrating them into general public health.[5]

For these reasons a permanent infrastructure (as outlined in Chapter 20) should be promoted at the outset: and not left until mass campaigns are far advanced; or, as is often the case, allowed to take second place to hospital construction.

The relative value of mass campaigns and general public health is often discussed as if they were antithetic; whereas they should be complementary. Success in one should lead to development in the other; the elimination of malaria, yaws or typhus gives immediate economic and health benefits, so that, freed from these debilitating diseases, the whole life of the community takes an upward surge. The demonstration of a cure in a manner so dramatic helps to convince people that there is something in scientific medicine, and such a demonstration may be more successful in replacing folk treatment and beliefs than attempts to diffuse modern practices of preventive medicine and their theoretical justification (Erasmus)[11] (see Chapter 6). To begin with a mass campaign may well be best, providing always that steps to develop a permanent infrastructure are immediately put in hand and purposefully pursued.

c. *Practical aid with long term objectives*

WHO contributions to the development of a permanent infrastructure of health throughout the underdeveloped and developing worlds have taken second place to other more spectacular means to combat disease. Nevertheless, WHO has played a part in developing general public health through demonstration projects, giving the opportunity to try out new techniques best suited to the social conditions of the country; and to train new types of auxiliaries, such as home visitors, health assistants or village workers, as in Indonesia, Burma and India (see training of auxiliaries p. 204). Such schemes aim to train staff to cover all the needs of a public health scheme, including the collection of data, and ultimately to establish viable structures, which can continue unaided and provide the nucleus for multiplying health units in other parts of the country. Counterparts are trained to take over from WHO specialists when they leave.

WHO demonstration projects for public health have been most successful in 'special public health', where the object is to provide a service for individual diseases, or for special, so-called vulnerable, groups of the population. Many hundreds of such schemes have been set up for mother and child, ante-natal care, school health and tuberculosis control. For their direction they need a medical specialist in the particular subject, e.g. paediatrician, obstetrician or tuberculosis officer. They can operate from a central clinic, demonstrating the techniques of social and preventive medicine, based upon the epidemiology of the condition, or the group involved: preventive examinations, visiting for advice in the home, vaccination and immunization, contact tracing etc.

Special public health projects carry some of the disadvantages of the mass campaign, in that they tend to establish separate kingdoms, which later resist integration into a permanent infrastructure for general public health (see Chapter 20).

Demonstration projects for general public health have been established to a much lesser extent, partly owing to the cost and difficulties involved (but see Chapter 20). Some of the difficulties which this type of demonstration project has to meet can be seen in the story of the Larissa Model Health Area, which WHO established in 1959 in conjunction with UNICEF in Thessaly, Greece.[6]

*The Larissa Model Health Area.** The principal objective of the scheme was 'to assist the government to reorganize public health throughout Greece, based upon health units giving preventive and medical care and health education'.

The project (with the exception of occupational health) constituted a blue-print for a general public health service for Greece as a whole.

The constituent *nomoi* (Larissa, Trikkala, Karditsa and Volos) were to continue to be administered separately, under an area director at Larissa. Whole time staff would consist of a deputy director, a director of studies, a medical director of PIKPA, a microbiologist, a sanitary engineer, a chief nurse, a health educator, a medical statistician. Part-time specialists in tuberculosis, mental health, maternal and child health and chronic and degenerative diseases were to be appointed jointly with the upgraded Larissa hospital.

The area director would coordinate the work of various ministries and voluntary agencies, rationalize the use of staff; ensure the provision of sanitation, vaccination and follow-up of infants and children; establish health centres in town and country; encourage general practitioners and hospitals to promote health; organize regular meetings of staff; and publish a periodic bulletin of information. The public health infrastructure would contain two types of health centre, each with a physician, midwife and public health nurse, one having 6 beds (5–7,000 population). There would be satellite health posts, with one physician acting alone (2,500–3,000 population). The PIKPA mobile units were to be used, under the authority of the area director, for consultation in paediatrics, mental hygiene, school health, dental health, tuberculosis and for epidemiological investigations. A public health laboratory, a training institution, a central or regional hospital with special units for premature babies, chronic diseases and geriatrics, would be provided. A committee in Athens, with national and international members, meeting twice yearly, would receive the director's report and approve the budget and, by means of a subcommittee, would supervise training and research. A local committee at Larissa of prefects and nomiatroi, with representatives of ministries and institutions, would help guide the project.

* The Greek demonstration area centred on Larissa, appropriately included the traditional birth place of Aesculapius, Trikkala. This area had already benefited from much international aid through agreements with WHO (1951), Technical Assistance (1956), UNICEF (1957); with free medical care, based upon fixed centres, in rural areas (1955); with a well developed scheme, under a voluntary agency (PIKPA) for maternal and child health; but otherwise with a rudimentary public health structure.

Despite early promise in the Larissa nomos, the project was slow to get off the ground and did not cover the whole area until five years had passed. Progress slowed and eventually came to a halt and, in some respects, the scheme regressed. After ten years it was less well staffed than at the outset, with no deputy director, medical statistician, PIKPA director, nor hospital consultants, and half the complement of sanitarians. The chief public health nurse, heavily involved in treatment in the Larissa health centre, was not available to supervise public health nursing throughout the area. The hospital had not been upgraded.

The director, working single handed, deputizing for specialists who had not been appointed, and lacking a senior sanitary inspector to supervise the work of the auxiliary sanitarians, had little opportunity to fulfil his proper rôle. The absence of the medical statistician and of supporting staff prevented the demonstration of systematized collection of vital, and health, data. Health centres were poorly staffed, lacking doctors, nurses and midwives. A few did excellent work in maternity and child welfare, but few of the staff were trained to do social and preventive work. Some integration of school health was achieved, but none with PIKPA, which retreated to the towns, continuing to give preventive care to mothers and babies without involvement in curative care. The transfer of PIKPA mobile units to specialized fields did not take place.

A *spirit of public health* permeated the organization, despite disheartening events, staff appointments never made, discontinued or left vacant, lack of support and even, it would seem, lack of interest in high places. The tone of the service and the respect in which it was held showed how much could have been achieved in a more favourable climate. The public health laboratory, sanitary engineering, the mental health service and the training school at Pharsala, all in the hands of dedicated men and women, contributed. The laboratory was the mainstay of environmental hygiene, although the part-time microbiologist had not been able to do field studies. Sanitary engineering in the Larissa nomos had brought water to 90 per cent of households. Mental health clinics served most of the area, with psychiatrist, psychologist and nurse engaged for the greater part of the first ten years; the nurse had been abroad twice with fellowships to study mental health services elsewhere in Europe, before being inexplicably transferred to tuberculosis visiting. The Pharsala Institute, with part time lecturers from Athens and no health centre in its neighbourhood for teaching field techniques, and short, mainly theoretical courses in the philosophy of public health, had become highly respected, not only in the demonstration area, but throughout the whole of Greece.

Failure to carry out the plan in its entirety was due partly to the fact that integration of the four nomoi was never achieved and, seemingly, without reorganization of the local government structure itself, never could be; partly to an exaggerated idea of what was possible and perhaps to lack of definition of what was intended; partly to inadequate payment of field staff, of whom only the general practitioners received supplements for working in the demonstration area. Only the dedicated or those with other means, or those willing to work in private practice after hours were available from among the specialists, and few could be recruited. Nurses, after the compulsory year of practice, left for better paid work in hospital.

But chiefly the project fell by the wayside for lack of support from the government, which failed to implement the plan and to prepare for its extension to other parts of Greece. The main council had not functioned, with the exception of its scientific sub-committee, so that no machinery existed for furthering the interests of the project, implementing the agreed plan, getting staff appointed and preventing sudden changes of direction, such as the transference of staff without reference. Much of the reluctance of the Greek government to fulfil its part of the agreement was probably due to the sophistication of the project and the demands which it made for specialist staff. Had the project been more realistically costed at the outset, it would probably have been seen to be over-ambitious in relation to the level of development of the country.

You can take a horse to the water, but sadly cannot make it drink. Unless governments truly wish for a permanent public health infrastructure and are prepared to give it priority, the help of the international organization cannot alone bring it about. It may make blueprints and dream dreams, but the ultimate fulfilment of both lies not with WHO, but in the centres of power of national governments.

The nature of the infrastructure in most of the underdeveloped and developing countries, in terms of the services to be run and the staff required, is less sophisticated than that proposed in Greece. Model areas to deal with the most pressing problems, using a minimum of professional staff and large complements of auxiliary workers, have been successfully established in Egypt (at Qalyub, north of Cairo); in Indonesia (at Bandung and Jakarta); Thailand (at Chieng-mai and Chonburi); Burma (at Aung San, north of Rangoon); in India (at Singur); South America (at Espirito Santo in Brazil); as well as in many African countries and Malaya. The following details of Singur can be taken as illustrative:

The *Singur health unit*, jointly operated by the governments of India and Bengal for the past 30 years, situated 21 miles N.W. of Calcutta, originally covered 33 sq. miles, 62,700 people, 11,390 families in 68 villages. In 1955, the area was increased to 57 sq. miles with nearly 100,000 people in 105 villages and has since operated in six units each under the direction of a medical officer of health, with a staff of 4 sanitarians, 3 health visitors, 3 midwives, 2 dais and 2 servants. The area is used by the All-India Institute of Hygiene and Public Health for in-service training courses; between 1953 and 1972, 1,099 doctors, nurses, sanitarians and midwives from various parts of India were instructed in public health practice.[31]

The primary objectives, it was said, of the Singur health unit is to reduce readily controllable excess mortality and to build up a knowledge of vital statistics. The chief secondary objective is to build up a school health service. The work is governed by certain principles, e.g. (1) economic practicality, (2) interdependence of social services, particularly education, (3) the need to administer special functions by one administrative body, (4) the inevitability of compromise in short-term projects, (5) the need for scientific administration, and (6) the need for trained workers.

Self-help* provides much of the native force and is organized mainly through village health committees, co-ordinated by a 'unit committee' under the secretaryship of the rural medical officer of health. The village committees cover a population of approximately 1,000.

* For full details and references see *Self-Help – its Uses and Limitations in the Field of Health* (1955) **2**, No. 1. London: Central Council for Health Education.

Each committee consists of five members elected by the village with a sanitary inspector as secretary. Each member of the village committee is responsible for the supervision of one of five routine health activities (vital statistics; epidemic control and smallpox vaccination; environmental sanitation; maternity and child welfare; malaria control). The scheme provides for the training of laymen in all villages to discharge their special functions, e.g. in the case of maternity, a young married woman, preferably the daughter of a practising dai (1945). See ref. 14, Part 4.

Sample surveys of morbidity were conducted in 1944 and 1957 (877 families chosen at random from 26 villages, i.e., 5,352 persons or 7·3 per cent of the population (see Chapters 24 and 25)). Malaria had been eradicated, but other forms of sickness (diarrhoea and dysentery, smallpox, liver disease, tuberculosis, hookworm, malnutrition) all preventable, had increased,[18] eloquent testimony both to the need for public health and the difficulty in its practice.

Two factors contribute to success in these 'grass roots' operations, illustrated by Larissa and Singur namely, (1) relative lack of sophistication, or at least careful adjustment to the state of development of the country and (2) perhaps most important of all, continued unstinting government support. With varying degrees of sophistication, this form of *general public health organization* can be established everywhere. It is to this that we should look for solutions to many of the world's most pressing health problems; and it is to such a fundamental need in the underdeveloped and developing world that Part Six of this book is devoted.

Training for long term public health

Long term public health calls for trained staff; medical, para-medical; professional and auxiliary. The preparation needed and their use in service is examined in Chapter 20. Here it is only necessary to outline the ways in which WHO seeks to help in this difficult task. *Aid in training professionals* is given in three ways:
1. by posting consultants to places of higher learning
2. by sending teachers and others for further training
3. by establishing in-service training courses at convenient centres locally.

Countries wishing to set up departments, institutions, universities or medical colleges, may seek WHO's help in deciding on the practicability or suitability of such a step. This was the case with the proposals for medical colleges in Kuwait and Jordan. But the more frequent use of consultants for training is by service in medical colleges and other institutions. Doctors, nurses, midwives and sanitarians are posted to establish departments and train counterparts, often giving years of devoted service. A senior midwife and a nurse from countries with well developed midwifery services began a midwifery school in Bali, in the early 1950s, to train midwives for the islands east of Java, where modern midwifery was unknown in any form except that of Mother Gamp. In Saudi Arabia, help was given to establish nursing schools at Huffuf and proposals were made for establishing a course for professional nurses at Dammam hospital.[4] In India help in creating departments of social and preventive medicine resulted in dynamic changes in teaching. The lessons learnt in the medical college of Nagpur in the fifties, when India was beginning to build a complete system of 115 such colleges to cover the whole country, were used to establish similar departments throughout. The teaching was based on field work in defined areas around the colleges, beginning a process which in turn has helped to enlighten the developed world, where medical education over the centuries has become unduly clinical. WHO's aid in this, as in other fields, has been enzymic in action, a small inoculation leavening a larger mass. Sending professionals for further training abroad (see p. 203), as noted in the Larissa demonstration area in Greece,[6] has been exceptionally fruitful. The need to staff training institutes with teachers of their own nationality (as, e.g. nurse tutors with teacher training certificates for nursing colleges) has often been met by fellowships for training abroad. At Ege University in Turkey, it was hoped to solve the problem of a nursing director of the university nurse course by sending a graduate nurse for further training to Europe or North America (see p. 203).

In-service training courses for professionals have been established for specific purposes in many strategic centres either to serve one country or, often, a region. Courses were held in health statistics in Kabul (1953), in industrial health in Alexandria (1959), in poliomyelitis control in Prague (1961), for medical supervisors in the Phillipines (1962), for medical librarians in Beirut (1964–5), for medical records officers in Bangkok (1965), foci of infection in USSR (1966), epidemiology of tuberculosis in Prague and Rome (1966). Teachers are supplied also for short courses in existing institutions, as in the teaching of public health to post graduate doctors in the school of public health in Ankara. More than 40 per cent of all projects, not including fellowships, have been concerned with education and training.

Aid in training auxiliaries is given mainly in the establishment of institutions[6] in which to give formal courses. WHO appoints the full time staff, directors and lecturers, and helps in finding and training counterparts. The training of counterparts is a first consideration in all such schemes, with the object of building up a staff from the same culture and speaking the same language. Professionally qualified counterparts may need further training which cannot be obtained in the country itself. For nursing schools, adolescents can be selected for continued education with a view to sending them abroad later for full nurse training and nursing tutor's certificate, a process which can take up to eight years. The numbers willing to undergo long training are limited and after completion counterparts tend to leave for more attractive work. It has often happened that WHO's assistance in running training colleges, begun on a temporary basis, has had to be prolonged.

The problems of institutional training do not end when the institute has been taken over by the mother country. Differences of opinion in high quarters and between departments as to the best course of action in what is still a new and relatively unexplored field; budgetary miscalculations; staff deficiencies and many other problems, call for advice. The institute at Gondar, after being taken over by the University, was involved in disagreement with the ministry of health as to the true nature of the training to be given, and, in addition, found itself in conflict with the philosophy of the country from which, subsequent to WHO, it had accepted aid. In Somalia, after eight years of WHO aid, the whole concept of training was radically altered to its manifest detriment; the institute was converted to provide in-service courses for training hospital staff as 'pairs of hands'; open selection had given place to 'priority for government employees'. Saudi Arabia encountered difficulties in organizing field training in the Ryad, Jeddah, Huffuf and Safwa institutes established on the WHO plan.[4] For all these, and similar problems in auxiliary training institutes throughout the world, WHO, when asked, can provide consultant advice.

The subject of world health, perhaps more than any other, has a healing quality. Through discussion comes understanding. In a world torn with psychological dissension and suspicion of motives, the World Health Assembly may well be one of the vital sources of world peace.

> This is the thing, this truly is the thing.
> We dreamed it once. Now it has come about.
>
> *Edwin Muir*

19. The Limitations of Internationality in Health Affairs: an Assessment

Logistics

The World Health Assembly is an *international* public health authority; but not *supra-national*. WHO must work *for, with,* and *through* governments, each being responsible for the health of its own nationals. It has no magic remedy except goodwill and cannot do the job alone. It responds to the request for help from the countries themselves; and in consequence, its scope and usefulness depend upon the expectations, resources, and values of the countries which it serves, and which must contribute a considerable proportion of the money required. Since, except in limited fields of demonstration, it is debarred from active public health work, it functions as a catalyst to foster the development of public health services and to build up international collaboration where this is necessary to success. Or it may be likened to a wise physician with a large family of sick patients scattered over the globe, who, for the most part, must bring about their own recovery. Thus we come down immediately to earth. Health may be a fundamental right irrespective of economic or social conditions, but it is none the less dependent upon them. The nations that look to WHO for guidance will sooner or later be forced to examine their own social and economic framework. This applies to all countries, not only to the developing and underdeveloped ones.

It was therefore inevitable that WHO, as presumably any other international body, would be least successful when it put on its field boots and went out to crusade for a more effective world health structure among the nations themselves. In the quiet of its study, WHO has done a gargantuan service to mankind. This is very much the pattern, although on an improved scale, of previous international bodies. We are therefore left to ask, given that the difficulties are great, why has WHO not been more successful in promoting health within the terrains of its individual members? In an attempt to answer this question, of immense importance to the future of the movement, the following suggestions are made.

Herculean labours

The coming together of the nations has been a remarkable gesture of goodwill, but it is easy to exaggerate the extent to which it can be translated into public health practice. The budget of the organization is not large. 115 million dollars is soon spent among 3,800 million people, when eight out of ten harbour parasites, live in danger of deadly diseases, or suffer from malnutrition. The means at the disposal of WHO have been necessarily limited, and should not be over-estimated. The tasks facing WHO, even in the limited form of helping others to help themselves, have been bewildering in their complexity. Spurred on by the successes of science, with so much to do and so few facilities, there has been a constant risk of overstepping resources. Many who have studied abroad return to disillusionment and frustration. Ideal schemes evolved by experts lie neglected on the desks of administrators, overworked and harassed by massive sickness, lacking the machinery of government or education, or without the doctors, nurses, sanitarians, and teachers to put them into practice. The road to health often cannot be engineered without other social services, such as education and agriculture. Perhaps too slowly we learn that the experience of the developed world cannot easily be translated, without trial and adaptation, into practical measures in less developed areas.

So much depends upon considerations of social and economic well-being, which often bar the road to progress. Sound local units of public health, for example, may tax the resources of underdeveloped countries to the limit and can be brought about only slowly. The advice of experts achieves nothing in itself; the establishment of a statistical machine, a venereal disease or tuberculosis service, or more widely of a sound public health administrative system, is easier to talk about than to achieve. Again, public health depends much upon a knowledge of the incidence and prevalence of disease, current, reliable, and comparable, which is not easy to get, without the social structure that is part and parcel of development and which is generally lacking. Although all may agree upon common forms of collecting data, many years must elapse before this relatively simple need is satisfied. Lack of organization inhibits accuracy and in turn uncertainty reduces efficiency. It is easy to complete the circle and return to where you started.

The impact of bilateral aid*

The work of WHO is complicated by direct aid from individual governments. A UN agency has no political strings; it does not seek to enhance the prestige of any nation. It brings no financial rewards to any but the recipient of its favours. Bilateral aid differs in all these respects; it expresses political aspirations; it aims to improve the image of the donor; and it looks to exports without which it is often withheld. Bilateral aid in the field of health at best fulfils tasks better done by the international agency – as when mass campaigns are continued bilaterally after WHO has withdrawn from lack of funds, an unhappy reflection on the seriousness of international aid. At worst, it confuses by duplication and overlap – as when advice on administrative reorganization was given to a Middle Eastern country in parallel with WHO (see p. 160).

Multinational secretariat

WHO has suffered from its multinational nature and the restrictions which this places upon recruitment to its various hierarchical levels, so that excellence has sometimes given way to expediency in the choice of staff to comply with the unwritten rules of international representation.

---

* Aid has been called 'bilateral' when it operates between two governments by mutual agreement, independently of international organizations.

Political bias

The organization, as a piper, has had to play those tunes which its political masters in the Assembly were prepared to pay for, and the choice of tune often depended on prejudice and emotion rather than on a scientific approach to international health. The remarkable weapon of the mass campaign, about which much is said elsewhere (p. 162), has been used with more emotion than reason. Jenner would have been disappointed with the delay in bringing about the eradication of smallpox; ophthalmologists everywhere will have wished to see mass attacks on onchocerciasis, which causes blindness throughout the Volta river basin; and paediatricians will have regretted the long delay in applying mass techniques to the common children's diseases for which immunization has been perfected. All but the most sanguine of epidemiologists must have questioned mass campaigns against leprosy in advance of the means 'to sever the chain of causation in one relatively simple operation, or at most in a limited series of such operations repeated at intervals' (p. 163); many consider that subjects of importance, such as accidents, have been neglected for lack of emotional appeal. There was more emotion than reason in the malaria eradication scheme which at the outset won approval in the Assembly, over smallpox, for immediate action.

The flags that fly in your mind's eye from the roof of the headquarters' building, as you approach along Avenue Appia in Geneva, display all too clearly this emotional approach and the divided loyalty of the secretariat to which it has led for they are the flags of individual campaigns most dear to the hearts of member nations. The flag of *general public health,* which above all else the world needs, if it does not seek, is signally lacking. Nor is there a flag for *population limitation,* without which all else will be undone and public health lost in a 'pestilential heaping of human beings'.[32]

Hippocratic constitution

The subject of population control illustrates an essential weakness in the constitution of WHO, based as it is upon the hippocratic tradition. The subject, raised at the outset in an impassioned speech by the delegate from Norway, was ruled out of order by the Chairman, Andrija Stampar, himself probably more aware than anyone in the Assembly of the great dangers of overpopulation. WHO, to its credit, set out to study human fertility and, in a long series of technical reports from international scientific groups, it has been able to throw light on an almost completely unexplored subject (see Chapter 8, refs. 12–24). On this basis the Assembly agreed late in the 60s to offer advice on family limitation in the interests of the health of mother and child, i.e. to any nation asking for it. But the mass attack on the problem, comparable to that against malaria, has not been and, seemingly, never can be, undertaken by WHO.

Unreality

More serious perhaps has been the unreality of much of WHO's work. During the course of 25 years, its course has been shaped more by the visionary than by the practical man of affairs. Harsh ecological truths and socio-anthropological barriers to action have often been ignored.

Unreality has been WHO's chief weakness, symbolized by the malaria eradication scheme upon which money, time and effort has been unstintingly spent
in the belief, seemingly, that the basic laws of ecology and social-anthropology
would be lifted to allow a magical disappearance of the disease. Some might
say that the organization has tried to teach the underdeveloped and developing
worlds to run before being able to walk. The lessons which should have been
applied to the problems of these areas, so much in need of help, had already
been learnt by the developed world, particularly those countries in the Anglo-
Saxon orbit, where the health problems 150 years ago had been much the
same as those to be found in the underdeveloped world today. The chief lesson
was that much could be done to deal with a host of environmental hazards by
relatively simple means. The first need was for a 'vehicle', (infrastructure of
health, see Chapter 20) through which to apply preventive techniques. Once
created, it could be staffed by auxiliaries, with relatively little basic education,
'in-service trained' for supervising construction of privies, protecting water
supplies, collecting vital statistics, controlling insects, ensuring cleanliness in
food handling and preparation, effecting immunization etc. In the course of
150 years scientific weapons had immeasurably advanced both in range and
effectiveness. It must have been clear that the underdeveloped and developing
worlds needed just such a machine, with teams of auxiliaries, some 'institution
trained', but mainly trained 'in-service', directed from district, regional and provincial levels by experienced medical epidemiologists.

It is ironical that WHO gave of its best in a gigantic effort to create an effective
machine for the eradication of one particular disease, malaria, but signally
failed to do the same for the whole of public health, dealing with the numerically, and significantly, greater burden of disease.

WHO's obsession with mass campaigns should have been paralleled by at
least an equal concern for general public health. In the first place mass campaigns,with their military precision, concentration on a single end, and highly
scientific basis, could not act alone, nor necessarily, if left to themselves, would
they be lasting in their effects; and where successful, they would leave a multitude of other problems unanswered. Penicillin can cure yaws, bejel and pinta,
rife in Africa, the Near East, and South America; chlorinated hydrocarbons
of various kinds can kill many of the insect vectors and so help to abolish
malaria, typhus, and other insect-borne diseases; BCG vaccination may well
do the same for tuberculosis. This is a dazzling prospect for newcomers to
public health. Not for them, or so the uninitiated think, the hard road of sanitary
reform, along which Edwin Chadwick drove his people during the last century.
People may live in over crowded hovels where the tubercle bacillus thrives and
yet, it is thought, be saved by BCG. In a world where 1,900 million lived in
malarial regions, and nearly half as many under threat of yaws, the hand seemed
inexorably to reach, metaphorically speaking, for the DDT spray and the
penicillin syringe. It was a temptation to throw into such campaigns of eradication a large part of the slender resources of the organization. But when the
jeeps left, habits remained, and we have, sadly perhaps, to accept that health in
any community cannot be entirely secured with a syringe or a dusting machine.

When DDT spraying is discontinued and the penicillin umbrella withdrawn, there remains the everpresent risk of renewal by importation from outside or by transmission from uncontrolled residues within; these risks can only be met by traditional public health epidemiology.

Second, mass campaigns, although of tremendous significance to the world, have, in terms of the wide spectrum of human illness, a relatively limited field of action. The great bulk of disease and ill-health is in fact outside the scope of the mass campaign, including nutritional, viral, bacterial, protozoal, helminthic and fungus diseases within the field of primary prevention and practically the whole field of secondary prevention (Conference on the application of science and technology for the benefit of less developed areas).[36] All such can be combated only by traditional methods of public health.

It was equally obvious that in the operation of such an infrastructure of health, doctors trained in the traditional medical schools of the developed world, clinically orientated and ill-equipped to direct auxiliaries trained for house to house work, were likely to be more of a hindrance than a help. Waiting for sufferers to attend at health centres could never be more than a partial answer to the abundance of disease due to faults in the environment, which distinguished the underdeveloped from the developed world in the mid-twentieth century.

Administrative direction of the health infrastructure at district, group, regional and central levels, by doctors sufficiently versed in the art of social and preventive medicine, provided an equal challenge. Doctors trained as undergraduates in traditional medical schools inevitably proved singularly ineffectual. *Creating the infrastructure and training doctors and auxiliaries to work in it called urgently for attention, possibly before all else.*

The same failure to deal with essentials can be seen in WHO's relative unconcern about the problems of collecting data at ground level. The means to obtain data about disease and death in the underdeveloped world, where doctors were few and far between, were almost universally lacking. When health planning depended upon valid data, if it was not to work in the dark, an effective alternative to medical certification had to be found. When doctors didn't exist, or, as generally, crowded into the towns leaving the countryside to its own devices, everything depended upon training auxiliaries for the work. For this they need an abbreviated code of diseases, easily understandable and unambiguous. For want of this relatively simple instrument, basic data has been left at the mercy of the ignorant and illiterate.

Lack of understanding and undue waste

The reasons for the failure of WHO to give priority to the infrastructure for general public health are not far to seek. Perhaps the most significant was the failure of many world leaders at the time WHO was created, to appreciate the full implications of such a fundamental need. The developed world had itself not universally developed this facility, leaving health problems to be resolved by rising standards in social and economic development. Some members of the Assembly, and even heads of departments in the organization itself, had no clear idea of what was meant by an epidemiological approach to all disease under the direction of doctors with special training in the problems of health in a community. Second there was the time factor. This type of infrastructure for general public health cannot be brought about by methods applicable to mass campaigns, since it requires time for changes in habits, for the development of discipline and for growth and development in government and social affairs. To have made this the first plank in the platform would have meant that WHO accepted that the health problems of the underdeveloped world were not to be immediately resolved by their own dramatic intervention; and this did not suit the mood of the Assembly. Had a substantial fraction of the enormous sums spent on malaria been expended in establishing permanent general public health services the world might be a healthier place today.*

Failure to appreciate the significance of general public health and undue haste to do doughty deeds has in turn led to lack of co-ordination. Sectional interests have held sway rather than an overall concern for health plans, designed to meet total needs of each individual country. Projects have tended to proliferate and to self-perpetuation. As Richard Jackson said in his study of the capacity of the United Nations development system,[17] 'programmes do not reflect real needs of developing countries', depending more upon 'agency salesmanship' than on priorities.

Bureaucracy

WHO, by its regional structure, has escaped many of the disabilities of undue centralization, which its member states too often display, but not altogether those inherent in any organization which, as the years pass, slows in its movements and stiffens at the joints. Richard Jackson said that the UN with its specialized agencies was a 'disproportionately old and bureaucratic organization' with 'a bureaucratic undergrowth which strangles action'. From this he inferred that the organization was 'incapable of controlling itself' and 'in the strictest sense of the word unmanageable'. WHO, as one of the UN's most distinguished 'specialized agencies', cannot escape these strictures. The secretariat has multiplied according to Parkinson's Law and gives the appearance of sinking beneath a weight of paper, sufficient, in some countries with an overloaded post mail, to be recycled without distribution. Too often verbiage befogs meaning and jargon clothes the obvious with spurious importance. Projects are 'impact orientated', when, if undertaken at all by a responsible organization, they should be 'effective' by unspoken rule. Prolixity numbs the senses into a false sense of purpose and calls urgently for Sir Ernest Gowers' *Plain Words*,[14] the syllogism of Macaulay and the perfectionism of Balzac. Like many organizations grown to maturity, WHO has come to live too greatly for itself, multiplying special units according to bureaucratic whim, so that the sight of the wood is lost in the trees.

A beginning has been made, nothing more; the goal of mental, physical, and social health for all mankind lies far ahead. But WHO, with its limitations and imperfections, represents the belief that mankind can escape from ill-health to a better life, and that scientific knowledge is international.

* Expenditure on malaria, in the years 1964 to 1969, amounted to between one sixth and one seventh of the total budget; after this it declined to about one fourteenth in 1973.

Part Six: A Permanent Framework for General Public Health for Underdeveloped and Developing Countries

20. The Creation of a Public Health Structure

General principles

It is not easy to find in the study of public health practice any set of principles which can be generally applicable in the establishment of a *permanent framework*. What works well in one country may fail in another. Unification or diversification, centralization or decentralization, state or voluntary agency, whole-time or part-time health officers, have all in different ways caught the imagination of able rulers.

The ideas about the administration and organization of public health, which have been growing in recent years may not, and indeed cannot, be generally applicable in a world in which geography, needs and customs vary so greatly, but they help in a critical analysis of existing services and in the establishment of new ones.

Four concepts concerning the permanent framework have had general agreement and should be aimed at in all countries:

1. *The need to give preventive medicine primacy in administration*

It has been said that 'primacy of preventive medicine is to be maintained by having health-minded rather than disease-minded persons responsible for overall planning and the direction and allocation of community resources' (Grant, 1947).[15] Where the hospital has been included in the administration this offers the best opportunity of preventing hospitals from becoming autonomous, with uncontrolled vested interests in curative medicine. It is the health officer rather than the hospital officer who should plan.

2. *The need for unity or control*

It has been said that 'when a special function is to be undertaken, it shall be undertaken by one governing body of the whole community needing the service';[15] again: 'developments in public health make it essential to co-ordinate all measures of prevention, care, and restoration under one system of health service' (WHO 1952).[21]

One system covering all functions which influence health in a community may be impracticable. But the three services which come within the immediate sphere of the doctor, hospitals, medical care by the general practitioner and public health, can be administered together. This measure of unity should always be sought despite the obvious danger of too great emphasis being laid upon hospital care, 'when preventive medicine often receives meagre attention'.

Even under one system of administration careful attention must always be given to the way in which different parts of the service work together. Lack of coordination in central and local departments, inadequate working arrangements between hospitals, general practitioners and public health, disjointed efforts by voluntary bodies, are everywhere limiting factors. It is not unknown for one organization to be undoing the work of another. There are many answers to this particular world-wide problem, but none is a sovereign remedy. Perhaps the most effective is the well-trained health officer, operating at central, provincial, and local levels, who can work effectively in the field of human relations. Some part of the answer lies in a clearer definition of functions as between authorities and at different levels.[21]

3. *The need to unify curative and preventive medicine*
  The Dawson Committee in Britain said in 1920:

> Preventive and curative medicine cannot be separated on any sound principle, and in any scheme of medical services must be brought together in close coordination. They must likewise be brought within the sphere of the general practitioner whose activities should embrace the work of communal as well as individual medicine.[16]

The linking of curative and preventive medicine is of importance both in hospital and in field work. Its most important expression is in relation to the work of the general practitioner in the health centre, where medical care, based on the family unit, can go hand in hand with health promotion, prophylaxis, health education, rehabilitation and 'the stimulation of local interest in public health'.

Half a century after Lord Dawson of Penn chaired the committee which made this pronouncement, it has to be admitted that the marriage of preventive and curative medicine at the level of the health centre has not so far greatly advanced the cause of prevention throughout the underdeveloped and developing worlds. The greatest difficulty, from the point of view of prevention, has lain in the excess of illness which presents in most of the developing world. This swamps preventive work and health centres, e.g. those initially established in Turkey[5] function chiefly at the level of dispensaries. A further considerable handicap has been the difficulty which many nations have found in providing those general practitioners who are to work in health centres, with the necessary postgraduate training in social and preventive medicine to enable them to undertake preventive programmes successfully. The adaptation of mass campaign techniques to operate from health centres, with skilled direction from higher levels, now points the way to further advance (see p. 192). As part of such a development, mobile teams for home visiting, by medication for intestinal infections and infestations and other devices, can reduce the volume of sickness which overburdens the centres.

4. *The need for local government*
  The development of some form of local government is essential in a *permanent framework*. As Haven Emerson said (1948)[14]: 'The health of the nation is based on the competent performance of established health functions at the local level of government, where local initiative, responsibility and resources are involved by the power of local public opinion'. Weir in his analysis of rural problems in Egypt, interpreting the same philosophy, pointed to the needs

among economically depressed and illiterate populations for autonomy of action at the village level, with village councils.[20]

Such local bodies must have legal backing. Public health thrives on the support of the people, but also calls for sanctions. Some of India's community projects, begun with enthusiasm, fell away for lack of legal enforcement. The evaluation report of 1954 said 'the keeping of the wells clean was seen to be indifferently cared for' and 'the advent of the monsoon was marked by an outbreak of cholera'. When 'a small fee was proposed' for maintaining the spraying of DDT, few would have it.[18] These findings, the report said, underlined the need 'for making statutory bodies responsible for maintaining such services'.

The need for local government, as an essential component of the infrastructure of health, is one of the chief reasons why the establishment of a permanent framework is both slow and difficult. This fact, added to others discussed in the *limitations of internationality* (p. 179), is one of the reasons for WHO's preference for mass campaigns, which it could organize without involvement in local politics.

Local boards of a sophisticated character exist in the developed world, either 'elected' by public franchise, spending money mainly collected locally, as in Britain,* or 'selected' by the government and spending money allocated from central funds, as in parts of the USA and various countries in Europe. Local government in these sophisticated forms is not easy to create, depending, as it does, on the slow evolution of education and social awareness. The less developed must rest content with local boards which constitute the peripheral organ of a centralized machine, with delegated powers and relatively little autonomy.

It is the continued existence of this simpler form of local health organization which makes it necessary to define, and distinguish clearly between, the functions to be performed at the centre and those which must be left to the periphery; for it is only when this distinction has been grasped that proper delegation of powers can be brought about. The importance of this aspect can be seen in the many statements made in recent years emphasising the need to distinguish between the functions to be performed by the ministry of health and those which lie elsewhere in provincial, regional or district offices. Shubbar Hasan said about Jordan:

Distinction is not made by the Ministry of Health between matters of principle and policy on the one hand, and routine administrative operations on the other.[23]

The rest of this chapter is devoted to setting out the principles upon which such definition and distinction of functions should be made; outlining the nature of the work to be performed when a proper division of duties has been made; and examining the vital question of how to staff the permanent framework of Public Health.

---

* The reorganization of health services in the U.K., referred to on p. 121, has limited the involvement of 'elected' councils to matters of environmental hygiene; all personal health services being, in 1974, united in the jurisdiction of 'selected' boards.

Central health administration

The functions of the central authority should be strictly limited to high policy matters, programmes, plans and budgets, technical guidance and accountability. The centre should limit its activities in policy making to matters concerning the whole country, i.e. major departures from protocol, capital expenditure and appointments of high level staff. It should assess efficacy, efficiency and suitability of all that is being done in the regions, with inspections and continual re-appraisal; and above all, it should plan and count the cost. In Jordan consultants in public health administration recommended a maximum degree of decentralization with 'centralized control through reports, periodic inspections, audit procedures, performance evaluations, programme budgets etc.'[27]

Planning

The first and immediate need is for a *health plan*. The range of possible developments in the field of health is so great, while resources are so limited, that developing countries find themselves in constant danger of muddle and frustration resulting from unplanned activities. Confusion repercusses throughout the services; for those away from the national controls, working in hospital or in the field, with little if any power to guide events, it is frustrating to witness plans go awry, services halting and monies spent overgenerously here and niggardly there. The permanent framework can come about *effectively* only as part of a National Health Plan, scientifically designed, economically sound.[30] The health plan should ensure:

1. that a balance is struck between curative and preventive medicine. This alone will make possible the development of a health infrastructure and also ensure a balance between care for in-patients and of sickness in the home.

2. that the priority of certain diseases, age groups and occupational groups be decided upon and used as a firm guide to action.

3. that the most economical instruments (staff and materials) be chosen to meet the objectives.

As Socrates Litsios has said: 'the health plan must be periodically "evaluated" to determine effectiveness and relevance'.[31]

All programmes must be related to needs and cost and they can never be more than a compromise between what a nation would like and what it can afford. Year in year out, choices have to be made, e.g. between services for home care or hospitals. The most striking deficiency in most administrative arrangements is lack of planning and inadequate costing. It is sometimes difficult to see why particular hospitals have been built; why some services have been developed and others neglected; why little is done to prevent a disease, such as kwashiorkor, while providing facilities for its treatment in hospital. It is manifestly unsound to establish a hospital system to care for illness that need never have occured. The infrastructure which gives the means to tackle public health problems at the point of origin, should be given high priority in all planning. It should come before hospitals or at least in parallel with them. The underdeveloped world, harassed by sickness, may rush too easily to hospital construction. Hospitals will not eradicate infestations with worms, which lower the stamina of millions, will not stem the onset of kwashiorkor with its frightening hazards for child life, nor will they prevent rickets in the sun-drenched lands of the Middle East. It requires great wisdom to follow the lead of Professor Stampar in establishing *institutes of hygiene* and *health centres*, as he did throughout the republic of Croatia. But those who do reap a rich reward. Britain in the last century, when the health picture was little better than that of the underdeveloped world today, did not build hospitals, except as a by-product of charitable activity. It built drains and set up public health departments, under the lash of Chadwick's whip. It is undeniable that the infrastructure of health throughout most of the developing world is weak and calling urgently for improvement, much more immediately than hospital construction. Consisting of simple buildings, this infrastructure can be brought into existence at relatively little cost, and, with determination, foresight and planning, rests within the capacity of every country.

The existence of a national plan carefully costed is essential to all training schemes, so that students when graduated can fit into the appropriate part of the service for which they have been trained. When this is not so, as with auxiliaries in Somalia (1968),[8] the results are lamentable. The building of the infrastructure consisting of health centres and health posts, needs to be synchronized with the training of teams of professional and auxiliary workers to staff them; their relationship to existing 'in-service' personnel must be settled in advance; and one part of the service must not be unduly developed at the expense of another.

The national plan is often indefinite or incomplete, so that it undergoes changes which upset the the original balance, leading to curtailment or even postponement. Budgetary overstrain can be disastrous, as was the case in Somalia,[8] where hospital construction, with direct aid from several countries, absorbed all available funds. Not only should the plan be within the resources of the country, but it must allocate funds equitably between hospitals and the field infrastructure. In view of the great importance of training in all developing countries, the cost of staff should be estimated, making allowance for yearly increases, which improving education and better supply of teachers make possible. Planning should be a major function of all sections of the central authority and each director of a division plan for his own services each year.

One reason for failure to plan may lie in the absence of any senior person specifically charged with the function of planning in an understaffed headquarters; or it may be that no doctor on the central staff has the training needed for examining the phenomena of disease in the mass.

Planning and administration call for special training in the principles of the subjects involved, particularly epidemiology and sociology. For this purpose postgraduate courses must be established for the training of a sufficient number of physicians to run the country's services.[28] As an interim measure intensive in-service courses can be organized in most countries (see p. 202).

A *planning committee* is needed within the ministry itself 'to develop health policies within the framework of present and new enabling legislation and to draft plans for their implementation.[27] This should have a statutory composition, meet at fixed intervals under the chairmanship of the chief of the department or the minister of health, and be required to decide priorities within the total budget. To avoid later opportunist adjustments to the plan, it should be changed, if accepted by the minister, only after reconsideration by the planning committee in formal session.

A *council of health*, with statutory rights and duties, will be needed as an external committee to advise both the minister and the planning committee. Such a committee is more than a 'meeting of minds' within the ministry itself; it involves doctors, nurses, and other health workers *from outside the ministry* and it gives a chance for the voices of the profession to be heard in matters affecting health affairs generally, about which they feel strongly and in which their opinions can help to keep plans, programmes and budgets in balance with reality. Service on the council should be statutory with fixed seats changing annually. It should elect its own chairman, meet at regular prescribed intervals, and report direct to the minister through the secretary, who might be the chief of the department. Its views cannot be binding on the minister, but none-the-less they can help to strengthen and coordinate the services.

A *central planning body* with representation from other ministries is also needed to plan all the services in unison. This is a much wider issue. Health planning must 'form part of a rational organization and deployment of national resources',[30] so that it becomes 'an integral part of economic and social development'. Only in this way can the health plan be realized against the background of the realities of national development. In this way, for example, the education services can work in harmony with the health services, designing courses and recruiting students in higher education in terms of the immediate priorities and practical possibilities of the health plan.

Where the infrastructure of education is in advance of other community developments, as in Jordan[11] (see p. 209) adolescents can be frustrated for want of opportunities of further education or advancement. The infrastructure of health, if developed concurrently, would help to solve this difficulty. Where two central departments, as in Spain (Direccion General de Sanidad and Seguridad Social) are each developing services for hospitals and general medical care, it is impossible to avoid overlap and duplication. Of this, it was said in 1967: 'it is most important to eliminate without delay the artificial divisions separating the two services'.[4] To meet these and many similar issues, a central planning authority can draw up a national plan of community development, formulating coordinated schemes, getting agreement of political heads, and periodically evaluating the plan.

The Chief Medical Officer, or permanent under-secretary, is ultimately responsible for formulating proposals for his department to go forward to the minister. He should write annually an account of the health of his country in which he will consider the main problems, social, industrial, economic, environmental, which it has to face. He should hold meetings of professional staff and seek, by reports and visits, to obtain first hand knowledge. Professional meetings give the opportunity to learn what those working in the field are experiencing and to impart the general lines of policy. Meetings with regional medical officers, nurses, midwives, sanitarians and hospital staff can do much to further the work of the department and should be held at fixed intervals with a formal agenda.

Control from the centre over the work of the peripheral infrastructure may be helped by the creation of a division of 'field service operations' or 'district affairs'. This gives a direct line of communication to the periphery for all important matters of policy. The medical director of such a division must be able to handle all matters, preventive and curative, on behalf of the chief medical officer, calling in other sections for consultation.

A strong clear and well informed leadership by the chief medical officer is only possible with *delegation* within the ministry itself. The chief must be able to confine his work to a small fraction of the total administrative business. Directors of divisions, with full delegated powers, should refer for his consideration only such matters as need his specific authority, and then 'with full documentation', i.e. with all relevant data and proposals for action.

Professional staff (doctors, nurses, pharmacists, midwives, dentists) working in the central office should be given full authority to communicate on professional matters, directly and in their own names, with colleagues in the infrastructure.

The chief medical officer's relationship with his political head varies with the state of development and philosophy of the country. Executive power tends to be concentrated in political hands in developing countries, with the advantages of speedy decisions and the disadvantage of lack of continuity in a changing political scene. With increasing development and complexity of services, the advantage lies in giving administrative control of day-to-day affairs to the chief medical officer, and retaining to the minister the task of interpretating the policies of his department to the government and of securing an effective allocation of monies. In this event the chief medical officer acts as the highest civil service authority and the penultimate in matters of high policy, programmes, plans, budgets, technical guidance, and accountability. He gives continuity in the changing political scene.

Peripheral health administration*

An effective infrastructure for health must be woven like a fabric throughout the nation. In this fabric the hospital, albeit indispensable, is only an element, part of a wider whole, within which a team of professional workers is deployed into the heart and home of the people. The infrastructure of health has been defined as *'the organized collection of peripheral units capable of providing certain basic health services ... to cater for the most urgent needs of the population'*.[34] It is the most peripheral viable organ of administration; designed to undertake day-to-day activities in the field, both curative and preventive, under the direction, with varying degrees of autonomy, of higher policy-making bodies. It consists of *groups of local health units* (as in Fig. 20.1) each covering

* The functions of the health infrastructure are well described in 'Basic Health Services', a joint UNICEF/WHO document (1965).[19]

G*

say 250,000 people; 4 groups constituting a *district* and 5 districts a *region*.

Within the group, each *local health unit* (perhaps 50 to 100 thousand people) is designed to provide basic health services for its area.

Local health units can best coincide with the boundaries of local government in other matters, but care must be taken to find means of overcoming the limitations which arise from the use of local government areas, as the scope and sophistication of public health services advance (note the difficulties in USA and UK p. 124).

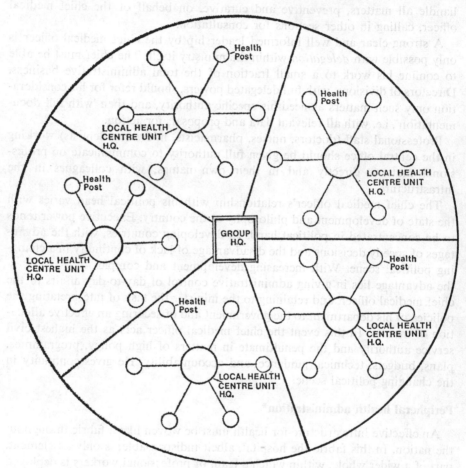

Fig. 20.1 Health infrastructure; peripheral unit. A group of five local health units, approximate population 250,000.

The infrastructure of health should be directed by a physician with postgraduate training in epidemiology, sociology and administration, variously styled director of health, health officer or medical officer of health; he should be an expert in the organization of health services with special consideration for prevention and promotion of health in the community.

Few countries have found it easy to train sufficient doctors for this delicate work. Generally speaking, this difficulty is so great that it is impractical to use doctors for direction below the district level, i.e. one million; for groups, i.e. 250,000 and for the local health unit itself, i.e. 50,000, it is best to think in terms of direction by auxiliaries with special training in the elements of epidemiology. The local health unit, through which the day-to-day activities will be conducted, must look for much of its motive force – as for planning, technical advice, finance, hospitals, laboratory services, research, special services for eradication – to the group, district and regional levels of the infrastructure. Control over its day-to-day activities, to ensure steady progress and a fair measure of uniformity over the region as a whole, can be ensured by visits of inspection from higher levels, by grants-in-aid, and other financial devices.

Health centres

Each local health unit should have at least one health centre staffed with physician, nurse, sanitary inspector and auxiliary helpers; satellite health posts, covering villages or groups of villages can be staffed by an auxiliary nurse or midwife for multipurpose functions (see p. 208). The health centre will be concerned with conditions not requiring hospital care, the relationship being directly with home and family, with *continuing* medical and nursing care in the health centre and at home, and with care in childbirth by midwives or by village women with in-service training. Care should be based on attention to social factors in the home, at school and at work and, through the confidence engendered, it can provide the atmosphere most conducive to health education. Preventive services in maternal and child health, school health, industrial health and in the control of infections and animal borne disease should be based on the centre and closely related to clinical care. Health centres should be responsible for collecting and validating the basic vital and health data, which is indispensable for national planning. In the case of non-medically certified deaths and infections, visits to the home by specially trained auxiliaries will be needed. Instruction in the use of the international death certificate and an abbreviated code of causes of death and disease (see appx 6) are essential for validity and objectivity. Schemes of data collection will need supervision from district level. For fuller discussion of the statistical needs of underdeveloped countries (see Chapter 29).

Prevention of disease

It is to the infrastructure that we must look for the means to prevent illness and to remedy abuses in the environment which are the cause of so much illness throughout the underdeveloped world. With present knowledge most of this disease could be prevented, if the means could be found to 'deliver' the wide range of preventive techniques, some long established but many of recent date, which we now possess. Nothing illustrates better the need to apply knowledge which we already have than the continued existence of diseases due to faulty sanitation. In some areas, 50 per cent of prevalent disease can be ascribed to this cause (see Chapter 3). Pure water supplies, hygienic disposal of human waste; cleanliness in food handling, good ventilation and the avoidance of overcrowding have all been shown, by bitter experience in the developed world, to be overriding considerations. These needs call for the lessons of environmental hygiene at the level of village neighbourhood and home. We possess the means to immunize children against most common and often lethal infections of childhood. We have developed the mass campaign to a fine art, and this could be put to use in the infrastructure, not as a time limited temporary expedient, but as a continuing process, in a setting where passive detection, as a natural development of clinical care, would reinforce consolidation and maintenance. When seen in this light, it is difficult not to regret the years which have passed without the establishment of permanent infrastructures of health in those regions of the world where public health has come so late on the scene.

It is no longer a question of 'give us the tools'; we have the means; what we need is the facility to bring them to bear. It is this aspect of prevention which presents the greatest difficulty. As Cockburn has said about immunization; 'it is necessary to look for the means of 'delivering' ... and 'the development of such means is not simple and straightforward'.[13] The health centre, as we have seen earlier, tends to become inundated with sick people and to revert to a dispensary, with little time or inclination for undertaking purposeful and dynamic schemes of prevention. The physicians practising in the centres rarely have sufficient training in social and preventive work to enable them to supervise such operations. For this work some form of postgraduate training in an institute of community medicine (see p. 202) is essential and few countries have been able to organize such courses.

Mobile teams

The solution to the problem of providing dynamic schemes of prevention lies in the establishment of mobile teams of auxiliaries to work from health centres under team leaders, with supervision and technical guidance from group and district levels. The basis of this work will lie in *home visiting*.

Collection of specimens for surveys, and of vital and health data, reporting infections and pregnancies, following up cases, census taking, first aid and much general sanitary work, all call, in one way or another, for home visiting. Duties in general sanitation can include latrine construction and supervision, insect control and disinfestation. First aid in the home can include medication for diarrhoea and parasites; vaccination against smallpox and oral vaccines against poliomyelitis; field work in the control of intestinal parasites; application of ointment in trachoma; and follow-up of leprosy and tuberculosis. Detection, surveillance, supervision, contact tracing and home treatment for all diseases which are the subject of mass campaigns, call for house to house visiting. The great bulk of the work of mass campaigns can be handled by multipurpose visitors working from the health centre or health post, trained to recognize trachoma in its various forms, early cases of leprosy, minor manifestations of yaws; who can make house to house enquiries for fevers which might be malarial, take smears for the examination of malaria parasites, and supervise the treatment of trachoma by teachers, parents, older children and other selected lay workers – subject to the confirmation of diagnosis, state of development and supervision of treatment by experts at higher levels.

Home visiting must also play a part, perhaps the most important rôle, in countering the upsurge in population by teaching the importance, as part of a general programme of public health, of *limiting the family*.

Although some preventive schemes will need to be concerned with one particular problem, there is much to be said for conducting home visiting programmes by means of multi-purpose auxiliaries, in which form home visiting can be more acceptable, less disturbing and in many ways more efficient. A coordinated approach makes it easier to deal with defaulters and to overcome resistance to public health work. In trachoma campaigns, non-attenders often come from poorer and more trachomatous families and may be more easily discovered when a home visitor covers all or most of the field work; and visits for *any* purpose can provide a useful check on the ophthalmic state of the family. Visits to advise mother and child may be used to follow up tuberculosis, or detect fever as an indication of incipient malaria.

Home visiting on this scale, particularly when it includes simple techniques for dealing with worm infestations and intestinal infections can do much to relieve health centres of the excessive burden of sickness, which turns them into dispensaries for the sick.

Involvement of the people

Health programmes can be truly effective only with the understanding, support and participation of the people. Without these, as so many authorities have said, no lasting advances in public health can be made.

This is a chief reason why the infrastructure should be part of local government which involves important members of the community in the solution of their own problems. *Health cannot be imposed upon a people; it has to be won in partnership with them.*

To this end an infrastructure of health, properly staffed, has much to offer, since it brings public health down to the people. This it does in 4 ways:

1. It demonstrates that continuous oversight by a health officer and staff is capable of building up protective measures and that these can be maintained against adverse influences.

2. It stimulates voluntary effort, indispensable to development of health services. In its simplest form villagers can be trained for simple tasks and self help. The more sophisticated can take part in government and social activities; such involvement takes many forms – local government by election in Britain, social participation of public and doctors in Scandinavia, soviets in the USSR, voluntary councils in America, village committees in India, and no doubt in a variety of other ways.

3. It is the ideal means to promote health education and to enlarge understanding thereby.

4. It creates among the health staff themselves a greater understanding and sympathy for folklore and customs and by so doing greatly increases their ability to practice their various skills successfully.

Levels of infrastructure

Five levels of infrastructure can be distinguished in different parts of the world:

Grade 0. Little or nothing in the form of service below the level of central ministry or region (e.g., Liberia or Mauritania).

Grade 1. A rudimentary network of treatment points or dispensaries, without social or preventive functions, generally linked to a distant district hospital. Epidemiological cover is lacking and supervision is by hospital clinicians without post-graduate training in public health (e.g., Togoland).

Grade 2. A system of 'health posts' or 'district sub-centres', grouped under a health officer at the district level. The health officer is usually engaged in private medical practice and the health posts are manned by auxiliaries with the possible addition of a midwife (e.g., Nepal).

Grade 3. A system similar to the above, but with a whole-time health officer at the level of the district and with 'health centres' covering 1 to 3 hundred thousand population. The 'health centres' contain auxiliaries, para-medical workers, nurses and general medical practitioners; they have a number of 'health posts' or 'district sub-centres', say 10 to 15, dependent upon them for supervision (e.g., India).

Grade 4. A system of whole-time health officers at the level of the 'group' (250,000) or the 'local health unit' (50–100,000) with a full complement of general medical practitioners, health visitors, midwives, social workers, etc. Health centres and district sub-centres may or may not exist in the developed countries.

A minimum infrastructure for general public health should lie somewhere between grades 3 and 4.

Common failings in the infrastructure

Public health in the form made possible by such an infrastructure has enduring qualities, covering a wide spectrum of disease; not solely that capable of attack by mass campaign, but attacking root causes, involving people in their own health problems, uniting preventive and curative medicine, coordinating home visiting, and dealing with both primary and secondary prevention. But the great possibilities which it has to offer are at the mercy of two common failings which, once a satisfactory infrastructure has been established, can gravely limit its success. These are 1. *inability or unwillingness to integrate special schemes for individual diseases with general public health in the health centres* (see mass campaigns p. 168) and 2. *failure to delegate adequately from centre to periphery*. These important aspects will be dealt with in detail in the following pages.

Integration of mass campaigns

Integration of mass campaigns into the permanent infrastructure of health is best achieved, as now shown to be possible in the smallpox eradication scheme and in the development of immunization against the common childhood diseases, *at the outset* by making use *to the greatest extent possible* of the existing health centres. The campaign direction remains in the hands of experts at district, regional and central levels, with teams of auxiliaries recruited and based upon health centres for field work. Such a marriage of mass techniques with the permanent health infrastructure *from the outset* disposes of many of the problems which have arisen from dichotomy and, as it now represents the official policy of WHO, should lead to greater harmony in future between the two forms of public health.

The problems of integration which are discussed in this section, therefore, relate to schemes which have been developed over the past years and which have resulted in two types of administrative structure unrelated to each other.

Special schemes for public health relating to individual diseases, or to vulnerable groups of the population, show a natural desire to continue to operate independently, directing their own affairs and employing their own staff. Nevertheless, integration with public health in a well established infrastructure is essential if the benefits of coordination are to be secured. This applies particularly to auxiliaries trained to operate in single purpose campaigns, against yaws, leprosy and particularly malaria which too often continue to work independently.

Integration[24, 25, 26] can take two forms, a fusion of the field work of more than one single purpose campaign, and a fusion of malaria and other single purpose campaigns with general public health.

Fusion of single purpose campaigns presents no more difficulty than that inherent in the rival power complexes of the hierarchy. The skills involved in various types of mass campaigns require much the same level of in-service training and education. In contrast, the fusion of mass campaigns with general public health, poses more delicate questions; the adequacy of infrastructures, notably in the case of malaria, is brought into question; in particular the dangers inherent in lowering standards of surveillance, of exacerbation in areas of freedom and of epidemic return in areas of consolidation.

The fear of losing hard won freedom from malaria has often determined governments to operate malaria services independently, even after a permanent public health service, capable of handling all mass campaigns, has come into being. This was the case in Ethiopia in 1969 when funds necessary for the development of the infrastructure were absorbed in maintaining malaria eradication services, directed by agricultural experts, in regions already staffed by health officers trained in general public health at the institute in Gondar.[7]

Malaria services, based upon house-to-house visitation are themselves well designed to undertake general public health. In Turkey, where malaria teams covered 95 per cent of the country, integration could be seen to provide an immediate and effective service of house-to-house visiting, undertaking a wide range of basic public health. It was said that integration would have enormous advantages 'not only for public health, but also for malaria surveillance[5] in that it would maintain an adequate malaria service when the consolidation phase had been reached and add the advantage of passive detection by health centre staff', and further that 'nothing found in general public health, not even the village midwife, achieves such regular, systematic and intimate contact with households'. Malaria surveillance officers, supervised by district heads, with weekly and monthly programmes, have been shown to be capable, despite low standards of education, of undertaking a wide range of duties involving visits to the home. In the Mersin province of Turkey, under the enthusiastic leadership of Dr Hayri Hanlioglu, the malaria surveillance officers were trained to do all the ground level work and this was done 'with the support and appreciation of the people'.[5]

Integration, therefore, has much to offer to public health. In Turkey, it was said that 'many of the grave and intractable health problems of the country could best be dealt with by incorporating the malaria service into general public health'. But from the point of view of malaria surveillance, integration cannot be satisfactorily achieved unless a sufficiently strong health infrastructure exists. An impeccable machine for case detection involves an infrastructure not less than grade 3.[24] Simpler types of infrastructure can cooperate with mass campaigns, but they cannot be relied upon to take over consolidation and maintenance.

The difficulties of effecting a take-over owing to inadequacies of the infrastructure, can be met in two ways:

1. *Where little or no infrastructure exists* or only a rudimentary network of dispensaries without health officers at district level, general practitioners in health centres, or sufficient auxiliaries for home visiting (as in Liberia or Togoland), by first undertaking *pre-eradication programmes.*[22] This is easier said than done, since a pre-eradication programme involves the building of a sufficient infrastructure where little or none exists, seeking to accomplish rapidly what should have been in the process of growth from the outset. At this level of infrastructure, it would be more realistic for a well developed malaria service to take over general public health than vice versa. None-the-less the pre-eradication philosophy at least recognizes the reality of the situation and calls attention to the fundamental need to develop a permanent general public health infrastructure.

2. *Where infrastructures of at least grade 2 exist,* integration can be brought about by a two stage operation. The first step will be to bring about integration *at the periphery* in a single local health unit, or in a group (see Fig. 20.2). Sufficient time must be allowed for in-service training of staff, both those to engage in a wider range of field work and those who are to direct the new service at provincial, regional, district and group headquarters.

Public health directors, who are to take on malaria surveillance, will need in-service training in a malaria institute. Malaria directors, who will enter the general public health service at any level will need training, in the principles of epidemiology, sociology, and administration, in short courses in the school of public health, or in a community medicine institute (see p. 202).

For the field work, either the staff of the infrastructure is trained in-service to take on additional duties of malaria surveillance; or malaria surveillance officers can be trained to extend house-to-house visits to include general public health duties; or a combination of both. The process of taking on new functions should be arranged step by step. Where the malaria surveillance staff are used

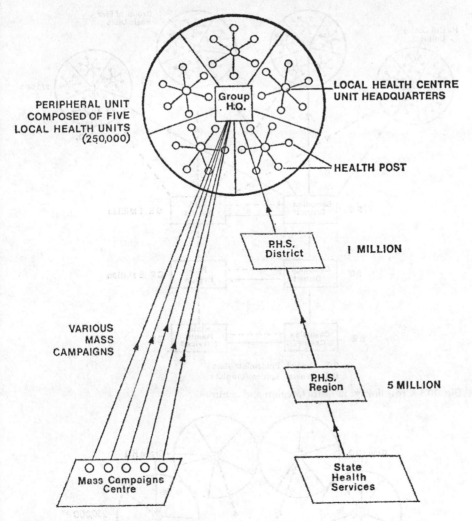

Fig. 20.2 Take-over by peripheral unit.

the *long term aim* should be to replace the field workers with auxiliary nurses, and the district supervisors by male professional nurses.

The second stage, as shown in Figures 20.2, 20.3, 20.4 and 20.5, involves transfer of control in the hierarchical structure at different levels up to the centre. This should be done gradually with formal decisions based on local study before each successive step.

Prior to integration crosslinkage should be established at each level of command; so that counterparts in the permanent service are established and trained in preparation for the final transfer. At the level of the district (1 million) the special epidemiologist will hand over to a general epidemiologist (or health officer); at higher levels, i.e. region and centre, special epidemiologists will almost certainly need to be retained for an unspecified period of time and, indeed, possibly permanently.

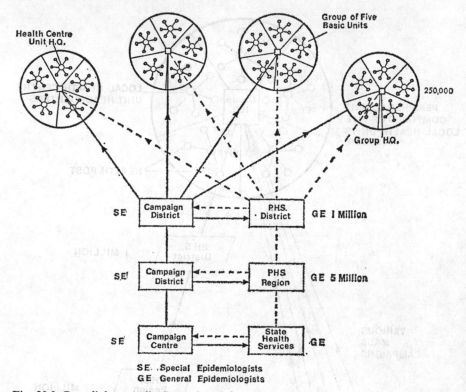

SE   Special Epidemiologists
GE   General Epidemiologists

Fig. 20.3 Cross linkage at district, region and centre.

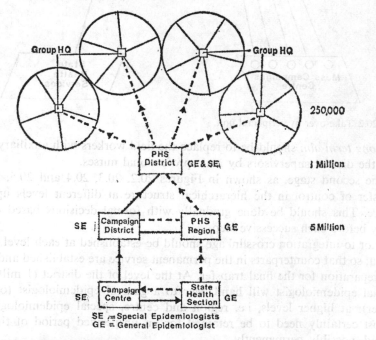

SE = Special Epidemiologists
GE = General Epidemiologist

Fig. 20.4 Take-over at district level.

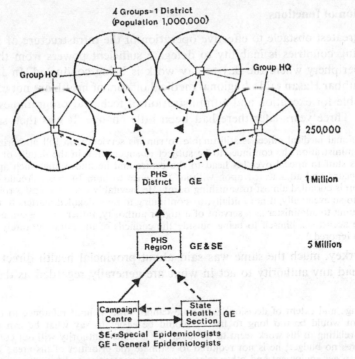

Fig. 20.5 Take-over at region.

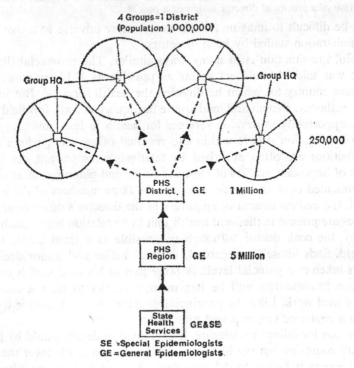

Fig. 20.6 Take-over at centre.

Delegation of functions

The greatest obstacle to effective operation of the infrastructure of health in developing countries is inability to delegate sufficient powers from the centre to the periphery where the day-to-day work is being conducted. In Jordan in 1962 Shubbar Hasan said: 'regional medical officers of health are not effectively responsible for execution and administration of technical programmes in their areas'.[23] Three years later there had been little change. It was then said:

The regional medical officer is still unable to run his services with full authority for day-to-day administration; he continues to be subject to supervision in the details of his work; he expects staff to appeal over his head to the centre and he knows that such appeals will often be heard and adjudicated upon without reference to him. In these circumstances, his jurisdiction is curtailed almost to vanishing point. He inevitably takes the easier road; indeed he must do so eventually, if not initially, by continuing to refer detailed matters to the centre, by continuing to administer as a servant of a higher authority, rather than as an independent agent. He accustoms himself to being outside the councils of the ministry, rarely consulted and often ignored.[3]

In Turkey, much the same was said about provincial health directors, who hardly had any authority to act in what are generally regarded as day-to-day matters.

The range and extent of decisions which he cannot take without reference to the central department would be too long to list; it would be easier to say what he can do. Many decisions relating to his work seem to be taken by a higher authority without consultation. He prepares no budget; he is not required to estimate the priorities of his area; he has no authority to get equipment and other relatively minor necessities and he cannot appoint his own staff. Any hospital matters go automatically to Ankara. It is frequently said that the chief function of a provincial director is that of a post box.[5]

It would be difficult to imagine circumstances more adverse to a live progressive administration staffed by keen directors.

In Spain, the situation is in many ways similar. The provincial director of health, it was said: 'should act as far as possible as if his province was an independent country for which he directed the health services'. But in fact he had little authority, a small and inadequate headquarters staff, few field workers and little opportunity to develop services for health in his community.[4]

Lack of delegation occurs within the regional office itself, where those in senior positions are often absorbed in relatively unimportant detail to the exclusion of important matters of regional policy and planning; most observers have commented upon the waiting queues, the large numbers of documents to be signed, the endless stream of enquirers at the director's office door. Similar disabilities are present in the local health unit in its relation with health centres. In Turkey, the ocak doctor 'although responsible as a team leader for work in the field, finds himself unregarded, with all major and minor decisions in his affairs taken at provincial level'. A large part of his field staff is controlled from group headquarters and he has no opportunity to plan a coordinated scheme of field work. Like the provincial director, the ocak doctor feels himself to be a neglected cog in a vast machine.[5]

The reasons for failure to delegate, if examined in detail, would be found to differ in all countries; but the ill effects will be the same, whatever the origins. The chief enemy is failure to delegate from the centre. This acts like a chain reaction. The centre occupies itself with detail for which the provincial director should be responsible; the provincial director in turn usurps the functions of the district or group director, and he in turn those of the health centre. In these circumstances, the remedy must be to reverse the process by beginning decentralization from the centre. But sound administrative systems are not born without travail. The practice of centralized power and decision often rests in long established custom, itself resistant to change. In many countries socio-anthropological studies of the hierarchical processes at work are needed to determine the proper course of action.[3]

Staffing the permanent framework of public health

Professional staff

All public health *ultimately* depends upon fully trained professional workers, doctors, nurses, midwives, and sanitarians, who can staff the infrastructure of health. A profession has been defined as: 'a vocation in which a professed knowledge of some department of learning is used in its application to the affairs of others or in the practice of an art founded on it' (*OED*) and also as 'a calling requiring specialized knowledge and often long and intensive preparation, including instruction in skills and methods, as well as in the scientific, historical and scholarly principles underlying such skills and methods, maintaining by force of organization or concerted opinion high standards of achievement and conduct and committing its members to continued study and to the kind of work which has as its prime purpose the rendering of high service' (WID). By general agreement the term professional covers all those trained in places of higher learning, including a variety of technical and other institutes, whose entry level demands at least the completion of secondary schooling; in a few instances the level may be lower, but rarely less than 10th grade. The range of professions is considerable (nearly 100 in Britain) and levels of attainment vary greatly.

The training of sufficient numbers of professionals for work in public health has proved to be a difficult task for developing countries, dependent, as they are, upon inadequate infrastructures of education, with too few institutes of higher learning, lack of teachers and of eligible students. Yet remarkable progress has been made in many countries since the Second World War. In India with a total of 105 medical colleges the number of doctors is now about 112,000 at the rate of 2·1 doctors per 10,000 persons, comparing favourably with the developed world.

But the problems of staffing have depended not only upon numbers, but also upon willingness of the doctor to serve in the infrastructure, away from hospital and centres of population; and upon his ability to fulfil the tasks which the special circumstances of the infrastructure impose upon him. All countries, including those that have been most successful in training doctors, have found it difficult to staff health centres, isolated and remote from centres of learning, and it has been even more difficult to provide staff with the necessary skills. This is true of all field staff, but particularly of doctors working in administration and as general practitioners for whom something more is required than what can be obtained in undergraduate training, even in the most modern medical schools such as Haceteppe in Ankara. Many developing countries have succeeded more easily in solving the problem of numbers than they have that of outlook. This is basically a challenge to the universities. As John Grant said in 1947: 'the first step in the demonstration of new forms of medical service is in its establishment by the teaching hospitals.'[15]

Most developing countries, once they have begun the creation of an infrastructure of health, find that general practitioners do not sufficiently appreciate the need to combine preventive and curative medicine, nor the significance of a team operation in which they provide the leadership. It was this deficiency which helped to halt the progress of the demonstration public health area in Thessaly, Greece (see p. 170),[12] and it had much the same effect in slowing up the development of public health in the nationalized provinces in Turkey.[5] Lack of training in administration, as seen earlier, has been an equal handicap. In many countries there is a lack of administrators in the central and regional headquarters with a sufficient understanding of the techniques of social and preventive medicine. Much of the work of the Turkish nationalization scheme, an exciting venture with great hope for the future of public health in Turkey, has been nullified by the lack of doctors with these skills. Many directors had no more instruction than that given in the undergraduate training, and the output of postgraduates from the school of public health in Ankara had been a mere handful. The same problem exists in many countries in different forms for all professional staff recruited for work in the field.

The special training of graduates and undergraduates needed to equip them for work in the infrastructure and in administration at headquarters can be met by the development of *Institutes of Community Medicine* in all medical schools. Each institute will need to have one or more field training areas in which the health problems of the community, its epidemiology and techniques of family health care can be demonstrated. A field training area can conveniently cover one or more local health units (50,000 population, see p. 205); the constituent health centres and satellite health posts should be specially staffed for teaching purposes, with, in particular, general practitioners on the staff of the college medical faculty who can teach '*family health care*', as a combination of preventive and curative medical care based on the home.

Every country has it in its power to establish such field training areas as, e.g. at Pharsala in the Thessaly demonstration project, where, in a period of ten years, some 1,400 doctors, midwives, sanitary inspectors and nurses were given short courses of training for work in different parts of Greece.[12] The chief difficulty lies in equipping health centres for teaching family practice, both for lack of graduates able to undertake teaching and failure of the universities fully to appreciate its importance. This was the chief weakness of the Greek training area (see p. 170).

For the doctor who is to take up administration, a two-year training course is needed in the principles of: (1) epidemiology, (2) sociology and (3) administration and planning. This has traditionally been given in schools of public health, generally distinct from the undergraduate medical school, many established by the Rockefeller Foundation in chief centres of population. This admirable expedient has served magnificently to demonstrate the possibilities of postgraduate medical training in public health in various parts of the world, but it no longer meets the increasing needs of greatly expanding infrastructures of health. With the establishments of *institutes of community medicine*, it should be possible for all medical schools to undertake postgraduate teaching in public health. Government grants will be needed to encourage graduates to undertake administrative work in sufficient numbers to staff the infrastructure.

The training of the professional nurse as a public health worker, ideally one public health nurse to every 5,000 persons, should be a function of all schools of nursing, with public health integrated into general nursing training given in post certificate courses. Training of the public health nurse has been slow to develop even in the developed world. In many countries, e.g. Spain,[4] the public health nurse does not exist. The WHO demonstration area in Thessaly, Greece, in the first ten years of existence, was able to secure no more than a bare minimum. Until 1960 Greece, considered by many to be fully or even over doctored, had only one state nursing school giving integrated training.[12] In Turkey with the male 'saglik memuru', deeply rooted in Turkish social history, like the 'practicante' in Spain, trained in a 4 year nursing course, but practising in everything but nursing, the public health nurse only exists at auxiliary level.

Professional male nurses are needed for both hospital and field, and their training should be encouraged. Hybrids, such as the 'saglik memuru' and 'practicante' are best avoided and should in future be channelled into the practice of nursing.

The university trained nurse graduate is now to be found in limited numbers, in most parts of the world, with considerable impact upon the status of the profession. In the developing world she is invaluable for directing nursing in hospital and field work and for teaching in nursing schools. University nurses can replace doctors as directors of nursing schools and so help to establish nursing as a profession, in parallel with, and not subservient to medicine. The Chair of Nursing with its bachelor degree in nursing, such as that at Manchester University in Britain, points the way. But training for the university nurse has encountered difficulties in both developed[32] and underdeveloped[1] countries. The course at EGE university in Turkey, which started in 1955, 'to prepare administrative nurses, teacher nurses and public health nurses at university level' was in 1972 still directed by a doctor (on a part time basis) in a faculty which did not seem to appreciate the importance of nursing as a profession. The curriculum was hospital centred, with little emphasis on the social aspects of disease and it lacked field training of any sort. Practical training in hospital was gravely handicapped, as was to be expected in a country which, in 1972, had six doctors to one nurse, by inadequate staffing in the wards chosen for teaching; in the surgical department, wholly devoid of nurses, student nurses themselves gave the only nursing in ward and theatre. As the nursing image had a low profile in the country generally and graduates could aspire to little or no career, students tended to enter from the bottom of the admission scale.

Auxiliaries

Throughout much of the 'developing' world, a quarter of a century after World War II and the creation of WHO, lack of professional staff remains a serious barrier to progress and one which only the passage of time can remedy. If the standards of professional work, as evolved in the developed world, are to be retained, some alternative for staffing has had to be provided. Inevitably attention has focused upon the auxiliary, who, in the form of dresser, tamarjee and the like has been a familiar innovation wherever medical services have had to operate in countries lacking an education infrastructure. The damaging effects of lack of staff in otherwise ambitious schemes, as e.g. the nationalization scheme in Turkey, has been so great that many would regard auxiliary training as constituting a first priority and certainly one which should keep in balance with the development of the health infrastructure. It was said of the Turkish nationalization scheme that its extension should be made *dependent upon* an adequate supply of paramedical workers, mostly of auxiliary status.[5]

Auxiliaries in the field of medicine, with formal training, have long been used, e.g. feldshers in the USSR and sanitary inspectors in Britain; and the extension of this system, both logical and practical, has sought with varying success to meet the widespread, grave and often overwhelming need for preventive and curative care throughout the world.

The auxiliary has been defined as *'a paid health worker with less than full professional qualification in a particular field who assists and is supervised by a professional worker.'*[35] The professional is distinguished by the extent and quality of his learning, performance, ethical conduct and disinterested service; the auxiliary by a lower entry level, a training which is essentially more practical and a measure of responsibility in varying degree limited. Supervision after graduation is essential and where this is lacking, from want of the appropriate specialists, ward sisters, qualified technicians and medical specialists in different fields of work, the standards inevitably decline.

The dividing line between professional and auxiliary is, however, far from clear cut; it is further blurred when, for reasons of national prestige, or varying interpretation of professional status, the products of government training schools (as e.g. the health colleges in Turkey or the nursing schools in Libya) are locally regarded as professionally trained; when a more orthodox interpretation, considering levels of entry, nature of training and need for supervision, would rate them as auxiliaries.

Auxiliaries can be categorized in terms of the *field of work, the character of work,* or *the nature of the training.* The field of work may be in hospital, where auxiliaries can work either in the care of the sick, or in special departments, e.g. theatres, laboratories, anaesthetics, radiography, pharmacy; or outside hospital, where they can work as single purpose or multi-purpose technicians in health centres, in mass campaigns, in public health laboratories, malaria detection centres, health offices or in environmental hygiene. The character of the work will vary between 'assistants (or substitutes) to professionals' – doctors, nurses, midwives, sanitarians – and 'technicians' in, e.g. mass campaigns or in vital and health statistics. The nature of the training can be 'on the job' or alternatively in formal whole time courses.

Auxiliaries trained in institutions

It is necessary to distinguish between auxiliaries trained in institutions, constituting a sub-professional, and those pairs-of-hands trained in-service. An institute provides the equivalent of a boarding school, or junior technical college, with lecture theatres, library, canteen and residential quarters, with the advantage of continuous contact between staff and students in and out of the classroom. Libraries help students to use leisure time in further study and organized games help in the development of the team spirit. Where students are drawn from sparsely populated countryside, residence is of value in the development of sociability.

A reasonably sound schooling is indispensable for a formal course in a training institute, as distinct from in-service or on-the-job training, which can be given in one form or another to practically anyone, irrespective of educational background. A sound training in an institution cannot be ensured with anything less than six years schooling. It is well to recognize the built-in difficulties which limit the numbers who can be given formal training. The limitations imposed by the educational infrastructure are considerable; thus in Libya (1968) it was possible to get only a handful of applicants with six or seven years schooling. It is better to proceed slowly, maintaining standards and advancing with the stream of lively young minds, rather than filling voids with the half educated. Educational systems are advancing rapidly with better opportunities for recruitment every year that passes. There are other reasons for caution, dependant on the very general lack of facilities for practical training and supply of teachers. Recruitment of teachers is limited by language difficulties and by international competition; practical training depends upon the availability of departments properly staffed in which to teach. It is certainly unwise to imagine that large numbers of institutional trained auxiliaries can be produced, as it were out of a hat, as some reports seem to suggest.[29]

The educational level at entry will vary with that of the professional to whom the auxiliary will act as assistant, so that one type, say substitute doctor, may have an entry level higher than that of a professional, say sanitarian. The experience of Ethiopia suggests that the entry for the auxiliary doctor should be *matriculation* i.e. university entrance and in any event not less than 10 years schooling. The quality of the end product rises disproportionately with the level of entry; and length of training must necessarily increase with the weakness of the educational background. Sufficient time must be made to remedy lack of schooling. *Courses in institutions should in no circumstances be less than three years, and in view of the greater opportunities for character training during residence, should be residential.*

Auxiliary training relies heavily upon *practical exercises* for the teaching of techniques; it follows that an institute needs to be able to organize field practice under its direct control. Guidance in practical work is essential and much is lost when students practise without it, with no one to answer questions, elucidate difficulties or even to determine that practical exercises are completed satisfactorily. The Ryad Institute, taken over from WHO in 1964, suffered in this respect.[10] A whole time member of staff should take responsibility for this aspect of the institute's work.

Lack of auxiliaries usually goes hand-in-hand with weakness of the services themselves, so that the need for practical training is not easy to satisfy; well staffed wards, laboratories, pharmacies, anaesthetic units, etc, may be lacking and above all else in importance, field training units. In recent years improvements in hospital nursing and in the organization of special units, such as central laboratories and WHO schemes for malaria, tuberculosis and other diseases, have helped to provide good practical experience, but the weakness of field training remains to be solved in most countries. Good field training units, complete with health centres and satellite health posts, in which it is possible to demonstrate : (1) unified public health in action, (2) unified home visiting and (3) family health care by general practitioners, as in Ethiopia, are few, and in many countries such as Somalia and Saudi Arabia, in 1968, they were still on the drawing board, or in proverbial pigeon holes.

The institute can be established, independently or attached to a hospital, anywhere with proper facilities for practical training. The direction should rest in the hands of a medical doctor with post-graduate training in the principles of epidemiology, sociology and administration, himself able to play a part in the teaching – preferably native to the country, if initially acting as a counterpart to a WHO consultant.

Success in training auxiliaries has varied greatly from country to country. A study of the institutes in the Eastern Mediterranean (Ethiopia, Somalia, Saudi Arabia, Libya) in 1968 showed considerable variations in range and types. No country had produced a full range of auxiliaries for work in hospital and field.[6] In Saudi Arabia, the hospital team was most complete and in Ethiopia and Somalia, the field team. Libya alone had trained the male nurse and Ethiopia and Somalia, the auxiliary doctor. The training of auxiliary midwives had encountered difficulties in Libya, Ethiopia and Somalia, largely due to lack of facilities for practical teaching in domiciliary midwifery. Auxiliary sanitarians were prepared in depth in sanitary engineering in Ethiopia and over a broad field of environmental hygiene in Libya. In Saudi Arabia the sanitarians specialized in the third year in one of four subjects, quarantine, community development, malaria and municipal work. Each country trained in some form the auxiliary nurse.

In view of the need for sound systems of collection and compilation of vital and health statistics, and of the deplorably low level of records in so many parts of the world (see p. 217), it was surprising that none of the four countries was training an auxiliary to be stationed at strategic points in the infrastructure for the supervision of this difficult task. The importance of an auxiliary statistician is greater where non-medical certification exists (see p. 285), where the international certificate of death is not yet in use, and particularly where lay reporting calls for follow-up from health centres.

No attempt had been made to train health educators as such, a wise empirical decision, since all field staff should be able to do their own health education. To make this possible courses should present the philosophy and techniques of the subject adequately. Work in the field can then be given in planned programmes guided by a limited number of professional health educators at central and regional levels.

Auxiliaries trained in institutions should not be unduly specialized, as were the sanitarians in Saudi Arabia, since this gives a narrower base to knowledge, limits mobility and opportunities for advancement, and lowers status. A clear distinction is advisable between different types of auxiliary to avoid hybrids, such as the mixture of doctor and nurse seen in many early schemes, e.g. in the form of 'health assistants' in Yemen.[9]

The auxiliary doctor. Experiments have been made in various countries to train an auxiliary doctor. In Somalia, the Mogadishu institute set out in 1959 to train a team of three auxiliaries, public health nurse, sanitarian and 'health officer', to work together in health centres 'in small towns and rural areas'.[8] The health officer, who would play the rôle of the doctor, was required to have intermediate education at least grade 8; by 1967, 40 health officers had been trained in three year courses. The training then came to an untimely end 'owing to budgetary difficulties', which made it no longer possible to guarantee employment to the graduates. Employment was further complicated by the continued existence of 'medical assistants' (trained under a longstanding apprenticeship system) without any attempt to define either the field of work or the relationship of the two parallel auxiliaries. No health officer worked for long in a health centre; a few worked as senior sanitarians. The 1963 national plan made no mention of health centres, keeping in existence the ambulatories already staffed by medical assistants. Thus the project to train an auxiliary doctor failed essentially for lack of planning.

In Ethiopia, Gondar college was similarly established to train a team to work in health centres (health officers, nurses, sanitarians and midwives).[7] Unlike Somalia by 1967 the college had staffed 68 health centres, giving a thin cover for the whole country. By this time the college had been taken over by the university at Addis Ababa and the training had lengthened out to four years, with entrance requirements approximating to those for the university and a bachelor of hygiene degree. These developments reflected the realities of the Ethiopian situation, where the problems of rural practice, isolation for the doctor and difficulties of travel for staff and patients, are so great as to beggar description. The four year course allowed a better grounding in the basic sciences and more effective teaching in both clinical and social and preventive medicine. The gap between the training of a medical graduate and the auxiliary had narrowed to the point that the question was being asked as to whether it was any longer necessary to train an auxiliary at all.

Gondar and Mogadushu illustrate the complexities and uncertainties which surround the training of the auxiliary doctor, for which there can be no immediate answer. It may well be that, even when doctors become available in greater numbers, health centres 'out in the bush' will exist in conditions too discouraging for the medical graduate. Or it may be that frustration among the auxiliary doctors, as in Ethiopia, will lead to undue wastage, as they feel themselves to be poorly paid doctors and leave to complete medical training, or to find better paid jobs in industry. For Ethiopia at least the need exists for someone to work in the health centres with the training, status, and qualification similar to that produced in the Gondar college; and for these a channel of advancement to graduation as a doctor must be devised.

The auxiliary nurse is needed equally in hospital and in the infrastructure. In some countries, e.g. Saudi Arabia, for cultural reasons it is the male assistant nurse who is in most demand. The auxiliary nurse in hospital can work under the supervision of a ward sister, or in special departments. In the field he or she can form part of the health centre team or man, as a multipurpose worker, the satellite health posts. For this latter, the auxiliary nurse provides an excellent expedient, capable of greater use in many countries, such as Ethiopia, India and Turkey, where the areas covered by the health centre can be very great. For this purpose students are best chosen from outlying areas, to which they can return after training, practising in their home country. Students are generally admitted with 5 or 6 years basic education and sometimes, as in Turkey, 2 to 3 years after leaving school. It may be convenient, as was recommended for Ethiopia,[7] to establish schools for auxiliary nurses in the region where the students live.

Schools for female nurses tend to be established independently of the institutes, reflecting the need for nursing to be accepted as a separate discipline, and to build up its ethos. Separation makes it less easy for the auxiliary nurse to understand her place in the field team, a weakness which can best be remedied by the use of the field training area jointly with other auxiliaries. The same applies when nursing auxiliaries are trained, as can conveniently be done, in schools of professional nurse training.

Institutes for auxiliary training can also be used for training certain types of professional, e.g. sanitarians and laboratory technicians, with the advantage of bringing them into contact with auxiliaries during training; and also giving the chance of advancement to professional status for selected auxiliaries, who can remedy their educational background in evening or special classes. *The role of an auxiliary should not be regarded as a 'dead end' and all schemes for auxiliary training should make concrete plans for further education to professional status.*

Auxiliaries can never be more than a second choice and the first objective, wherever possible, should always be to train professional workers. For many countries now lacking certain types of worker owing to late development as, e.g. sanitarians in Greece and Spain, the training of a professional rather than an auxiliary is preferable, providing there are sufficient applicants for higher institutes of learning and a reasonably well developed infrastructures of health. The decision as to which step to take will depend on local circumstances, as illustrated in Jordan,[11] where staff was needed for health posts, or district sub-centres, to undertake the following range of duties: (1) first level care under medical guidance; (2) health education; (3) first level sanitary hygiene; (4) tuberculosis and malaria control; (5) collection of health and vital data; (6) maternal and child health promotion; (7) school health; (8) vaccination and immunization; (9) early detection and follow-up of the mentally ill.

Such responsibilities must often be undertaken by auxiliaries, even in isolated country districts and under distant supervision, but circumstances in Jordan favoured the use of professionals. Villagers had become sophisticated by access to the doctor, midwife and MCH clinic and were unlikely to be satisfied by another 'tamarjee', for whom they no longer had much respect. But, even more important, since some 9,000 adolescents left school annually at 17 years of age (population 1965/66 2 million) it was reasonably assured that there would be sufficient applicants who could benefit from a professional training and equally certain that students with 'university entrance' would not be satisfied with auxiliary status, offering little prospect of advancement. Jordan, therefore, took the decision to enlarge the professional nurse school, already well established in Amman, deepening the teaching of public health and opening the nursing course to males, who would be most suited to work in a sparsely populated countryside.

Auxiliaries trained in-service

For much of the world, formal training in institutions cannot be established for more than a small proportion of the staff needed to work both in hospitals and in the health infrastructure. The need for ground level staff, to prevent services from folding up altogether, makes it quite indispensable to employ many workers with little education as 'pairs-of-hands', and for these training 'in-service' or 'on-the-job' is the only answer. Just as Charing Cross hospital in London, at the time of Edwin Chadwick and Shaftesbury, had to be staffed with 'watchers', often recruited from the streets,[2] so to-day many a hospital in the developing world would have to close its doors, if denied the services of women with little or no education. Courses, to raise standards of bedside care, limit the risks of cross infection, and rationalize the nursing procedures, can be organized within the hospital. For this the use of the university trained nurse, as in Chile, can be of great help.

Programmes of training 'on the job' outside hospital are also widely needed, e.g. in training auxiliaries for work in health centres, mass campaigns and other field work, and for retraining field workers for multi-purpose functions, as at Mersin in Turkey.[5]

Courses given in-service, consisting of 100 hours of instruction (including 40 hours practical), can be organized and conveniently given in selected hospitals to cover a continuous month or spread over a year. A course can cover the following topics:* elementary knowledge of structure and systems of the body (10 hours); medicaments and injections (6 hours); general principles of first aid, prevention and treatment of shock; artificial respiration (2 hours); the circulatory system and treatment of haemorrhage (6 hours); treatment of fractures and head injuries (4 hours); infection and its spread by air, water, milk, flies, dust, excreta, contacts, food (15 hours); foodstuffs necessary for

---

* Publications of the Red Crescent and St John's Ambulance Association can be used as textbooks.

growth and maintenance of health (12 hours); record keeping and reporting (5 hours); practical work in sterilization, dressings, treatment of minor ailments and infections (20 hours); observation of the work of a trained nurse, a trained midwife and a trained sanitarian (20 hours).

Modifications will be needed to meet the needs of various types of auxiliary and even simpler syllabuses can be devised for village workers, self-helpers and those engaged in simple forms of home visiting.

Part Seven: The Measurement of Health

21. The Purpose of Vital and Health Statistics

William Farr, in 1875, concluded his 35th Report with the following words:

The great source of misery of mankind is not their numbers, but their imperfections, and the want of control over the conditions in which they live. Without embarrassing ourselves with the difficulties the vast theories of life present, there is a definite task before us – to determine, from observation, the sources of health, and the direct causes of death in the two sexes at different ages and under different conditions. The exact determination of evils is the first step towards their remedies.[80]

In 1975 we may no longer be so complacent in the belief that there is no misery for the world in numbers (see Chapter 8), but we must still agree that public health has 'to determine, from observation, the sources of health, and the direct causes of death'. One means to this end, as Farr was implying, is by statistical enumerations. Thus we learn how the community lives and dies, in much the same way as dissection of the human body, and pathological studies, have been the basis of clinical medicine. Indeed, since Farr wrote these words, mortality statistics, by showing what diseases were taking heavy toll, and in what circumstances, have quite transformed the Western world.

Vital and health statistics serve three main purposes; for research, organization, and planning.[56] For research they are needed virtually throughout the whole field of medicine and surgery. Many valuable discoveries in recent years have been achieved through statistical inquiry, such as the relationship of carcinoma of the lung with smoking (see p. 268), and the association between cardio-vascular disease and certain habits of living. For organization they provide clues as to what causes disease and what preventive measures are best applied. They provide the only measurement of health in the group. From the point of view of world health, this is our only means of weighing up the state of health of peoples in different parts of the world and the magnitude of the problems which face them.

An understanding of what diseases exist in any community, and how they are distributed, if unhappily not always attainable, must yet always be of the greatest value in planning services, both medical and public health; and those allied social services, housing, insurance, welfare. The greater the development of a country, and the more complex its services, the more the need for strict accounting. No longer can it be assumed that expenditure of money on health is its own justification. This belief motivated the Canadian Sickness Survey:

In order to avoid the possibility of haphazard spending and to provide a sound basis for planning the type of health insurance which would be most suited to the actual needs of the people of Canada, it was necessary to know a great deal more about how much illness was actually occurring, what were the characteristics of the persons and families experiencing illness, how much it was costing, to what extent existing health services were being used and

H

by whom and for what reasons, and a host of similar questions about which little or nothing was known. This was the stimulus which resulted, early in 1950, in agreement by all provinces to participate in a nation-wide sickness survey . . .[30]

It should be a fundamental consideration of all health administration that such accounting should be done. Much more accounting is needed, if national administrations are to make the best of their resources. The data will enable the health planner to determine priorities in the allocation of funds and to obtain maximum returns with minimum cost. [93, 106, 114, 116] The example can be given of an underdeveloped country with virtually no statistics of any kind, no census, no morbidity nor mortality reporting whatever, wishing to begin a malaria control campaign.

Aside from general impressions, gained from the patient-loads of its physicians and the continual processions of funeral cortèges, the country would not know the extent of its malaria problem and would be hard put to formulate an intelligent control plan.[15]

Obviously no country wishes to spray all habitations throughout its territory. It needs some measurement, in terms of incidence and mortality, of where and to what extent malaria is distributed. When the control or eradication programme is under way, it will need statistical measures of its effectiveness; when once the disease is eradicated, if it is to be kept in check, the need to know where fresh cases are occurring becomes even more urgent.

There is also a need to measure the effects of existing programmes – an operation which is now only too rarely undertaken. Doctors, civil servants, and politicians assume all too readily that existing smoothly working administrative schemes are conducted to the best purpose. In fact, many may already have served their time; others may need radical alteration; most need considerable adjustment. The National Health Service in Great Britain raised many such important issues:

Why did the introduction of the National Health Service in which every child could have a general practitioner make so little difference to the School Health Service? What were the appropriate roles of School Doctor and G.P.? Did children in Leeds, Leicester, and Exeter still run three times the risk of losing their tonsils as did children of Manchester, Bradford, and Gloucester? . . . Who did the industrial medicine in the great majority of factories and other work places where there was little or no industrial health service?
The last 25 years have seen many studies to explore these and other vital problems arising out of socialized medicine.

It is also too easily assumed that a service in one part of the world will be equally effective elsewhere; that what is done in England or the USA can be done to equal advantage in Central Africa. This is sometimes true. But more commonly it is false. To know what services are needed, and how they are meeting current needs, demands a skilled application of vital and health statistics. This may be called operational research, or administrative tactics – the name hardly matters.

Statistical measurements must always have been of importance, but in the modern age they have become indispensable. Vital and health statistics are the eyes and ears of the community health doctor. They are virtually his only means of knowing the nature of the problems which face him. Society everywhere throughout the world is changing fast: motor cars, smoking, women going out to work, secularization and changing rôles, penicillin and other antibiotics to be bought in a village store, and many and varied hazards of a rapidly developing industry; all these, and much else, are interacting with one another to change the health picture and the health needs. The studies of sickness absenteeism, which were made possible by National Insurance (see p. 256), revolutionized ideas about the major causes of community sickness. Bronchitis caused about 2,200 days of sickness absence per 1,000 male workers and psychoneuroses and psychoses about half that amount annually in the UK over the period 1962 to 1968.[96] Statistical studies in Malaya have shown the rise of infant mortality in rice-eating countries during times of plenty with decline in times of scarcity of food; and in Sri Lanka, the differences in mortality rates at different ages during the past 25 years. What are the proper services to meet such demands?

Studies of reproductive performance according to age or type of birth were equally challenging. Late foetal deaths for 'elderly primiparæ' in Great Britain in 1949[56] ran at over twice the rate of all others; the rate of neonatal deaths among multiple births was over five times that of singles; post-neonatal deaths in infants of 'young mothers with relatively large families' three times that of all others. In what way should public health services be adjusted to meet such phenomena? Studies in social class differences of mortality and morbidity (see p. 235) provide one of the most effective means to maintain health in a dynamic and ever-changing society. What the professional classes can achieve should not necessarily be beyond the capacity of others; and the diseases, such as coronary thrombosis, from which the professional classes suffer unduly, need not be their inevitable lot.

Much of this will be reflected back upon the national political machine. National statistical services should provide adequate statistics, including vital statistics, which can be a basis for informed national decisions on economic and social matters and which meet international responsibilities in the field.[63]

Expenditure on medical statistics, it has been said, has 'the character of an investment, from which a full return may be expected only over a period of years. Although doctors, hospitals, and others are naturally concerned more directly with the immediate needs of their patients than with the future health of the community, or with providing the means for a health audit of the country, it would be wrong that they should, therefore, neglect the part they can play in providing for the future.'[65]

Thus, vital and health statistics should be one of the first steps in the pursuit of health throughout the world. (See also Uses of Epidemiology.)[56]

22. The Availability of Vital and Health Statistics

Vital and health statistics are means to an end – to build up each nation's health. International comparisons of the health of different regions of the world can help to point the way, but the chief value must always be national. The first objective of any nation must be to produce satisfactory records for its own use, according to the nature and stage of its own economic development. There is hardly one record which is essential to every nation; not even the registration of vital events, births, deaths, marriages, divorces, adoptions, will have much use, for example, in a nomadic society. The greater the development of the country, generally speaking, the wider the use of vital and health statistics; but the needs of different countries will always vary.

Article 64 of the Constitution of WHO states that each member 'shall provide statistical and epidemiological reports in a manner to be determined by the Health Assembly'. This calls for uniformity, in materials, methods, and tabulations, for a minimum set of statistics.

Vital statistics

Vital statistics are *the facts systematically collected and compiled in numerical form, related to, or derived from, records of vital events*. Data used for health purposes have been limited largely to mortality (deaths and foetal deaths) and natality; but increasingly, with the growth of social medicine, use is made of other vital events, marriages, divorces, and more rarely annulments, adoptions, legitimation, and legal separations. General and specific death rates, natality and nuptiality, the state of the population, its rate of growth, its characteristics and geographical distribution are the first essentials. Morbidity data, and other information collected by public health personnel on living conditions and environmental factors, for example, nutrition, are increasingly emphasized, usually under health statistics (see p. 219).

Mortality has been a subject of study for many centuries, at least back to the sixteenth century, when London recorded the numbers dying weekly in the city, in what were called Bills of Mortality, obtained by house-to-house visiting. It is to these records that the father of vital statistics, John Graunt, and his associate, Sir William Petty, looked, in the following century, for the studies, which showed the increase of mortality in town over country, with a higher rate of male over female births and the greater mortalities of childhood (1662) (see page 87). Many others in succeeding centuries, including the Heberdens, Short, Greenhow and Percival, studied the births, deaths and marriages maintained in the ecclesiastical parish registers in England and Wales, and elsewhere throughout the West. But it is only in comparatively recent times that registration in any country has been able to provide a reliable framework for statistical analysis.

Although the nucleus of a registration system is one of the earliest developments of government in any area, yet international comparability of vital statistics, the oldest type of statistical compilation, has not yet been achieved. Vital statistics, even in developed areas, are subject to inaccuracies. In 1954 Moriyama reported that death rates in a number of counties of the USA were much lower than could be accounted for 'on the basis of known mortality levels and age distribution; in many small areas, incomplete registration makes it impossible to interpret the death rates'.[55]

The less the country is developed, and hence in those territories with the greatest problems, the more defective are the vital statistics; the greater the need the less the supply – a phenomenon much less marked in the fields of finance, trade, industry, and production. In 1953, Fales said that no country in SE Asia, other than Sri Lanka, had adequate records of vital statistics on a nationwide basis, even for demographic purposes.[18] This remains true today, and in other parts of the underdeveloped world, where some data are available, their quality is deficient.

The UN Demographic Yearbook classifies vital statistics in the following three categories:[92]

1. Data stated to be virtually complete, i.e. representing at least 90 per cent coverage
2. Data stated to be unreliable, i.e. less than 90 per cent coverage
3. Data concerning which no specific information is available.

In 1956, statistics were available for only 168 statistical areas out of 214.

Of these, 58 were recorded as 'complete', 56 as 'incomplete' and 54 unknown and almost certainly non-existent. Nineteen had statistics referring to only part of the territory and in 24 they referred only to certain ethnic groups.

Vital information of the simplest kind was available[75] for only half the world's population.

130 reported total live births, covering 1,242,448,000 people or 50·5 per cent of the world's population; 131 reported total deaths; 108 reported total infant deaths, covering 1,148,729,000 people, or 46·8 per cent of the world's population.[86] For the years 1951–5, 38 million births were registered (42 per cent of 90 million), and 16 million deaths (33 per cent of 47 million).

Where vital events are said to be completely registered, this of course relative, the information which is tabulated varies greatly.

Up to 1954, of 58 areas covering 1,229,076,000 people (i.e. about half of the 1954 total), only 7 classified deaths by age, sex and occupation; only 22 recorded occupation for the father and 24 that of the deceased.[86]

Total figures of births, deaths, infant deaths and late foetal deaths only could be said to be generally available.

In the remainder of the world in 1954, covering over 1,200,000,000 people, the data for vital statistics were even more incomplete and often non-existent.

The changes in the subsequent 15 years were not very great. In 1971, 35 per cent of the world population lived in areas with relatively complete data for live birth (cf. 27·7 in 1950); 33·7 for general mortality (cf. 28·3 in 1950); 33 for infant mortality (cf. 27·6 in 1950); 30·6 for deaths by cause (cf. 22·3 in 1950); 33·9 for live births by age of mother (unknown in 1950). No information was available in all these aspects for about half the total population (52·6 per cent deaths etc). The proportions with reliable data for live births had increased significantly in Africa from 2·1 to 17·4, and in South America from 10·0 to 33·0; but for the underdeveloped world as a whole reliable data remained minimal.[60]

The statistics of infant mortality, long regarded as a good index of unhealthiness of localities in the developed world, are generally quite unreliable elsewhere. Little distinction may be made between live births and still births; and the definition of first birthday can also vary considerably, it may be taken from the date of conception and not from birth, or periods of time may be measured by successive harvests, or the first birthday may be dated from some conspicuous festival.[17] More serious perhaps is the fact that the population against which the rates are calculated may be guesswork, or that only a proportion of the vital events may have been recorded, thus giving a distorted result. Africa, particularly the tropical zone and Asia, particularly East, are most defective in their returns; here not more than 10 per cent of events are registered.

Deficiencies are partly due to the fact that the need for vital records develops only as school systems, pensions, social security, and other social measures require people to declare their age. Compulsory registration is difficult to introduce, with any chance of success, much before the corresponding certificates are required at various stages of an individual's life; until, for example, age must be known on entry to school or employment or at death for insurance or inheritance claims. And sad to relate, the appreciation of good vital and health statistics leaves much to be desired. 'Many administrators today not only do not obtain adequate statistical data . . . but have come to regard them as unnecessary.'

Foetal deaths. No country has ever reported all foetal deaths, although it is known that 14 have adopted the new definition (see p. 231). In 1971, foetal deaths were recorded relatively completely for only 10·6 per cent of the world's population.[60] Late foetal deaths are subject to so many difficulties of interpretation and recording that the statistics are of little value for international comparison, although, where they exist, they are useful for long-term analysis in the country itself. In 1972 they were recorded for 114 countries,[14] but the Demographic Yearbook regarded only 33 as reliable. The ratios per thousand live births ranged from 40·4 in Mauritius, 8·2 in Denmark, 7·4 in Czechoslovakia to 7·2 in Luxembourg.

The criteria for viability of the foetus vary much. The minimum period of gestation most frequently specified is 28 weeks. But in 12 countries the gestation period is 26 weeks or more (Belgium, Bulgaria, Colombia, Egypt, Finland, France, Italy, Liechtenstein, Luxembourg, Mauritius, Netherlands, and Venezuela); in three countries 20 weeks (Panama, Philippines, and United States) and, prior to 1953, in Japan 3 months. Confusion also arises over the use of calendar and lunar months. A few countries make confusion worse by including as late foetal deaths those babies that die shortly after birth, either within 24 hours (for example Cuba), or before registration (for example Pakistan, Algeria).[28]

Even under highly efficient registration systems many late foetal deaths can escape registration. It is sometimes difficult to identify incompleteness, particularly where late foetal deaths and live births are both under-registered. Perhaps the most that can be said is that the information in countries where most confinements are medically attended is more complete than in others. The value of such information to public health is so great that every country should give the matter serious consideration.

Health statistics[112]

Health statistics have a wider connotation than vital statistics. They cover three measurements: *of the state of health*, chiefly morbidity data, which relate to the distribution of illness (as distinct from mortality) in the population; *of factors affecting health*; and *of items of service*, all, or most, of which are to promote health, to protect the health of the community, or to treat sickness. Health statistics, therefore, are a means to measure not only health, whatever that may mean, but also factors influencing it and the steps which a community takes to produce it.

Measurements of the state of health. The sources of morbidity data are more varied, and less stereotyped, than those of mortality data. Many arise as a by-product of the development of services. Generally speaking, the more developed the country, the richer will be the possible sources, although this does not mean that the material will be used. The main sources can be listed as follows:[99]

1. Surveys by individual inquiry (for example, home visiting) (see p. 266)
2. Mass screening
3. Census enumeration: a. of sick persons, b. of certain defects
4. Notification of communicable diseases
5. Registration of certain diseases (for example, cancer, rheumatism, etc.)
6. Certification of certain conditions (for example, for special benefits such as food allowances)
7. Road accidents
8. Industry and occupation: a. accidents, b. diseases, c. absenteeism
9. Armed forces: sickness and recruitment records
10. Insurance schemes: a. social security – voluntary and statutory, b. life and sickness insurance, c. voluntary health pensions funds, d. pensioners and veterans
11. Medical and nursing care: a. hospitals – in-patients and out-patients, b. general medical practice, c. home visiting and nursing service, d. special clinics and hospitals, agencies, e. health and welfare centres (maternity, infant, and pre-school), f. educational institutions (routine inspections, sickness, absenteeism).

Measurement of factors affecting health. The sources of information for an assessment of the factors affecting health and of the means to health are to be found in *analyses of the use and development of public health services*, as, for example: (a) maternal and child health services, the number of centres, of mothers attending, of individual consultations; (b) tuberculosis service, the number of dispensaries, sanatoria, beds, patients admitted; (c) venereal disease services, the number of centres, the amount of contact tracing, etc.; (d) environmental sanitation, details of services; (e) health education, courses of instruction; (f) vaccination and immunization, numbers protected.

Measurements of items of service and estimates of services available for medical care, as, for example: (a) general and special hospitals, numbers and beds; (b) mental and mental deficiency hospitals, numbers, beds, vacancies, patient admissions and discharges; (c) doctors, dentists, nurses, pharmacists, sanitarians, and veterinarians, numbers; (d) family expenditure for each of the various types of health service. There are others which can be devised for particular inquiries.

The assumption which lies behind the statistical study of service is: the more the better. Thus, if Jordan has say 4,000 hospital beds occupied each for 300 days, there would be 1·2 million hospital days or 600 per 1,000 inhabitants, as compared with perhaps 4 times this amount in the United States. The axiom is true only in a general sense. Services tend to be concentrated in towns and to be lacking in rural areas. In some instances, liberal provision of services, for example, sanatoria and dentists, may be an indication of bad health. Many variables in population, age and density, communications, efficiency and skill, and in the continued prevalence of controllable but uninhibited health hazards also need to be taken in account in any assessment made. Perhaps, also, the use made of services is a better indication of health than their mere presence.

The data for health statistics are obtained from records which are made for statistical or other purposes connected in one way or another with the administration of the health services; they are not registered documents and the persons involved, generally speaking, have no interest in the validity of the data or its recording. This has many repercussions on the validity, completeness, and accessibility of the data.

Availability of health statistics. Health statistics are scattered among many government departments; for example, the Ministries of social welfare (national insurance returns, hospital statistics), of defence (army, navy, and air force health statistics); and of education (school medical inspection, numbers of students and graduates in medicine and in allied professions). Many of these are accurate, as those for hospitals, staff, investigations and data from clinics; but there are often difficulties to be overcome in obtaining comprehensive data. The fact that health and welfare in many countries are the responsibility of provincial and municipal authorities, and that the relevant statistics are often not uniform, or on occasions not even available in the central government administration, complicates studies, particularly in countries with a federal organization. In addition, the most advanced countries have decentralized forms of government; and many private or voluntary organizations, hospitals, clinics, etc., do not furnish statistics to the national authorities. To compile a complete list of existing health statistics in any one country often requires many months of search in publications and reports and in correspondence with national administrators.

In June 1953, WHO sent out a questionnaire to all member-states in an attempt to learn to what extent health statistics were available in various countries.[75]

The information was summarized under 11 headings (excluding notifiable diseases): (1) morbidity data (all illness and special); (2) infirmities (blind and deaf mute); (3) medical and public health personnel; (4) hospitals (number, beds, smallpox); (5) immunization and vaccination (diphtheria, B.C.G., other); (6) maternal and child health centres; (7) tuberculosis (pulmonary, nonpulmonary); (8) venereal diseases; (9) drug addiction and alcoholism; (10) mental health (hospitals, institutions for mentally subnormal children); (11) homes for incurables and aged.

Few countries answered fully. Of the 95 returns listed, 28 only gave sources of morbidity data. Planned surveys of sickness were conducted by Canada, Japan, England and Wales, Scotland, Northern Ireland, Sri Lanka, and Denmark (see Surveys, Chapters 25 and 26). Otherwise there was little available, except records of communicable diseases and some information from hospitals, insurance, and school examinations. But questionnaires of this character are notoriously difficult to fill in, as they are to frame, and it may well be that the actual position was better than indicated.

In 1965, a questionnaire, returned by 98 countries, showed limited improvement, particularly in hospital data, but little evidence that the data collected reflected the needs of the area; traditional and often outworn practices were too often adopted. By 1971, further limited improvement had taken place, particularly records of health personnel and health establishments, which 'had greatly improved in quantity and quality'.[60] Other health statistics, including morbidity, remained defective or absent.

Underdeveloped countries are again at a disadvantage with health statistics, yet their need of these is even greater. If the many hazards to health 'are to be combated successfully, certain basic facts concerning them must be recorded with precision, and the assembly of the necessary facts must not be limited to records of compulsory notifiable diseases if gaps in existing medical knowledge are to be filled'.[17] The most important single criterion for the underdeveloped world must be *relevance*. They need to collect data *relevant to their particular problems* and moreover sufficiently flexible to remain relevant as the problems change.[71]

The stage is well set upon which to play one of the world's most fascinating stories – how the human being lives and dies.

H*

23. The Standardization of Recording

1. The development of national committees
2. Certification of cause of death
3. Standardization of diseases, injuries, and causes of death
4. Practice and procedure of a vital statistics system
5. Classification by occupation and industry
6. Classification by social class
7. Census enumeration
8. Health indicators.

1. The development of national committees[100]

In an effort to get greater comparability between the nations, the 6th International Conference for the Revision of the International List of Causes of Death (1948) recommended that all nations should establish *national committees*, which could work on problems of an international nature, and improve the production of national statistics.

Many of the means of collection of national statistical data are of a relatively primitive character: in many circumstances unsuited to the production of current, reliable, and comparable data, upon which health organizations depend for the development of services and the United Nations for its analysis of world health conditions. Furthermore, it has often been overlooked that vital statistics and population are closely related; and that, in order to relate vital statistics to the corresponding population, both must cover the same area and use the same definitions and classifications. There is a similar failure to recognize the interrelationship of health and vital statistics.

National committees are designed to help in assessing needs for vital and health statistics, the recording of the minimum core, the free flow of information, and the co-ordination of the activities of diverse agencies; to make vital and health statistics of greater practical use and appeal; to stimulate statistical studies and the training of personnel; to assist in the implementation of international recommendations; and, possibly their most important function, to bring users and producers of statistics into a closer working partnership.

The functions should normally be advisory and consultative, in response to requests from the appropriate government authority, and membership should include administrative, professional, and lay persons concerned with the collection and analysis of health and vital statistics and with the various uses (medical and social) of such statistics; for example,
a. at the national level, persons from governmental and non-governmental institutions and

agencies concerned, from the medical profession, from the universities, from research institutions; and

b. at the regional and local levels, persons from local and regional governmental and non-governmental institutions and agencies concerned with the collection and use of such statistics, and other competent persons concerned with the specifically regional or local aspects of such collection and use.

The national committees working within their own framework have begun the long uphill task of bringing satisfactory schemes into operation, relating population to vital and health statistics, helping to bring together the work of many departments, studying health statistics in relation to family structure, social, economic, and occupational backgrounds, and assisting schools of medicine and public health in the problems of education.

The first international conference of national committees held in London in October 1953, was attended by 28 members states and associate members of WHO; and the second, in Copenhagen in 1973, was attended by 59 states.[100]

2. Certification of cause of death

The international death certificate

In countries where medical certification is possible, either in whole or in part, there is need for uniformity, both in completion of the death certificate and in its interpretation. Particular difficulties have arisen from an increasing tendency to enter more than one cause, together with a diversity of systems of arbitrary rules by which the primary or underlying cause has been selected for statistical use. Certificates stating only a single condition seldom present difficulties. Such certificates, however, form a diminishing proportion of the total, owing to various factors, or a combination of them: such as the rapidly decreasing incidence and fatality in many countries of acute infectious disease, the rising average age at death, and the increasing proportion of deaths from multiple chronic conditions. In 1928, a certificate, almost identical with the form introduced in England and Wales in 1927, was recommended for international use by the Cairo Commission of the International Statistical Institute. The purpose of this was to make it possible to select *the underlying cause* of death without resort to arbitrary rules of selection. In 1948, the 6th Decennial International Revision Conference designed the following certificate for general use (again confirmed by the World Health Assembly, 1967).

Where several conditions are present at death, the classification of cause now largely depends upon the order in which the certifier enters them on the certificate. The *underlying cause* of death, which appears on line (c) is

1. the disease or injury which initiated the train of morbid events leading directly to death,

or

2. the circumstances of the accident or violence which produced the fatal injury.

The instruction to physicians on the use of the international form points out

INTERNATIONAL FORM OF MEDICAL
CERTIFICATE OF CAUSE OF DEATH

CAUSE OF DEATH I		Approximate interval between onset and death
Disease or condition directly leading to death*	(a)	....
	due to (or as a consequence of)	
Antecedent causes	(b)	....
	due to (or as a consequence of)	
Morbid conditions, if any, giving rise to the above cause, stating the underlying condition last	(c)	
II		
Other significant conditions contributing to the death, but not related to the disease or condition causing it	....	....

* This does not mean the mode of dying, for example, heart failure, asthenia, etc. It means the disease, injury, or complication which caused death.

that the responsibility for indicating the course of events now rests upon the certifier:

Since he is in a better position than anyone else to decide which condition leads directly to death and what antecedent conditions, if any, gave rise to the direct cause. It is a new principle in mortality statistics that they shall represent, as nearly as possible, the opinion of the doctor who knew or saw the patient as to what was the underlying cause of death; previously, automatic precedence of one condition over another was often given regardless of the sequence in which they were recorded on the death certificate.[52]

The importance of this homily can be judged from Logan's statement that it was not until 1940, thirteen years after the introduction of the form, that 'certifiers were using the form carefully enough for the order of the statement to be used to select the underlying cause of death for tabulation in preference to the old system of selection by rules'.[45]

Difficulties of continuity

The introduction of the international certificate has created its own problems of how to maintain continuity in subsequent years, when diseases have been displaced from positions of priority which they have held under rules of precedence. As an example, all systems of rules of precedence, dating back to pre-insulin days, gave preference to diabetes, then often fatal, over most conditions, except acute infections, cancer, and violent causes. Since diabetes has ceased, except in a few instances, to be considered as the underlying cause of death, the effect of the change in the certificate on the incidence of diabetes as a cause of death has been considerable. Thus, immediately after the change in Canada, in 1949, deaths attributed to diabetes were reduced by 45 per cent. It is important, in countries where such sudden artificial changes take place in morbidity rates, that the appropriate adjustment should be made in past statistics to enable a continuous and comparable picture to be presented. Many other difficulties of continuity result from the refining process of international standardization, for example, those which arise from adjustment in definitions, as with foetal death (see p. 231), or alterations in denominators and numerators, as has occurred in maternal mortality. It is one of the tasks of the WHO centre of classification of disease to advise nations about them.

Instruction to doctors in certification

Despite the use of the international form of death certification, ambiguity, vagueness, and other faults in its completion still complicate the preparations of mortality statistics. In the USA in 1954 perhaps 20 per cent of the medical returns were not properly made (Moriyama.)[55] Doubt, for example, may arise from the physician's failure to specify clearly the underlying cause, as where death has been certified as due to 'diabetes due to chronic rheumatic endocarditis', two unrelated conditions. This particular difficulty, which affects all countries in the world without exception, can only be met through the education of doctors. The booklet *Medical Certification of Cause of Death: instructions for physicians in the use of the international form of medical certificate of cause of death* is recommended for use in medical schools.[52] This should enable medical students and newly qualified practitioners to understand that the death return is a valuable document.

It is, however, to established practitioners that we must look if more immediate improvements in the quality of mortality statistics are to be achieved. One means to this end is the inclusion of 'explanatory notes and suggestions to practitioners' in the issues of books of forms, so that a medical practitioner called upon to give a death certificate always has at hand some written guidance. In England and Wales books of forms also include an alphabetical list of undesirable terms, with a note of the further information which should be supplied and a number of examples of how the form should be used.

There are many other ways of approaching the established practitioner, as through the medical journals, society meetings, and refresher courses. The experience of England and Wales teaches one particular lesson:

That a large improvement in certification cannot be expected from a one-time application of a single method of instruction or propaganda. What is needed is the long continued application of many methods. Doctors in clinical practice are always ready to co-operate gladly with official requirements when they are satisfied that what is required of them really serves a useful purpose. Every opportunity must therefore be seized to remind them that a useful purpose is served by giving proper medical certificates of cause of death, and to explain to them clearly what is wanted of them.[45]

Much depends on doctors' attitudes, understanding, and beliefs. Moriyama[55] conducted a survey by personal interviews seeking the answer to such questions as 'What do you consider to be the value of certification?', 'What are the uses of death certificates?', 'Do you believe in the value of such procedures?' The answers to such questions give a better insight into the root causes of present inadequacies, and this method might be used with advantage in other countries.

An effective means of educating the doctor is through a system of personal inquiry from the central statistical organization. Such inquiries are probably general throughout the Western world; approximately three per cent of certificates are queried in this way in the United States of America and two per cent in England and Wales (10,000 inquiries to practitioners are sent annually by the Registrar General). Although such inquiries are more readily conducted in countries with well-developed medical services, they should be begun everywhere as soon as possible. The doctor should realize that somebody does scrutinize closely, from the medical standpoint, what he writes on his certificates. As an elaboration of this method an attempt should be made to single out cases of doctors who persistently return defective forms; these can then be interviewed in their own homes. In these ways constant effort can result in more or less uniform procedures being followed by individual certifiers.

Even under ideal conditions, however, the death certificate can do no more than register the physician's knowledge and medical opinion regarding causes of death – this will always be so whatever medical progress takes place. But in interpreting statistics derived from these reports it is important to know about reliability. For this the only means is to sample death certificates, and to check the diagnoses by going through hospital and autopsy records and interviewing the certifying physician.

Non-medical certification of death

The certification of cause of death presents difficulties everywhere, but these are greater in territories where there are few doctors, i.e., for large parts of the world including most, if not all, areas that do not reply to the United Nations questionnaires (see p. 217). In Chile, in 1954 it was said: 'a considerable proportion of diagnoses on death certificates are made by physicians who have not treated the patients ... or even worse by witnesses; there are usually no facilities for examination, and even diagnoses by physicians are likely to be inexact and unverified.'[70]

Non-medical certification of vital events is one of the chief causes of defects in national data, which no amount of sophistication in processing can remedy. For this reason it is imperative to build into the infrastructure of health adequate machinery for ensuring that non-medical certification is done with care and according to a set plan.

Nothing like a true picture of deaths can be obtained in such circumstances, but the results of simple procedures are by no means negligible. Although careful computing cannot give validity to data which never had any in the beginning, lay recording under skilled direction is certainly of value. We should bear in mind John Graunt's words, when he wrote of the London Bills of Mortality (1662)[21]

As for consumptions, if the searchers do but truly report (as they may) whether the dead corps were very lean and worn away, it matters not to many of our purposes, whether the disease were exactly the same as physicians define it in their books.

Two valuable expedients must in no circumstances be omitted: (1) the abbreviated list for tabulation and (2) the trained auxiliary at district level for general oversight of the scheme (see Chapter 29).

In rural areas, where compilation is done by headmen of the villages, special instruction will be needed. The village clerk acting for the headmen should seek answers to pertinent questions: (1) Was the patient ill for several days or for months? (2) Had he fever? (3) Had he diarrhoea? (4) Had he cough with spitting blood? (5) Did he die before he was old? (6) Did he die because of accident or murder? In the case of children: (7) had the child fever and/or convulsions? (8) Had the child swelling of the legs (oedema)? In the case of a young or middle-aged woman: did the person die in childbirth?

Indonesia may be taken as representative of developing countries in this respect. In 1957, it had approximately one doctor to 57,000 people, with little medical certification outside the large towns. A system of counting deaths, using headmen of villages, had been in operation from the end of the 19th century. A death certificate had been introduced in 1935 and extended to 13 regencies by the end of 1938, when the war and its aftermath brought registration to a halt until 1950. After this the towns of Java, with fair municipal services, appointed certifying officers to work from the health departments. In 1954, Bandung (population 802,105) had 16 certifying officers working under the direction of the medical officer of health.* In 1955, 447 deaths were recorded (11·7 crude death rate) arranged under 7 causes (less than the abbreviated lists in appendices 2 and 6). The situation remained much the same in 1974, by which time there was 1 doctor to 23,000 persons†

In India, the central statistical office is seeking to cover the country with model registration areas based upon primary health centres, covering not less than one million inhabitants, in which a specially designed scheme of lay reporting can be operated. In 1969, there were about 600 such areas. The manual of instructions issued by the Registrar General (A. Chandra Sekhar) is a valuable guide.

3. Standardization of nomenclature of diseases, injuries, and causes of death

The sixth revision of the International Statistical Classification of Diseases, Injuries, and Causes of Death,[49] largely the work of an Expert Committee under the chairmanship of Percy Stocks, Chief Statistician to the Registrar General of England and Wales, was adopted by the World Health Assembly in 1948. Since revised (1955 and 1965), it has been published in English, French, Spanish, Latin, German, Italian, Japanese, Greek, and Russian. Apart from its world-wide extension, the new classification achieved the hitherto unattainable ideal of fusing the codes of mortality and morbidity, which had so long been sought.

Abbreviated lists are available for special purposes: (see appendices 1 to 5)

List A – 'intermediate List of 150 causes for tabulation of morbidity and mortality.

List B – Abbreviated List of 50 causes for tabulation of mortality.

List C – Special List of 70 causes for tabulation of morbidity.

List D – List of 300 causes for tabulation of hospital morbidity.

* Personal communication from Raden Admiral Surasetja, Health Officer, 1957.
† Personal communication from Dr Gunaratne, Regional Director, South East Asia, 1974.

List E – List of 100 causes for tabulation of perinatal mortality and morbidity. Further abbreviations or expansions can be made to meet particular needs by varying the aggregation of the international code numbers. An unofficial list of 57 causes, resulting from an African seminar, for use by non-medical certifiers is given in Appendix 6. WHO is currently engaged on the preparation of official abbreviations for three different classes of lay certifiers: (1) laymen; (2) health centre staff; (3) public health administrators.

The new rules gave rise to many problems of interpretation and, as more countries began to use it, it became obvious that advice centres would have to be established for guidance. Four such centres have been established (London, Paris, Moscow, Caracas) charged with the continual study of the list for inconsistencies and inaccuracies, as well as of the means to collect, record, and tabulate data, and of the problems affecting comparability. The results of correspondence and consultation with those concerned with international classification have been incorporated in the following pamphlets: (1) *Medical Certification of Causes of Death: Instructions to Physicians*[52]; (2) *Amplification of Medical Certification of Cause of Death: Inquiries to certifiers concerning incomplete or vague statements.*[1]

Training of Coders. In developed countries particularly, and elsewhere when the International Classification comes into use for mortality and morbidity, there arises the need to train coders for tabulation of data. To lay people unacquainted with medical terminology, ignorant of the structure and physiology of the body, and prejudiced by private theories and popular superstitions, the study of the international classification can be an exacting task, but one which leads to satisfaction in work and a surprising accuracy of application. Experience arising out of recent developments in the sickness surveys, schemes for cancer registration, and those for hospital statistics, has shown that it is necessary to give instruction in the coding process to record officers in hospital, statistical staff in government and public health departments, and in the central statistical office.

Courses for coders have been held in London, in Geneva, in the British West Indies, in Caracas, and in Santiago, Chile; a similar course for medical records officers was held in Bangkok (1965) and in New Delhi (1968). The general arrangement, as illustrated by those run by the General Register Office in London, is a course of one week of which two days are devoted to lectures and discussions and the remainder of the week to coding instructions covering the following main points: (1) the significance of the beginnings and endings of medical terms; (2) the names of the principal bones; (3) the layout of the classification; (4) the descriptive arrangement of the notes of exceptions and conventions for colons and brackets; (5) undesirable terms; (6) the use of code numbers which vary according to circumstances.

4. Practice and procedure in a vital statistics system

Registration

The origins of vital registration are to be found in the ecclesiastical rolls.

As early as A.D. 720 some such system seems to have operated in Japan. In the Western world records of fees received were kept, for baptism, compulsory in the Church of the Middle Ages, and for burials and weddings. Such records were deficient in many essentials; the date of registration rather than that of the event itself tended to be kept, and many vital events which did not concern the religious denominations of the parish in question were omitted. A regular system was introduced first in Spain in the fourteenth century when Cardinal Ximenes, Archbishop of Toledo, required parish registers to be kept. In 1501, Germany began regular and continuous registration at Augsburg. Thomas Cromwell, Vice-General, is said to have introduced a compulsory system of ecclesiastical registration to England in 1538, followed by France (1539), Sweden (1608), Canada (1620), Finland (1628), and Denmark (1646).[28]

Civil registration is said to have been begun by the Incas in Peru; being without written characters they intertwined coloured strings and knots to record the facts. Massachusetts, then the British colony of Massachusetts Bay, introduced legislation for civil registration in 1639. France followed with the Napoleonic Code in 1792. The civil section of the Napoleonic Code was destined to influence strongly the development of vital registration throughout Western Europe, Latin America, and parts of the Middle East, which came under French influence.

A state system of registration in England and Wales began in 1837, when the clergy were relieved of functions previously placed upon them, and a new machinery with a general register office in London, and local registries, was instituted under the direction of the Registrar General. Registration became compulsory in 1874. At this time also a doctor's signature was first required on all death certificates. A certain measure of secrecy was introduced in 1926, giving effect to the recommendation of the Royal Commission on Venereal Disease (1916, Cmd. 8189). The Births and Deaths Registration Act (1926), re-enacted in 1953, states that:

The doctor in attendance during the person's last illness shall sign a certificate in the prescribed form stating to the best of his knowledge and belief the cause of death and *shall forthwith deliver the certificate to the Registrar.*

The advantages are often lost when the doctor 'delivers' the certificate by handing it himself to the relative.

Vital statistics depend greatly, perhaps too greatly, upon registered documents, i.e. documents filed for legal purposes, in which the informant generally has an interest in the validity of the data and their recording. For this reason alone it is important that such documents should not be overburdened. Even the first priorities may unfortunately be too burdensome for underdeveloped countries in which remoteness, illiteracy, lack of understanding of the purposes of vital records, and lack of qualified personel to complete reliable certificates combine to make such a service impracticable.

Comparability between nations calls for the adoption of uniform systems. Unfortunately this could only be achieved if the whole world could establish a common registration system, with a direct relationship between vital and health statistics through the use of the same area, definitions and classifications.

It is equally necessary for the authority responsible for vital statistics to be in close working partnership with those responsible for the census. All, or most of this, is possible in the developed world where registration has been in operation for many years. The first report of the Statistical Commission of the Economic and Social Council of the UN outlined *Principles for a Vital Statistics System* in 1953, as if the underdeveloped world, if made aware, could immediately follow in the footsteps of the developed world producing sound statistics, with legal machinery and codes of behaviour of the same standard.

The experience of 20 years has had a sobering effect, which is not surprising in view of the inadequacies of the data produced for half the world, as outlined in the last chapter. The revised *Principles For a Vital Statistics System*, which the Commission produced in 1975[63], is an attempt to meet the particular problems of the underdeveloped world, setting out in simple terms, clearly and precisely, what should be their immediate aims. The Commission hoped that this 'would assist individual countries in the production of a wider range of vital statistics than has existed up to now'. The use of this revised version could be the basis of a more realistic approach to vital statistics than has been possible before and it should be compulsory reading in the higher echelons of any health infrastructure.

Every country should strive to establish an efficient system of civil registration for the advantages, both legal and protective, which it carries to individuals; for its administrative advantages; and for the unequalled support which it can give to the compilation of worthwhile statistics. Because of the fact that 'registration of vital events for legal purposes is an almost universal requirement', statistical processing of the record of registration has become the accepted or conventional method of producing vital statistics. Nevertheless much can be done by the intelligent use of field surveys (see Chapter 26) and by means of sampling[71, 112] (see Chapter 25). It is in these last two expedients that the chief means to collect worthwhile data in the underdeveloped and developing world is to be sought. (For discussion of difficulties in underdeveloped countries see Chapter 29).

The selection of topics to be investigated in a vital statistics system needs to be realistically adjusted to the capacity of the country. *They should be needed; acceptable to the people; within the capacity of the average respondent to answer easily; and not likely to arouse fear, prejudice, or superstition.*

Live births statistical report items (¶ = priority)

All live-born infants should be registered, and counted as such, irrespective of the period of gestation, or whether alive or dead at time of registration; and if they die at any time following birth they should also be registered and counted as dead.

Live birth is the complete expulsion or extraction from its mother of a product of conception, irrespective of the duration of pregnancy, which, after such separation, breathes or shows any other evidence of life, such as beating of the heart, pulsation of the umbilical cord, or definite movement of voluntary muscles, whether or not the umbilical cord has been cut or the placenta is attached; each product of such birth is considered live born.[49]

Characteristics of the event or child
¶Attendant at birth
¶Date of occurrence
¶Date of registration
Hospitalization
¶Legitimacy
Period of gestation
¶Place of occurrence
¶Sex
¶Type of birth (single or plural issue)
Weight of birth

Characteristics of parents
Date of birth of father; if not
    available, age
¶Date of birth of mother; if not
    available, age
Date of marriage (for legitimate births)
Industry
Literacy or level of formal education
¶Number of children born to this mother
Occupation
Place of usual residence (of mother)
Status (as employer, employee, etc.)

Death statistical report (¶ = priority)

Death is a permanent disappearance of all evidence of life at any time after live birth has taken place (post-natal cessation of vital functions without capability of resuscitation). This definition therefore excludes foetal deaths.[63]

Characteristics of event
¶Cause of death
¶Certifier
¶Date of occurrence
¶Date of registration
¶Place of occurrence

Characteristics of decedent
Age of surviving spouse (if married)
¶Date of birth; if not available, age
Hospitalization
Industry
Legitimacy (for under one year of age)
Literacy or level of formal education
Marital status
Number of children born (for females of
    child-bearing age or over)
Occupation
¶Place of usual residence
¶Sex
Status (as employer, employee, etc.)

Foetal death statistical report items (¶ = priority)

Foetal death is death prior to the complete expulsion or extraction from its mother of a product of conception, irrespective of the duration of pregnancy; the death is indicated by the fact that after such separation the foetus does not breathe or show any other evidence of life, such as beating of the heart, pulsation of the umbilical cord, or definite movement of voluntary muscles.[49]

A definition of early, intermediate, and late foetal death in terms of duration of gestation was given by the 2nd Session of the Expert Committee on Vital Statistics (1950): early – less than twenty completed weeks of gestation; intermediate – twenty completed weeks, but less than twenty-eight; late – twenty-eight weeks of gestation and over.[98]

The length of gestation is still generally measured from the beginning of the last menstruation.[98] No recommendations have yet been made, however, for computing this period where the date of the last menstrual period is not known – a problem which arises not infrequently where calendars, etc are not available. Some more precise international measurement, by length or weight of foetus or size of fundus, would be an advantage.*

Registration of all foetal deaths irrespective of the period of gestation is a desirable goal, in spite of deficiencies in the criteria for abortion. As a minimum

* For late foetal deaths, Austria, Sweden, and the Federal Republic of Germany specify a minimum of 35 centimetres; Switzerland over 30 centimetres; and Czechoslovakia over 400 gram.

countries should register all foetal deaths occuring after the 28th computed week of gestation; these are late foetal deaths'.

Characteristics of event or product	Characteristics of parents
Cause of foetal death	Date of birth of father; if not
Certifier or attendant	available, age
¶Date of occurrence (of foetal delivery)	¶Date of birth of mother; if not
¶Date of registration	available, age
Hospitalization	Date of marriage (for legitimate
¶Legitimacy	pregnancies)
¶Period of gestation	Industry
¶Place of occurrence	Literacy or level of formal education
¶Sex	¶Number of children born to this mother
¶Type of birth, i.e. single or plural issue	Occupation
Weight at delivery	¶Place of usual residence (of mother)
	Status (as employer, employee, etc.)

The minimum record for foetal death certificates should be cause of death, and number of weeks of gestation; but for those countries which can secure additional data, whether on the registration certificate or by special inquiry from physicians or others, the following information should be obtained:

What conditions do you believe may have contributed to the death of the foetus (general health of mother, conditions of pregnancy and labour, conditions of foetus, placenta, and labour)?
Was autopsy performed and if so what cause was found?
What was the cause of foetal death in your opinion?
Additional data (duration of pregnancy in weeks, birth weight, time of death before or during labour, labour itself normal or manipulative instrumental or other operative procedure with details).

Compilation

Compiling vital statistics into tables is the means by which the significance of registration data can be examined. This is the means to study incidence, time trends, geographical variations, and their interrelationships. How much of this can be done will depend on the completeness of registration, upon staff and counting machinery, and all the other considerations which are discussed elsewhere in this chapter. There are immense possibilities which increase with the improvement in detailed recording (see p. 214); and particularly when data are studied in relation to social class, occupation, industry (see p. 236), and through other characteristics, ethnic, religious, and otherwise. It is of course, a mistake to try to run before being able to walk. But every nation should seek to perfect the recording, reporting, and collecting of data, so that compilation can be scientifically undertaken.

As the statistics of the British Registrar General have shown over the past 120 years, imaginative tabulation of data can be immensely rewarding. But in the circumstances where every nation's needs are so different and their capacity so varying, it is hardly possible to state precisely what an annual programme of tabulation should seek to do. Every country must examine its own possibilities, bearing in mind that the presentation of results is of value for international as well as national purposes. International comparisons can, of course, be helpful to individual nations as a pointer to national weaknesses. Comparability, above all else, must be obtained.

The procedure of tabulating mortality is set out in WHO Regulations 1 – 'Regulations regarding nomenclature with respect to diseases and causes of death (1948, amended 1965).[97]

The minimum goal for developed countries should be:

The provision of total monthly or quarterly summary counts of live births and deaths (and of foetal deaths, marriages, and divorces if these are included in the collection programme) on a time schedule prompt enough to provide information for administrative needs; and the production of detailed annual tabulations of such type and on such time schedule as will make possible their effective use for the scientific analysis of the interrelationship between demographic, economic, and social factors, for planning, operating, and evaluating public health programmes, and for other purposes as required. In so far as possible, such statistics should be comparable on an international basis and lend themselves to international analysis.[63]

The area of complete tabulation should be the whole country. Where this is impossible, complete tabulation should be secured for as many local areas as possible, with restricted tabulation from as much of the remaining territory as possible. The whole population should as far as possible be covered with separate tabulations for important groups which either cannot be registered completely, or are for other reasons outstanding. The compilation of statistics should be centralized. Tabulations should be by Gregorian calendar periods, by date of occurrence rather than by date of registration and, for the purpose of local statistics, by place of usual residence, i.e., of mother for births and infant deaths, and of deceased for deaths.

Generally speaking, data need to be tabulated for the country as a whole, each major civil division, and every important city. In terms of the few priority items distinguished by ¶ (see p. 230) the following tables can with advantage be prepared:

For deaths: by place of occurrence, by age, sex, and cause; by type of certification and cause; and, for selected diseases which are important as leading causes of death or which have significant seasonal variations, by month of occurrence. In the case of infant deaths tables should be prepared for: place of occurrence; place of residence of mother; age cross-classified with month of occurrence; sex cross-classified with age; and by cause of death. Foetal deaths should be tabulated by: place of occurrence; sex and period of gestation, and late foetal deaths (or stillbirths) also by sex and legitimacy; and by age of mother cross-classified with total birth order.

For live births: by place of occurrence; by attendant at birth; by month of occurrence; by sex cross-classified with legitimacy; and by age of mother cross-classified with live birth order. Confinement can usually be tabulated according to type of birth (single, twin, etc.) cross-classified with state of issue (born alive or dead).

5. Classification by occupation and industry

'If men knew the people', John Graunt said in 1662,[21]

it would appear, how small a part of the people work upon necessary labours and callings, viz. how many women and children do just nothing, only learning to spend what others get; how many are mere voluptuaries, and as it were mere gamesters by trade; how many live by puzzling poor people with unintelligible notions in diversity and philosophy; how many by persuading credulous, delicate, and litigious persons, that their bodies or estates are out of tune, and in danger; how many by fighting as soldiers; how many by ministries of vice and sin; how many by trades of meer pleasure, or ornaments; and how many in a way of lazy attendance, etc. upon others; and on the other side, how few are employed in raising and working necessary food and covering; and of the speculative men, how few do study nature and things! the more ingenious not advancing much further than to write and speak wittily about these matters.

He added:

> I conclude that a clear knowledge of all these particulars, and many more whereat I have shot but at rovers, is necessary, in order to good, certain, and easy government. . . . But whether the knowledge thereof be necessary to many, or fit for others than the sovereign and his chief ministers, I leave to consideration.

John Graunt would probably be astonished to find that his prophesy had been largely fulfilled and that the knowledge of how people work 'upon necessary labours and callings' has proved in the 20th century to be 'necessary to many' and 'fit for others than the sovereign and his chief ministers'.

Studies of mortality, morbidity, fertility, and other surveys to discover the way in which the comunity lives, are greatly enriched – as the International Labour office has emphasized[64] – by relating findings to the work in which people engage. The nature of the work, wherever it is performed, must contribute a major part of the strains to which men and women are subjected. Physically and mentally they are involved in the whirligig of working life. Men and women at work may be classified for statistical purposes in two ways: by occupation or by industry.

a. Industrial classification

For industrial classification, 'the industry in which any individual is engaged is determined, whatever his occupation, by reference to the business or economic activity in, or for the purposes of which, his occupation is followed'.[10] Much may be dependent on the industry in which the work takes place, but much may not – the grouping of individuals together, whatever their occupation, is of importance in itself, particularly from the economic standpoint. But there are other reasons; it is a very different thing to labour in the fields than at the steel furnaces. Industrial classification is based strictly upon the nature of the product, or, in the case of non-manufacturing industries, on the type of service rendered. No consideration of personal occupation enters into it.

The International Standards Industrial Classification[39] distinguishes:

Agriculture, forestry, hunting, and fishing
Mining and quarrying
Manufacturing
Construction
Electricity, gas, water, and sanitary services
Commerce
Transport, storage, and communication
Services
Activities not adequately described.

These divisions are subdivided into 'major groups' and 'groups'. Indices to the groups are *numeric*, containing approximately 10,000 entries, and *alphabetic*, consisting of 17,000 entries. These ensure uniform interpretation.

b. Occupational classification

Occupational standardization *distinguishes groups of people for which the basic common factor is the kind of work done*. Industry may contain many separate and distinct occupations, upon which the nature of the factory, business, or service, in which the work is done has no bearing. Clerks may work in any industry; navvies in a great variety of different undertakings from building to metal manufacture; a crane driver may work in a shipyard, an engineering works, or in building. Where the kind of work is too comprehensive – since it may include too great variations in skill, in physical energy, in environmental or in economic status, or in any combination of these – further subdivisions have to be made, to identify what are substantially separate occupations. The groups must, in any event, be large enough to justify separate enumeration, and they must be distinct in themselves and not dependent upon a parallel classification of industry.

The International Standard Classification of Occupations (see Appendix 8) has 9 major groups, 77 minor groups, and 283 unit groups, covering about 1,700 ocupations.[38, 64] This classification appeared in 1958 and was put to its first major test in the various national censuses held around 1960; it was revised in 1968.* For international comparisons of occupational mortalities and social class classifications based upon it, we may yet have to wait some years.

6. Classification by social class

Mortality, morbidity, and the use made of various services, can also be examined in relation to social stratification – a *prestige rating,* the grouping of people together in terms of the value which society places upon them. Any scale of values of this character must be arbitrary and is not likely to be universally accepted. But there is sufficient agreement to make measurement by social stratification a useful statistical tool. Many methods of devising such a scale have been evolved by social scientists, social anthropologists, doctors, and others – although not yet (1968) at the international level. For the particular purpose of vital and health statistics we need to examine three only, two American and one British.

a. *Evaluation participation*[94]

A method of placing individuals in one of the six classes by means of *interviews and observation.* What the individual says and how he acts provides the evidence for the class divisions, recognized by a particular community; it also reveals the place in these divisions which any individual considers himself and others to occupy. The final rating is obtained by matching the results of many interviews and taking the measure of greatest agreement. This research method can be used to check other methods; but it is costly and time consuming, and can have no real place in the day-to-day work of public health.

b. *Index of status characteristics*[94, 95]

A system of point valuation allots marks to the four chief characteristics which distinguish a man in the eyes of his associates: occupation, source of income, house type, and dwelling area. Warner says:[94]

For an accurate index of social class, each of the four characteristics and the points in their scales must reflect how Americans feel and think about the relative worth of each job, the

* The latest *British Classification of Occupations* was published by H.M.S.O. London 1970

sources of income which support them, and the evaluation of their houses and the neighbour-hoods in which they live. For it is not the house, or the job, or the income, or the neighbourhood that is being measured so much as the evaluations that are in the backs of all your heads – evaluations placed there by our cultural tradition and our society. From one point of view the four characteristics, house, occupation, income, and neighbourhood, are no more than evaluated symbols which are signs of status, telling us the class levels of those who possess the symbols. By measuring the symbols, we measure the relative worth of each; and by adding up their several 'worths', reflecting diverse and complex economic and social values, we get a score which tells us what we think and feel about the worth of a man's social participation, meaning essentially that we are measuring his Evaluated Participation or social class.

Each characteristic is subdivided into seven grades. The seven grades of income range from inherited wealth, which scores 1, to public relief or non-respectable income, which scores 7; housing from large houses in excellent condition scoring 1 to houses in very bad condition scoring 7; the dwelling area from 'superior region' to the 'lowest slum'; and occupation from 'high professional and proprietors of large businesses' to unskilled workers. A multiplying factor takes into account the varying importance of house, income, dwelling area, and occupation. Occupation is rated at 4, income and house at 3, and dwelling area 2. Thus the topmost score in this scale is 12; 4 for occupation, 3 each for income and house, and 2 for dwelling area; the lowest score is 84 (28, 21, 21, 14). A certain clerk (Mr Jones) with a salary, living in an average sized house in average condition, in a residential neighbourhood which is beginning to deteriorate scored:

	Rating		Weight	Score
Occupation (clerk)	3	×	4	12
Source of income (salary)	4	×	3	12
House type (average)	4	×	3	12
Dwelling area (below average)	5	×	2	10
				46

Six classes are used by arbitrary divisions with the range 12 to 84. Thus the two upper classes extend from 12 to 22; upper middle is 23 to 37; lower middle is 38 to 53; upper lower is 54 to 66; lower lower is 67 to 84. Mr Jones is rated as lower middle class.

c. Social class by occupation

The British social class grading uses the distinctions which arise out of working conditions alone. This arbitrary grouping dates back in substance to that of Dr T. H. C. Stevenson, the Chief Medical Statistical Officer, first produced in 1911, consisting of five classes: (1) professional, etc., occupations; (2) intermediate occupations; (3) skilled occupations; (4) partly skilled occupations, and (5) unskilled occupations. Its basis is the general standing of each occupational group within the community, economic circumstances not being taken into account, except in so far as they are reflected in occupation. The broad structure of the five social classes is as follows: *

* For the details of the British Social Class grading see Census 1951 Classification of Occupations, 1956, with amendments in Classification of Occupations 1960, H.M.S.O., London: Brockington (1965) Appendix, Social Stratification. In *The Health of the Community*, pp. 325–334, London: Churchill.

1. *Professional, etc.*
   Professional engineering, surveying, and architecture
   The medical profession
   The legal profession
   Scientists
   Ministers of all churches
   Officers of all the armed forces
   Literature
   Directors of business
(These are higher administrative and professional occupations and business
directorships.)

2. *Intermediate*
   Managing Directors and employers of business
   Various professional persons and officials
   Teachers
   Clerks (costing, estimating, and accounting only)
   Hotel and restaurant keepers
   Farmers
   Medical auxiliaries
   Proprietors and managers of wholesale and retail businesses
(These are persons responsible for initiating policy and others without this
responsibility but some responsibility over others.)

3. *Skilled*
   Clerical workers
   Shop assistants
   Personal service
   Foreman, superintending staff, and inspectors
   Skilled workers in:
      transport and communications
      minor professional and technical occupations
      civilian defence
      armed forces (other ranks)
      entertainment and sport
      wood and cane
      bricks
      glass
      coal
      chemical and allied trades
      metal manufacture and engineering
      textiles
      tanning, leather goods, fur dressing
      makers of textile goods and articles of dress
      makers of foods, drink, and tobacco
      paper, printers, and bookbinders
      rubber, plastics, and musical instruments

building, contracting, painters, decorators
agricultural craftsmen

(These are skilled workers with a special name, special responsibility and adaptability.)

4. *Partly skilled, i.e. workers on or in:*
   Agriculture
   Mines
   Metal industries
   Textiles
   Transport
   In service
   Various semi-skilled occupations

(These are semi-skilled or persons who are doing manual work which needs no great skill or training, but who are doing it habitually and in association with a particular industry.)

5. *Unskilled*
   Labourers
   Cleaners
   Other lowly occupations

(The use of the word unskilled does not mean of course lack of all skill).

The reliability of a social classification based upon occupation has been examined in a study in which 138 occupations were separated into 9 groups.[31] In 66 five judges differed no more than one grade and in 10 all agreed. A difference of 4 grades was observed for only six occupations; a difference of 3 for 19; of 2 for 37. In a further study, 30 occupations in 5 groups were graded by 74 members and friends of an Adult Education class. The median grading of the 74 returns compared closely with the standard. In 1,000 classifications obtained through representative organizations the average judgement of the general public differed from the standard classification (now in seven groups) in three instances only – farmer, coal hewer, and railway porter.

Thus occupations can be arranged in order of the social value ascribed to them in common acceptance, where the determining factors are the man's associates while at his job and their average standard. Yet no agreed scale could ever exist by which to rank all occupations. 'Farmers and farm labourers may agree on the social rating which each group affords the other. But such an agreement is far less likely to be reached by, for example, farmers and artists.[26] In the USA, it is said, people tend to class themselves as 'middle class' more frequently than in the judgement of independent observers. Some apparent discrepancies may represent no more than a difference in judgement as when the Registrar General placed actors and musicians (codes 835 and 836) originally within class 3, on the same level as stage hands (code 837), chimney sweeps (codes 876), and bath and wash-house attendants and managers (code 871) (they were moved in 1960 from class 3 to class 2)[10] Other discrepancies arise from the handling of occupational groups as units. Since each is assigned as a whole, there must often be individuals within the group for whom the resultant social class grading seems less appropriate. University teachers, including the Professors who are directors of University departments, are now better placed as professionals in class 1 than they were before 1960[10] as teachers within class 2. The main divergencies will be found in the central regions of the scale. Classes 1 and 5 are composed of individuals who would probably be assigned to the top and bottom of the social scale by almost any set of criteria. Bankers, company directors, and shipowners on the one hand, and street newspaper sellers and rag and bone sorters on the other, would, by common consent, appear at opposite ends of any scale.

The single criterion of occupation has many advantages in ease of handling; denominators can be obtained through the census and numerators through the returns from local registrars. Although no precise comparison has been made between the results of ISC and the Registrar General's classification or the International Standard of Occupations, it seems likely that the majority of individuals would find themselves in the same social class, whether their status was based on an 84 point rating, or upon a single judgement on occupation. Certainly Mr Jones, earlier quoted, would have been in class 3, in the British social class on occupation alone (unless a book-keeping clerk prior to 1960 in class 2).[10]

Nevertheless:

Although occupation may be a major determinant in social position (and, conversely, 'social position' a major determinant in the choice of occupation), it is by no means the only determinant, and no classification based solely upon that factor can be fully satisfactory. A more realistic result (bearing in mind the probable limitations) might be achieved by using education and occupation as double criteria; and when the next census is being planned the possibility of collecting, either for the whole population or by means of a sample, information on education and other criteria should be considered.[26]

Glass' suggestion has not yet been followed in Britain.*

The chief weakness of the social classification by occupation lies, not so much in the discrepancies of individual occupations – some are inescapable and, taking the broad view, insignificant – but in a five- or six-class social grading, which necessarily lumps together occupational groups of widely differing characteristics. Class 3, which includes skilled workmen, also contains the 'white collar' occupations; the shop assistants; and 'personal service'. Such a classification is often too broad for a detailed investigation of any one social factor.

Many expansions of the original social class grading can be made to meet the needs of particular countries. The five-class scale can be expanded or contracted, like the abbreviations of the International Classification of Diseases, Injury, and Causes of Death, retaining the code groupings, so that the effects of social class in mortality and morbidity and allied studies can be compared.

Standardization by socio-economic grouping

Mortality, morbidity and other attributes can be studied by socio-economic grouping, which groups together those with similar social, cultural and recrea-

* Cf. Kitagawa & Hauser (1960) *Social and Economic Differences in Mortality in the U.S.A.*

tional habits, while paying regard also to economic aspects. The Conference of European Statisticians' (1959)[13] 16 socio-economic groups are as follows:

1. *Employers and managers in central and local government, industry, commerce, etc. – large establishments:* Persons who employ others or generally plan and supervise in non-agricultural enterprises employing 25 or more persons.

2. *Employers and managers in industry, commerce, etc. – small establishments:* as in 1. but in establishments employing fewer than 25 persons.

3. *Professional workers – self employed:* self employed persons engaged in work normally requiring qualifications of university degree standard.

4. *Professional workers – employees:* employees engaged in work normally requiring qualifications of university degree standard.

5. *Intermediate non-manual workers:* employees, not exercising general planning or supervisory powers, engaged in non-manual occupations ancillary to the professions but not normally requiring qualifications of university degree standard; persons engaged in artistic work and not employing others thereat; and persons engaged in occupations otherwise included in Group 6 who have an additional and formal supervisory function.

6. *Junior non-manual workers:* employees, not exercising general planning or supervisory powers engaged in clerical, sales and non-manual communications and security occupations, excluding those who have additional and formal supervisory functions.

7. *Personal service workers:* employees engaged in service occupations caring for food, drink, clothing and other personal needs.

8. *Foremen and supervisors – manual:* employees (other than managers) who formally and immediately supervise others engaged in manual occupations, whether or not themselves engaged in such occupations.

9. *Skilled manual workers:* employees engaged in manual occupations which require considerable and specific skills.

10. *Semi-skilled manual workers:* employees engaged in manual occupations which require slight but specific skills.

11. *Unskilled manual workers:* other employees engaged in manual occupations.

12. *Own account workers (other than professional):* self employed persons engaged in any trade, personal service or manual occupation not formally requiring training of university degree standard and having no employees other than family workers.

13. *Farmers – employers and managers:* persons who own, rent or manage farms, market gardens or forests, employing people other than family workers in the work of the enterprise.

14. *Farmers – own account:* persons who own or rent farms, market gardens or forests and having no employees other than family workers.

15. *Agricultural workers:* employees in tending crops, animals, game or operating agricultural or forestry machinery.

16. *Members of armed forces.*

7. Census enumeration

For the calculation of rates, using mortality and morbidity data, it is necessary to know the '*population at risk*' which provides the denominator.

Census enumerations have been a feature of most civilizations throughout history, in association with conscription, collection of taxes, and other unpleasant events.[83] In modern times perhaps the earliest numerations were in the British and French colonies of Canada (1665) and in Iceland (1703). Census-taking in Europe dates from 1748 in Sweden and 1769 in Denmark. Most of the European countries followed suit in the latter part of the eighteenth century. The constitution of the United States of America (1790) prescribed a decennial census as a means for making a fair distribution among the States of seats in Congress. Britain did not take this important step until 1801, after a lengthy argument covering 50 years, as to the dangers of interfering with private liberty and contravening Christian teaching.[23] The apocryphal story of the excited Member of the House of Commons, who protested so indignantly, now echoes down the ages. 'I do not believe that there is any set of men, indeed any individual of the human species, so presumptuous or so abandoned as to make the proposal ... I hold this project to be totally subversive to the last remains of English liberty.'

A great change of outlook, making a study of this nature more acceptable to British people, had resulted from the publication in 1798 by Thomas Malthus of his *Essay on the Principles of Population*, in which he postulated that population must advance geometrically and food arithmetically, so that population must outrun supply unless checked by 'moral restraint, vice, or misery'.[48] English liberties have survived and perhaps been strengthened by the decennial census, which with unavoidable breaks has been held for the last 170 years.

Throughout the 19th century, most countries of the world took to this expedient. The USSR was late in the field (1897), Turkey still later (1927).[117] By 1973, few countries, Afghanistan among them, remained unnumbered. In 1971, the total aggregate population of the world with a complete census amounted to 3,481 million, a further 87 million were covered by sample surveys; and 39 million only went unnumbered, except for certain groups. In 21 years (1950 to 1971), the population covered by a complete census doubled (from 1706).[60]

Modern censuses provide not only information about the inhabitants, but also much detail about their living conditions – composition of families, race, religion, occupation, etc. The population commission of the United Nations[29] in 1948 gave a list of twelve items, as recommended subjects without regard to relative importance: (1) total population; (2) sex; (3) age; (4) marital status; (5) place of birth; (6) cititzenship; (7) mother tongue; (8) educational characteristics; (9) fertility data; (10) economic characteristics (total economically active and inactive population; occupation, industry, and industrial status; population dependent on various types of economic activities; agricultural population), (11) urban and rural population; (12) households. Approximately this minimum was effectively used in the 1950 Pan-American census. The topics recommended in

Principles and Recommendations for the 1970 Population Census (UN 1967) were more detailed (e.g. place of residence, relation to head of household, children living and born alive, school attendance, educational attainment).

During the past 50 years, particularly after the formation of the League of Nations, and more recently under the United Nations, there has been progress towards uniformity; so that today over eighty nations have more or less comparable census statistics. The number and nature of items included on the census schedule are many and they vary from country to country, and from census to census within the same country, according to national needs and interest, or previous census experience. Total population, sex, age, marital status, and economic characteristics are almost universally investigated; citizenship, place of birth, religion, education, language, race, physical and mental defects are frequently, but not generally included.

In underdeveloped countries where registration of vital statistics is least adequate the census is all the more important, because it provides the only source of information on such questions as fertility, mortality and migration.[28] In an African seminar,[69] the following minimum was suggested: (1) *de facto* or *de jure* domicile; (2) relationship to head of household; (3) sex; (4) age, or failing that, age group; (5) tribe or race (or citizenship where applicable). Further to these it was suggested that a high priority be given to questions on literacy, birthplace, and marital status; a lower priority to questions relating to economic status (occupation, industry, status), and lowest to questions on the total number of children born to each woman, and the numbers still living. Age may need to be estimated, and the population placed in physiological age groups: sucklings (up to two years), young (from weaning to puberty), adults (from puberty to menopause in women and longer in males), old people (past work).[17]

The advantages of refinement in census questioning to the compilation of vital and health statistics can be considerable. Occupation gives the population at risk for the calculation of occupational and social class mortality (see p. 236); and the number of rooms coupled with the persons living in the house makes it possible to calculate the density of living, either as an average of persons per room or in proportions living at various density levels. From this it is possible to determine the relationship of infant mortality and tuberculosis, etc., to the density of household living.

The census grows in importance. In spite of the increasing body of statistical data available from other sources and of the increasing use nowadays of other methods of obtaining necessary basic material for purposes of government, a periodical census of the whole population still remains a unique and indispensable instrument[11] (see Chapter 29).

8. Health indicators

Vital and health statistics provide the basic material for a judgement of health in a community; but the search for indices, or health indicators, has engaged the attention of statisticians since the time of Graunt, and is likely to continue to do so for many years. Health indicators may be either *compre-*

hensive or specific. Comprehensive indicators include: the proportional mortality ratio, the expectation of life and the crude death rate. A complete picture of health statistics would also make a comprehensive indicator. The proportional mortality ratio is defined as the number of deaths at age 50 and over as a percentage of total deaths (Swaroop). If everyone survives to the age of 50, the proposed index would be 100, and if no one does, it would be zero.[101]

Specific indicators are infant mortality and deaths from communicable diseases per 100,000, including all infective and parasitic diseases listed in the International Classification. Satisfactory specific indicators for health services and activities, calculations of the percentage of population receiving protected water supplies and having facilities for proper disposal of excreta, indices of mental health, of nutrition, etc, have yet to be devised.

Most indicators are in terms of the group – family, household, sections of the community, or in the population of the country as a whole (the macro-approach); assessments of individual health (the micro-approach), possibly by surveys (see Chapters 25 and 26), should be equally significant.

Indices of health should satisfy the following conditions: (1) records should be available on a national scale; (2) terms and procedures used in recording, classifying, and tabulation data should be comparable; (3) the indicator should reflect the effect of as wide a variety of factors influencing health as possible; and (4) if a choice is to be made from several indicators (in terms of (3) above), preference should be given to the most sensitive, i.e., the one which will best reflect variations.[107] So many existing indices fail in one or more of these requirements. More research is needed before valid and comparable indicators can be used effectively.

24. The Measurement of Morbidity

The significance of morbidity statistics

If the object of providing measurements of disease is to help reduce the ills, cost, and waste thereby caused, morbidity can supplement, and in some respects do more than, mortality statistics. They tell the story of the many diseases which do not lead to death, and yet produce immense suffering and economic loss. They tell us whether decline in mortality is due to change in frequency of a disease, or simply to a change in its outcome. They can be related more closely to the social conditions which cause disease and which may be at work long before death takes place.

They can help to detect new hazards early, such as thalidomide malformations; they can indicate changes in the frequency of diseases calling for special care, or in the relative proportions of preventable diseases and diseases calling for treatment; they help in the identification of cause, factors affecting incidence and natural history, and presymptomatic features; they show the strengths and weaknesses of preventive and therapeutic measures in diseases both acute and chronic.

They do more than mortality data to indicate where better facilities are needed and what administrative adjustments are necessary, particularly in the organized health services, which nations are now beginning to develop. In comparison with mortality we are surprisingly ignorant of essential details about the distribution of disease, and in consequence, of the services which are needed to handle it. We need to know about those who go to hospital and of those treated by general practitioners; about the illness that people have or think they have which do not take them to a doctor; and about absences from work and school; why the work done in different institutions differs; why some hospitals deal with more patients than others. We must know about the sickness resulting from cancer, and of course much else.

The development of recording systems, for illness at home, in hospitals, at work, and through general practice, is not an easy task; but it is one of the most important now facing the world. This will help in the special studies of particular problems *relevant to the circumstances of each country* which, as emphasized elsewhere, are so necessary.

The definition of illness

In contrast with death, a clearly defined event, illness is difficult to define. It may wax and wane; its manifestations may be indefinite or even subjective; it may endure for periods of varying length; and it may be repeated. The terms which are used to describe it are many and varied; for example, *sickness, illness, diseases, injury, defect, impairment, handicap, complaint, morbid condition.* Other terms in common use describe the particular episode rather than the illness itself, for example, *new, old, recurrent, sub-clinical, latent, manifest, continued, pre-existing, acute, chronic, relapse.* Still others describe the severity and duration, for example, *short-term, long-term, major, minor,* etc. So many terms cause confusion and interfere with scientific exactitude. The time has come for greater precision.

For the purpose of statistics, we cannot include all departures from health, such as were discussed in Chapter 1. Some more clearly defined boundary has to be found both for the starting-point of illness and what constitutes it; as well as for many variations on the theme of illness, which we need in order to measure it, such as *'new illness', 'recurrence',* and *'relapse',* and for the qualifying terms, such as duration and frequency, which help to define it. What the boundary line should be has not yet been internationally agreed. But national committees in Canada, Denmark, France, Norway, and the UK and the USA early submitted reports and recommendations.[99] For the present, the following definitions may provide a working basis.[78]*

Illness. A condition included in codes (001–795) of the International Statistical Classification of Disease Injuries and Causes of Death, 1948 (latest revision) and which caused some disability during the period of time to which the statistics relate. By disability is meant that the subject was "suffering from' it or was aware of its existence as something disturbing his state of health during the period.
New illness. An illness which 'began' in the sense defined above at some time during the period, and which was not a recurrence as defined below.
Recurrence of illness. An attack of illness similar to one experienced previously, any such previous attack having subsided at least one week before the present one began.
Continued illness. An illness present throughout, or terminating during the period, which had started before the beginning of the period.
Ill-defined illness. A symptomatic or undiagnosed complaint included in codes 773, 780–795 of the International Classification.
Minor ailment. Illness of defined diagnosis which does not customarily or did not, in fact, produce incapacity amounting to three days duration.
Injury. A condition produced by an external cause such as violence, accident, poisoning, or misadventure in applying a diagnostic procedure, and included in codes 800–999 of the International Classification of 1948 (as subsequently revised).

Since there are many concepts of what constitute illness, statistically speaking, there is no internationally understood starting-point. One definition put forward is that the start of the illness is the point at which either the subject began to be conscious of symptoms or some disability, or someone else decided that disease was present of a nature which could not continue to be ignored without danger to the patient. But this definition does not include residual conditions from past disease, or congenital abnormalities, unless they prevent the patient from living a normal life, or cause symptoms which he would describe as illness; nor would it include latent or early illness unknown to the patient, for example, incubating infections or unsuspected cancer.

Two frequencies of disease can be measured, namely, *prevalence* and *incidence.* Prevalence is *'the number of instances of illness or of persons ill, or*

* Broadly speaking these definitions, although not adopted internationally are still valid. Personal communication Dr Abe Adelstein, O.P.C.S., London, 1974.

I

of any other event such as accidents, in a specified population, without any distinction between new and old cases'. It may be recorded as a stated moment (*point prevalence*), or during a given period of time (*period prevalence*). Incidence is *the number of instances of illness commencing, or of persons falling ill, during a given period in a specified population*'. (For rates see Appendix 7.)

In both incidence and prevalence, it should be clearly stated whether the data represents numbers of instances of the disease, or numbers of persons ill; in recurring diseases, such as influenza, one person, may have more than one spell, just as in cancer one person may be affected in several sites simultaneously.

The following characteristics further distinguish incidence and prevalence:

1. Whereas incidence refers only to *new* cases, prevalence refers to all cases, irrespective of whether they are *new* or *old*.

2. Whereas prevalence reflects the situation existing at a given moment (point prevalence) or provides a picture of the situation existing over a given period (period prevalence), incidence is an index of a changing situation over a stated period of time. In other words, prevalence is usually a static concept, whereas incidence is always dynamic.

3. Whereas point prevalence can be determined by a single survey, incidence and period prevalence require continuous registration over a period of time. In practice, this applies mostly to notifiable diseases and to diseases recorded in hospitals, since for other diseases no permanent or continuous registration is available.

4. While prevalence and incidence may differ widely in the case of diseases of long duration, they will differ only slightly with diseases that run a rapid course. Thus, the total number of cases of cancer, old and new, recorded in a country over a period of one year (period prevalence) will obviously be much higher than the number of *new* cases registered.

5. If the incidence fluctuates, the fluctuations may not be reflected in the period prevalence when the disease is of long duration. Thus, a sharp decline in incidence may not be paralleled by a corresponding decrease in the prevalence, because the latter may be overtaken by a fresh rise in incidence. However, if a new treatment reduces the duration of a disease, even if the incidence remains unchanged, the prevalence will decrease until a new equilibrium is established. On the other hand, in chronic diseases that are incurable and ultimately fatal, a lengthening of the survival period will increase prevalence but not incidence.

An example of differences obtained through the expression of the frequency of a disease in terms of incidence and prevalence is given in Fig. 24.1. It is to be noted that, while for incidence over a long period (in this instance three years) the total number of cases represents the sum of the number of new cases for each of the shorter periods considered (5 + 6 + 5 = 16), this is not true for period prevalence (prevalence for the period 1960–62 is not 8 + 10 + 12 = 30; it is 8 + 6 + 5 = 19, since some cases stretch over two or all three of the years considered).

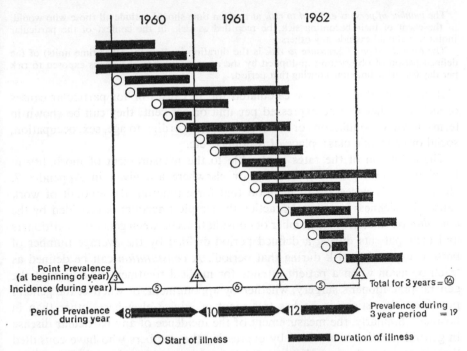

Fig. 24.1 Frequency of disease in terms of incidence and prevalence.

Units of measurement

It is possible to measure the illnesses themselves; the persons affected; the time involved; or the episodes associated with illness. The number of illnesses can be computed in three ways as: those which begin during a unit of time; those which were experienced at any time during it; or those present at a given point of time.[78] The persons affected can be measured in the same three ways. The time involved can be measured in days (or other time units) of illness during a period.

Commonly it is more convenient to measure not the sickness itself, but the episodes associated with it, for example, medical care, consultation, or absence from work. When this is done, the measurements may relate, for example, to spells of *sickness absence* or *in-patient care* or to numbers who *consult their practitioners*, who *attend out-patient departments* or who are *absent sick*.

The Statistics Sub-Committee of the British Registrar General's Advisory Committee, Britain's equivalent of a national committee, has suggested the following definitions for the words or terms used in these measurements (not yet, 1974, adopted internationally).[51]

The term *case* of sickness is intended to cover the whole course of one disease in one person, as far as that course is relevant to the particular inquiry concerned'.

A *spell* of sickness is a period during which a person is sick on one day (or shift), or on each of a consecutive series of days (or shifts).

The *duration* of a spell of sickness normally includes each of the consecutive days for which sickness is recorded. In measuring the duration of a spell of in-patient care, the day on which the patient is discharged should be counted as well as that on which he is admitted.

The *number of persons exposed to risk* at a given time should include all those who would, in the event of their becoming sick, be recorded as sick, in the context of the particular inquiry; it should exclude any others.

The *total duration of exposure to risk* is the duration in days (or other time units) of the defined period of observation multiplied by the average number of persons exposed to risk per day (or other time unit) during that period.

Rates of morbidity can be calculated for all causes or for particular causes of sickness; they can be expressed per unit or per cent; they can be shown in terms of whole populations or in subdivisions, according to age, sex, occupation, social or economic class, place of residence, etc.

The definition of the rates applicable to the measurement of morbidity in hospital, general practice, industry, or elsewhere are given in Appendix 7. Here it is only necessary to mention that for estimating the amount of work caused by sickness in general practice the simplest account is provided by the *consultation rate*, i.e., 'the number of consultations between general practitioners and their patients during a defined period divided by the average number of persons exposed to risk during that period'. A *consultation* can be defined as 'each occasion when a patient attends for medical treatment or advice at the general practitioner's surgery, whether by appointment, or when at the general practitioner's instigation he has treatment or advice elsewhere, other than in hospital'. Similarly, the measurement of the incidence of any particular disease in general practice is obtained by expressing the numbers who have consulted their doctor for the complaint at least once as a proportion of the patients on his list.

Notification as a source of morbidity statistics[85, 111, 112]

Notification is a convenient mechanism in day-to-day public health practice, for the control of epidemic and endemic disease. This applies to countries in all stages of development, including those in which full-scale eradication programmes are being attempted. Notification is one of the main defensive weapons in keeping at bay the depredations of bacteria and parasites. But it is as valuable in peace, so to speak, as in war, in epidemiological studies in the quiet of the office, which help us to keep a running account of the geographical distribution of infectious disease. The value transcends national boundaries for which the bacterial world has no respect.

As the circumstances in which infections flourish vary so widely, so also must the need for notification. The lists of notifiable disease differ greatly in different countries. Notification can never be made uniform and precisely comparable throughout the world. The time, trouble, and cost of operating it will always be the determining factors, so that where diseases are of little significance it would be unreasonable to impose irksome regulations. The notification of abortus fever may seem valuable in Norway and not in the United Kingdom, although it is not altogether clear why not. Nevertheless there is a strong case for agreeing a basic list of notifiable diseases common to all countries; such as that devised in a South American Seminar (1953). This list, justified by the severity, risk of spread (or both), the existence of control measures capable of universal application and other technical administrative reasons might be as follows:

Cholera, plague, relapsing fever (louse-borne), smallpox, typhus fever (louse-borne), yellow fever, diphtheria, encephalitis (virus), gonorrhoea, influenza, malaria, meningitis (meningococcal), poliomyelitis, rabies (human and animal), scarlet fever, syphilis, tuberculosis, typhoid and paratyphoid, typhus (murine), other venereal diseases, whooping cough.[85] Many consider also that medical and non-medical notifications should be distinguished and recorded separately.

If absolute uniformity is impossible, nevertheless the legal sanctions in which the process of notification is invested, and its close relationship to dramatic episodes with strong emotional appeal, give it qualities of particular value in morbidity studies. Common defects, which impair the usefulness of notification, both nationally and internationally, should as far as possible, be remedied. Among such common defects are *incompleteness, varying criteria for diagnosis, differing day-to-day procedures for correcting diagnoses and for avoiding duplication of notifications from more than one source, varying procedures for publishing data,* as, for example, where some classify by area and others by residence, some by sex and age, and others by general total, and *delays in notification.* A questionnaire to member states (1962) revealed that even the six 'quarantinable' diseases, with internationally agreed obligations (cholera, plague, relapsing fever (louse-borne),* smallpox, typhus fever (louse-borne), yellow fever), were not universally notifiable and even when notified were generally inaccurately reported.

Lack of doctors; their indifference, forgetfulness or unwillingness; ignorance, illiteracy, superstition of the population; lack of public services; non-medical notification; absence of standard forms of briefing, of scrutiny, of correction, of fees, of laboratory facilities; suspicions about confidentiality; failure to accept death certificates – all play a part in preventing proper notification.[85]

Some of these difficulties must be resolved locally by changes in administrative procedures, or by education of general practitioners. The fullest cooperation of the medical profession and health institutes alone can overcome incompleteness, while the development of correct procedures, which avoid duplication of notifications and which ensure that they are corrected for the final diagnosis, alone can do much to remove inaccuracies. But much can only be resolved by full international collaboration. The third report of the expert committee on health statistics (1952) recommended that the national committees of France, Italy, the Netherlands, the United Kingdom, and the USA make special studies of the problems involved.

The criterion for notification is of great importance. Here we must depart somewhat from our definition of illness as set out earlier (see Chap. 1). Clearly we cannot notify persons only by reason of the fact that they consider themselves to be sick. Nor could laboratory evidence alone justify a notification, unless the notifiable disease in question is clearly defined as such, as in the case of syphilis in pregnancy. The person recorded as having a notifiable disease should be 'suffering from' it, i.e. clinically sick. Recent developments in the

* Relapsing fever no longer ranks as a quarantinable disease (1974).

epidemiology of notifiable disease have only served to emphasize that any departure from this criterion is likely to lead to confusion, not only in statistics, but in administration. The finding of the causative organism in nose, throat, faeces, urine, or gastric contents does not constitute the presence of the disease; nor do thoracic shadows on a skiagram, or serum reactions to biological substances, *unless accompanied by signs or symptoms attributable to the disease.* We should resist using bacteriological, biological, and radiological tests as measures of notifiable disease without regard to what the subject is suffering from; although, of course, such special examinations may greatly help in the diagnosis of departures from normal health. The failure to make the distinction in statistical studies between the clinical presence of active disease and the detection of serological variations has led to confusion, as in statistical studies into the efficacy of BCG vaccination in preventing tuberculosis.

This narrower definition of illness for the purpose of notifiable disease does not reflect in any way upon the use of laboratory examinations in morbidity statistics in general. It is, of course, of great value to make statistical studies of serological and bacteriological reactions (Wassermann's, tuberculin reactions, and haemoglobin estimations) as determined by mass examination or otherwise. The positive tuberculin test in infants, like the positive Wassermann reaction, can help in the search for sources of infection.

Nevertheless, in view of the importance of carriers as sources of infection, there is a strong case for notification of the carrier, as such, with an internationally agreed definition to include: the presence of a specific microorganism; absence of recognizable symptoms or signs of disease; shedding of micro-organisms in discharges or excretions; liability as a source of infection; restriction to named diseases; and restriction to specific occupations.

Sub-clinical attacks of diseases, such as poliomyelitis, present exceptional difficulty, but the rules for their inclusion must be governed by the usual definition of notifiable disease. In each case an individual decision will have to be reached as to the presence of symptoms or signs which permit the diagnosis of a mild case of the disease. It may be necessary to record the incident as 'ill-defined illness'.

Notifications of non-infectious disease, such as cancer, congenital malformation, mental illness, often referred to as *registration* (see p. 258) play an important rôle in the establishment of permanent registers, giving information on prevalence and providing the basis of services for care.

The calculation of rates may help both in examining the distribution of notifiable disease and in indicating preventive measures. The notification rate, an inception rate (see Appendix 7), is:

the number of notifications during a defined period divided by the average number of persons exposed to risk during that period.

It may be applied to an *ad hoc* system of notification in a special survey, as well as to the statutory system. For the calculation of rates, notification must be known to be practically complete, or, if not, allowance must be made for varying completeness in different groups of the population. Nevertheless, incomplete statistics for a local area may be useful for comparisons over a period of years, provided the factors causing incompleteness are understood and remain unchanged.

The fatality rate may be sufficiently accurate to indicate substantial changes in severity or in efficacy of treatment, for a particular disease. But this rate will tend to be overstated, since the notification of cases must always be less complete than the certification of deaths.

Records of general practice[24, 25, 46, 60, 85, 101]

The study of general practitioners' records can yield rich sources of information which will help in three particular ways:

1. to examine the detailed working of general practice;
2. to measure the amount of work which different diseases cause in general practice; and
3. to estimate an incidence for many causes of sickness.

In this latter capacity they are likely to be among the most useful sources of information, but they cannot by themselves indicate the full incidence of sickness. Minor ailments for which people do not always consult their doctor will be under-stated; diseases usually treated in hospital will not be recorded after the initial consultation and reference to hospital. The household sickness survey (see p. 274) and studies of hospital records (see below) will provide some part at least of what is missing. Period prevalence rates will be subject to the idiosyncrasies of medical terminology in use by individual general practitioners and will generally suffer somewhat from being based upon small populations. For the calculation of rates (see p. 241) the population at risk must be known. This will be known in the United Kingdom, where there is a complete list of patients under the National Health Service Act who would normally attend each practice. Elsewhere the work of defining the population at risk in an individual practice, or small group of practices, may present considerable difficulty.

Experience in morbidity studies using general practitioners' records is still limited. Logan's studies 1951/2 and 53/4[24, 25] covered consultations and patient consulting rates per 1,000 population in terms of 200 different diseases and conditions together with a number of other calculations designed to show the details of work undertaken, such as how often patients consulted their doctors, the rates of admission to hospital, and analyses of sickness certificates given to insured patients. A larger inquiry covering half a million patients examined 280,000 clinical records[46] in more than 100 practices (May 1955 – April 1956), with a second national study in 1970–71.[60]

Records of hospital[112]

The use of hospital records for vital and health statistics has long been neglected, sadly so if we consider the immense significance of hospitals and the vast amount of valuable information which they must have had so easily to hand during the long period of their history. What records of past epidemics, what understanding of prevailing conditions in past times might now be our common knowledge, if hospitals had been accustomed to keep even relatively simple accounts of the patients who passed through their wards. What makes this defect even more difficult to bear is the fact that great minds in past times had recognized their importance and urged their close scrutiny. Florence Nightingale, in particular, understood their value; for, as previously mentioned, she submitted a reasoned statement on the subject of hospital statistics to the 4th International Statistical Congress held in London in 1870:

> With the view of rendering the present stores of observation useful, and of collecting all future observations on one uniform plan, tables have been prepared for recording, on one common form, all the facts of hospital experience.
> The forms will be submitted to the Congress. They have been already tried in several hospitals, and the results have been sufficient to show how large a field for statistical analysis and inquiry would be opened by their general adoption.
> They would enable us to ascertain the relative mortality in different hospitals, as well as of different diseases and injuries at the same and at different ages, the relative frequency of different diseases and injuries among the classes which enter hospitals in different countries, and in different districts of the same country. They would enable us to ascertain how much of each year of life is wasted by illness – what diseases and ages press most heavily on the resources of particular hospitals. For example, it was found that a very large proportion of the limited finances of one hospital was swallowed up by one preventable disease – rheumatism – to the exclusion of many important cases or other diseases from the benefits of hospital treatment.
> It has been shown that most of the cases admitted to the hospitals, where the forms have been tried, belong to the productive ages of life, and not to the ages at the two extremes of existence.
> The relation of the duration of cases to the general utility of a hospital has never yet been shown, although it must be obvious that if, by any sanitary means or improved treatment, the duration of cases could be reduced to one-half, the utility of the hospital would be doubled, so far as its funds are concerned.
> The proposed forms would enable the mortality in hospitals, and also the mortality from particular diseases, injuries, and operations, to be ascertained with accuracy; and these facts, together with the duration of cases, would enable the value of particular methods of treatment and of special operations to be brought to statistical proof. The sanitary state of the hospital itself could likewise be ascertained. The statistics of rare diseases and operations are still very imperfect, but by abstracting the results of such diseases and operations from the tables after a long term of years, trustworthy data could be obtained to guide future experience.[61]

Spent time has gone as irrevocably as spilt milk. These long neglected threads are now being gathered together to weave the fabric on which the story of man's suffering is indelibly printed. Hospitals everywhere can play a rôle in data collection; those in less developed countries are often the most reliable source of information on morbidity. Hospital statistics can help in three important ways: (1) in research to help not only in 'rare diseases and operations', which are as rare today as in Miss Nightingale's time, but also in our understanding of the cause of common afflictions; (2) in morbidity studies, at least of those conditions which lead to admission to an institution; and (3) in planning hospitals, both in the matter of their domestic details and in their relation to the health service as a whole.

The diagnosis of hospital cases can be made with the greater precision which results from laboratory and autopsy aids. Every effort should be made to take advantage of this. Each case should be recorded as follows:[99]

1. principal disease, injury, or other condition leading to admission

2. principal complication(s): the most important first and whether present at admission

3. principal accessory acute condition: whether present at admission

4. principal accessory chronic condition.

The entry under 1 should be the underlying cause, even if the cause of admission is entered under 2.

Identifying data to be recorded should include as a minimum: name, type, and location of hospital; patient's name, national identity number, hospital registration number, race, sex, and date of birth; dates of admission and discharge; information about service referring patient (general practitioner, consultant, other hospital, etc.). A special section should provide for deaths, indicating whether an autopsy was performed and the cause of death as entered on the death certificate.

Statistics for hospital planning

Statistics, which help us to understand the uses to which hospitals are put, are as essential as they have been neglected. The types of illness treated as out-patient and in-patient cases; the categories of persons admitted classified according to sex, age, civil state, occupation, duration of disorder; the period between the onset of illness and admission; the degree of conformity in diagnosis; the association between different diseases, can help to guide our plans for hospital construction. So also can the study of the hospital population help us to see hospitals in balance with other services. The information gained from the 1951 census in England and Wales may be cited as an example.[84] The 1951 census showed a preponderance in all hospitals of single, widowed, and divorced people over married – particularly in mental hospitals and those for the chronic sick over 65 years of age. Such an observation must give us pause. It raises vital issues, for example, the relationship of hospital to home care, which must some time be faced by all national planners.

Morbidity in hospital statistics

When we use hospital patients as a source of information about sickness in the community as a whole, we need to remember that hospital statistics are highly selective. They do not permit of generalization to the population as a whole, since they are necessarily restricted to those diseases which normally require admission to hospital and to those classes of persons who, for one reason or another, use the hospital more readily. Yet the numbers of various types of illness, classified according to the International List, and arranged according to age, sex, occupation, industry, and social class, can do much, by filling out other sources of morbidity, to present a picture of the community as a whole. For this reason alone it is important that such relatively simple recording, in collaboration with the health department, should be done in all hospitals. Hospital statistics should be produced at least annually; data should be collected through individual statistical reports completed on discharge of the patient; in long stay establishments the total of admissions and patients should be recorded on one fixed day in the year.[105]

When, however, we seek to calculate rates, using the hospital clientèle as

I*

a means to determine incidence, and prevalence, the proportions of sick from different causes, and other more difficult facts about community sickness, we encounter difficulties because of our inability to determine, except in unusually self-contained areas, the *population at risk*. For this and other reasons, the determination of incidence, and other more elaborate uses of hospital statistics in morbidity studies, must be undertaken with great care, even in countries with good statistical systems. Some hospitals, however, are in a better position than others to undertake the work. This is particularly true of reasonably self-contained areas where the whole population can be taken as the population at risk. In such cases rates of hospital morbidity can be calculated; a type of study which is much needed, both for local needs and as a general guide.

National Committees have been asked to aid the development of hospital studies in their areas, wherever there are hospitals with a defined population, and where the statistical machinery is available. The rates to be calculated are attendance rates for out-patients, and admission or discharge rates for in-patients. The out-patient attendance rate is 'the number of out-patient attendances during a defined period divided by the average number of persons exposed to risk during the period.' An out-patient prevalence rate (4 (a) in Appendix 6) may also be useful. The admission or discharge rate should be calculated on first admissions where more than one spell of in-patient care is normal. Rates 2, 3, 4, 5, 6, and 7 (see Appendix 6) help to give a picture of the hospital in relation to all diseases and total populations at risk in different sections. Thus the study by Avery Jones[42] of peptic ulcer in hospital showed, among much else, how duodenal ulceration was advancing as a hospital episode while gastric ulceration remained stationary. Again, in a study of mothers having babies in hospitals and nursing homes, Heady and Morris[33] showed that the over forties who had lost a previous child in labour and who had a higher peri-natal mortality rate were, contrary to expectation or wise practice, less often admitted to hospital. A comparable study by Baird[3] in nursing homes and hospitals showed that, in Aberdeen at least, the hospital was safer than the mother's own home and that the unknown causes of late foetal deaths and neonatal deaths were an important factor in the increased rates amongst the lower social classes. It is to such studies that we may look for a better understanding of the part played by hospitals in the health sources of a country.

For further details the reader should refer to the 8th Report of the Expert Committee on Health Statistics (1963).[105]

Records of sickness absence

1. *General considerations*

Records of sickness absence, particularly in services affecting large groups of the population, as in schools, industry, and insurance, provide a ready-made source of morbidity data which must command increasing attention. The relationship with work or with school has its own particular value in providing information of a type which general morbidity surveys can never satisfy; it is unique in the investigation of *wastage* through sickness. For many diseases, such as bronchitis and rheumatism, which rank high in the causes of incapacity, but which rarely lead to hospital care, except in terminal states, absence from work is one of the most valuable records.

As with other sources of morbidity data, records of sickness absence have their own peculiar limitations. They cannot give a measure of morbidity of the whole population, since by their nature they relate to a part only; nor of all sickness, even medically-attended sickness, since they do not normally cover absences of short duration. The certificates are usually for the use of lay people, so that they are subject to the unreliability of statements of diagnosis, as well as to the various factors which influence attendance. But checks can be made on the accuracy of diagnosis, for some of the more serious diseases at least, by examining employees on return to work. In London Transport in one such episode 75 per cent of the diagnoses agreed with that of the general practitioner.[67]

The units of measurement are those mentioned earlier and in Appendix 7. Particular advantages are likely to be gained by presenting the results in terms of age, sex, civil state, and various occupations within industry. The total spells of sickness absence beginning during the year and the total of numbers of days of sickness absence in any year can be presented for men, unmarried and married women in terms of age groups. Of particular value, where the numbers are large enough, are the annual inception rate in spells and the average annual duration per person, and from these the average length of spell.[76] These rates should be calculated in the same classes and groups. The sickness can also be classified according to diagnosis, using a simple grouping, based upon the international classification. In the analysis of sickness in London Transport a system of grouping into twenty broad diagnostic groups was used; a distinction was also made between absences of less than four days – for which lay certificates were often accepted – and those of four days or more for which a medical certificate was compulsory.

2. Records of sickness absence in individual industries

Sickness absence can be examined within individual industries where the rates of sickness can help in the management of the industry itself, in establishing standards for applicants in different types of employment, in determining the allowance to be made for sickness, or in seeking out causes of sickness and of absence and examining the effects of preventive measures. Such studies are of equal, if not greater, interest to medicine in general, and to the epidemiologist in particular, by establishing the relationship between occupation and disease.

The amount of sickness and absence varies substantially from one employment to another. It is of value to make comparisons between different industries, between different occupations in the same industry, between the same occupation in different industries, following the records from year to year. For this 'standards of sickness absence' are needed, which can be produced only by extensive statistical computations. *Health in Industry,* published by the London Transport Executive, was an attempt to provide such a standard.[34]

Among the clerical and technical staff in London Transport, 1950–2, sickness absence varied for different ages and according to sex and marital status. The average annual duration of sickness per person was 12·7 per annum in men aged 55 to 59, as compared with 5·3 at age 30 to 34; 16·4 per annum for unmarried women aged 55 to 59, as compared with 7·8 at age 30 to 34; and 14·8 for married women aged 55 to 59, as compared with 13·4 at age 30 to 34.[76] 'Women usually experience more sickness absence than men, age for age and job for job, and married women ... more than single.' The same might well be true for men and would justify the time and trouble needed to discover the marital status of male employees.

Every occupational group of men or women must be, to some extent, selected. Thus, rates in industry apply to a survivor population. 'The men who continue to work at the pit face (in a coal mine) are those who have survived the physical rigours of the task.'[67] They are to this extent selected even further than the initial self and employer selection. In order to understand this process, we must supplement information of sickness absence by other calculations, which measure wastage, i.e., rates for enforced premature retirement, job changing, or death in harness in different occupations. Thus, a study in the General Post Office showed that the wastage from premature retirement and death among outdoor workers results mainly from cardio-respiratory disease, which is 50 per cent higher than in sedentary workers.

The use of this new tool for establishing relationships between occupation and disease is in its infancy. Yet individual studies using occupational differences in sickness within industries have already helped to throw further light on the little understood epidemiology of degenerative disease. Thus coronary thrombosis, already shown by social class studies to follow a downward grade from the professional classes to the semi-skilled and unskilled workers, is now seen to pick out certain occupations for its most vicious attacks. Doctors, particularly general practitioners, have a greater liability, which appears to be declining with changing habits (less cigarette smoking and more exercise).[50] The sedentary worker in any industry is often more affected than his active counterpart; thus the post office clerk is more liable than the postman and the bus-driver than his conductor.[32, 57, 59] These studies, pursued in collaboration with pathologists, lead us, if they did no more, to a better understanding of the manner in which the heart muscle can be protected from arteriosclerotic disasters in the coronary arteries, by the development of collateral circulation[58] – and so again to fresh fields of investigation and some new material for health education. So also with such observations as the absence of relationship between lung cancer and garage work and the geographical variations in respiratory disease.[68]

3. Records of incapacity in social security systems[53, 112]

Statistics from this source, where they exist, are usually incomplete in coverage; only about 20 countries in 1974 had systems covering the whole country and even fewer the whole working population. The largest single example of the use of records of sickness is provided by the 'Incapacity Statistics' of the

British Ministry of Pensions and National Insurance which date from 1951 – these are themselves in a formative stage.

Incapacity returns suffer from several disadvantages as a source of statistics. Sickness benefit in the British scheme of social security is not usually paid for spells of incapacity of less than four days' duration. The diagnosis of the general practitioner in support of the certificate of incapacity for work is intended for the Ministry's lay officers; it is handed to the patient and may be available to the employer. Inevitably doctors may not always 'have recorded their diagnosis as precisely as possible'; sometimes they withhold the names of frightening or less creditable diseases.

The gigantic task of examining 20 million sickness records has been possible only with the support of the doctors who have responded favourably to the claims of this venture in acquiring morbidity data, essential both to the development of social services and to an understanding of the work of the medical profession itself. The Trades Unions pressed for the inclusion of occupation by the worker himself when making his claim and this is now entered on the medical certificate.

The analysis[53] is done by means of a sample made up of a random selection of cases derived from each local office of the Ministry, the selection depending upon the final digit of the National Insurance number of the claimant. The statistics are presented in terms of the special list of 50 causes for tabulation of morbidity for social security purposes with extensions.

The breakdown into occupation cannot yet be done satisfactorily, even for men, because of the inadequacy of the returns; and not at all for women, of whom large numbers are uninsured; and for those that are insured the population at risk cannot be calculated. Nevertheless such relatively simple compilations are of immense value in helping us to understand the relative frequency of illness as a cause of incapacity.

In 1962 there were in Great Britain 9,002,200 new claims to sickness benefit, cf. 8,995,700 in 1971/2. The number incapacitated (on the third Tuesday of each month) varied between a maximum of 1,352,400 in January to a minimum of 801,800 in August. The proportion of sickness in each age group was closely related to the size of the group; thus the 15 to 19 group had 18·3 per cent of the total sickness and 18·5 per cent of the population at risk; the 60 and over group had 1·3 per cent of the total sickness and 1·7 per cent of the population.

The spells of certified incapacity due to sickness (8,302,020 terminating in 1960/61) comprised in all 278·94 million days (199·88 million males, 79·06 million females). Of these some of the main causes were as follows:

1. Influenza, bronchitis, pneumonia, acute pharyngitis and tonsillitis, hypertrophy of tonsils and adenoids, quinsy, chronic sinusitis and the common cold together caused 3,447,920 spells totalling 62·18 million days.

2. Psychoneuroses and psychoses caused 221,180 spells totalling 26·25 million days.

3. Tuberculosis of the respiratory system caused 23,320 spells totalling 8·07 million days.

4. Accidents, poisoning and violence caused 671,020 spells totalling 19·04 million days.

5. Diseases of the stomach and duodenum (excluding cancer) caused 465,900 spells totalling 11·76 million days.

6. Boil, abscess, cellulitis, and other skin infections caused 221,860 spells totalling 2·76 million days.

The great decline in tuberculosis in the developed world (see Chapter 3) is equally reflected in the claims for sickness absence. On the 5th June 1953, tuberculosis was the cause of illness for 45,200 male claimants out of a total of 540,200 and rather more than half this figure for women (27,100). On the 30th May 1970, the total for both sexes had fallen to a mere 8,400 spells out of a total of 778,520. These details present another aspect of the impact of tuberculosis on an industrial society, even more revealing than the figures of notification or morbidity in hospitals and clinics.[53]

Cancer registration[8, 12, 35, 41, 66, 77, 98, 103]

Cancer is one of a group of diseases (with tuberculosis, mental illness, congenital malformations) for which notification needs to be supplemented by continuous supervision. For this process, which requires sophisticated medical and social services, *registration* is a more accurate description, if only because one of the aims is to build up complete registers.

Morbidity from cancer has been studied only in recent years – mainly because of the exceptional difficulties which it prevents. Tumour registration began in individual hospitals in the nineteenth century; but comprehensive cancer registration only recently. It began in Massachusetts (USA) in 1927 followed by New York State in 1940. After this it spread steadily: Denmark (1942), France (1943), England and Wales (1944), California (1947), Pennsylvania, New Zealand (1948), Norway (1952), Finland, Belgium (1953), Iceland, Israel, Netherlands (1954). The disease does not lend itself to traditional notification, i.e. reporting by law, if only because the great detail required, and the long process of follow-up, must be conducted through special centres.

In England and Wales the first steps in the introduction of a scheme for recording cases of cancer on a national scale were taken by the Radium Commission (1930 to 48), which controlled the supply of radium to radiotherapy centres. National registration proper began at the end of 1944, when the Ministry prescribed registration and case-abstract cards for approved local authority schemes (Cancer Act 1939). A conference, held in Copenhagen in September 1946, arranged by the Danish Cancer Registry, suggested that: great benefit would result from the collection of data about cancer patients from as many different countries as possible; that data should be recorded on an agreed plan so as to be comparable; that each nation should have a central registry to arrange for the recording and collection of data; that there should be an international body with the duty to correlate the data and statistics obtained in each country and to devise a terminology and methods of classification and tabulation to be used by all cooperating countries.

In 1950, the World Health Organization appointed a committee to consider the registration of cases of cancer, a sub-committee of its Expert Committee on Health Statistics.[98] The Committee recommended that efforts should be made to determine the total incidence of cancer in populations of sample areas within several countries during the year or period of years, using all available sources of information (for example, doctors, pathologists, hospitals, death certificates); and that cancer registration projects aiming at ascertainment of follow-up histories of patients be encouraged with a view to eventual inclusion in such registration systems of all persons affected by cancer – thus eliminating selective bias, so as to arrive at true morbidity, survival, and apparent recovery rates. It also recommended that the statistical classification of cancer should be based upon numbers 140 to 205 of the International Statistical Classification of disease, injuries, and causes of death.

The object of a cancer registration scheme is to obtain information about the incidence of cancer in relation to age, sex, and site; methods of treatment employed; survival in relation to the extent of disease when first diagnosed; and the interval between the earliest symptoms and the patient's coming under observation and treatment. The details of every case of suspected malignant disease must be entered on a *registration card* filled in at 'registering centres'. Centres can be either individual hospitals, or radio-therapeutic centres, acting for a group of hospitals, or area organizations responsible for all registration within their areas; they can be statutory or voluntary. Each registering centre should report to the General Register Office every new case of malignant disease encountered, by sending duplicates monthly. A registration card in duplicate should be completed for each case of cancer or suspected cancer, whatever the route by which it comes under observation, and in whatever way it is eventually handled. The card should be made out as soon as there are reasonable grounds for a provisional diagnosis of cancer. If a hitherto unsuspected cancer is discovered during treatment for some other condition, or at a post-mortem, this too must be registered. Registration in these circumstances makes it impossible, in many cases, to record a final diagnosis, but an indication of the first estimate of the situation should be entered under 'provisional diagnosis', even in indeterminate cases; for example, a doubtful lesion in the pharynx should be entered 'lesion pharynx – ? carcinoma'.

For every registration card an *abstract card* is sent later – whether the disease proved to be malignant or not, and whether or not it was treated. The abstract cards form the basis of continuous follow-up reports at intervals. They give additional information about the date and symptoms of onset, the state of the disease at registration, diagnosis, clinical findings, histology, and treatment. Every effort must be made to determine the first event, for example, cough, swelling noted, pain, bleeding, etc. Each case is followed up by calendar years from the time of the first main treatment up to 5 and then afterwards at 7, 10, 15, and 20 years. Registered cases which the corresponding abstract cards later show to be non-malignant are excluded. By checking abstract cards, with the aid of the index, cases registered by more than one centre can be detected.

Cancer statistics (1974) (classified according to the 1965 revision, in cooperation with the International Agency for Research in Cancer) are available in 35 countries. The rate of growth of cancer registration can be seen in the experience of England and Wales: 27,000 in the first year of registration (1945);[66] 49,810 in 1948; 65,597 in 1953; about half the total in 1967; and 'a little in excess of 90 per cent of new cases' in 1974.*

The full benefits of registration are yet to come. As they become more complete they will add increasingly to the data available for the study of regional and racial differences, which may well bring out environmental and possibly

* Personal communication Dr Abe Adelstein O.P.C.S., London.

preventable factors.[103] The significant differences which occur in the incidence of cancer throughout the world have been dealt with elsewhere (see Chapter 4). But we have also to be able to examine the significant local variations which exist in individual countries. In comparing cancer death rates with standardized rates for tuberculosis in certain of the counties of England and Wales, for example, it can be argued that the effects of local conditions 'must be almost as important for the one disease as the other'.[77] The high incidence of gastric cancer in North Wales, in marked contrast with the low incidence in the East, the South, and the Midlands of England, may be due to an environmental factor, possibly related to the character of the soil. It may be more important to study local differences, in countries where reliable statistics exist, than to probe into the phenomenon of almost total absence of cancer of the stomach in Java, which astonishes every medical visitor to Indonesia. Clearly we must hasten on with our statistical book-keeping. So much suffering and death, so much surgery, so much time of hospitals and doctors, might be saved.

25. The Use of Sampling in Morbidity Surveys and Public Health Investigations

The examination of vital events for a whole nation is a difficult and expensive business; so also is the process of extracting vital statistics from registration data, and, as is often required, the further step of asking additional questions on health matters. The difficulty and cost may be so great, particularly in underdeveloped countries, that the work of obtaining vital and health statistics may well in fact not be done. Any means of reducing the difficulties and cost involved must help, not only in the countries that have no complete census, nor any general registration system, but also in the developed countries, where the volume of detailed information sought may have become burdensome. For some part of the answer to this important issue we may look to *sampling*.[62] Sampling cannot replace registration in the legal sense, since it does not register everyone, but it can act as a pilot venture upon which to build a model for full registration later. For the production of statistics it can be effective, economical, relatively speedy, and a source of data of high quality.

Since for the whole nation we are intending to substitute part, the selection of the part is all-important; everything therefore depends upon the design of the sample. For this highly technical task 'It is desirable that a highly skilled mathematical statistician versed in recent sampling developments be charged with the task of sample design, the determination of sample size and procedures, the determination of estimation procedures, and the calculation of sampling errors.[31] Given expert advice, however, the task is relatively simple; and after the sampling unit has been established the operation can be conducted by local staff.

The smallest parts of the material to be sampled are called *elementary units;* the units which form the basis of the sampling process are known as *sample units*. The aggregate of the sample units selected constitutes the *sample*. Various refinements of the sampling process have been devised either to help to make the sample more representative, or to arrange the work in stages or phases. *Stratification* is the name given to the process of sampling when the elementary units are divided into groups and strata, each being sampled separately, so that a specified number of sample units is obtained from each stratum. In this manner it is possible to distribute areas in such a way that a number of different characteristics of the country, economic, ethnic, rate of growth, income levels, etc., have a chance of fair representation. The greater the use made of information about the characteristics of the country, the better the results of the sampling method. In *multiple stratification* the elementary units are divided simultaneously according to two or more classifications, geographical, quantitative, and qualitative.

In *multi-stage sampling* the elementary units are regarded as made up of a number of first-stage units each of which is made up of second-stage units, and so on. Thus each country may be divided into districts; each district into villages; and each village into farms. A number of districts is selected in the first stage, within each a number of villages in the second stage, and from each selected village a number of farms is selected at the third stage. *Multi-phase sampling* is used when it is convenient and economical to collect certain items of information on the whole of the units of the sample, and other items on some of these units, drawn as a sub-sample of the original sample. *Interpenetrating networks of samples* collect the information from the same domain of study in an independent manner – so that each sample would supply an independent estimate of the varieties under study. This provides a means of appraising the quality of the information. *Composite sampling* is the term given to the process which uses different methods of sampling for different parts of the material, for example, sampling human population in the rural parts of the country and households in the towns. For further details see *The Preparation of Sampling Survey Reports* (1950),[62] *Sampling Methods in Morbidity Surveys and Public Health Investigations* (1966) WHO *Tech. Ref. Ser.* No. **336** and the *Principles and Recommendations for a Vital Statistics System* (1973), chs. 6 and 7.[63]

In underdeveloped countries the fundamental design for sampling is a list of areas in substitution for the list of households or persons usually used, so that it is possible to select areas, which together are a miniature in every respect of the complete country. Each of these selected areas must be staffed for the purposes of registration, exactly as they would need to be in a complete registration system; there can be no saving in this. At the outset, birth and death data, the first priority, alone should be compiled. If censuses have been taken, the same registration areas can be used to obtain current figures, each year, by adjusting for births, deaths, immigration, and emigration. For the calculation of rates, estimates of population must also be provided. If these are not available from a relatively recent census, the sample registration areas can be adapted for census taking by the simple expedient of taking a sample survey within them. In making a sample registration scheme, to avoid bias, it is usual to exclude model public health areas, or to deal with them as a separate entity.

In countries with full registration, sampling by areas can be used to detect weaknesses, to examine procedures, to check for completeness, and to prepare for advance tabulations. Systematic sampling of the records obtained by a full registration system, or by other means, such as the census or sickness insurances, can be used to obtain information for research purposes, or to reduce to a manageable form the enormous task of examining large-scale returns. Thus the results of the examinations of sickness benefits by the British Ministry of National Insurance are presented in the form of sample analysis – an economical and effective substitute for complete analysis, or if desired as a means to obtain advance results. In the USA, a 10 per cent sample of deaths, systematically selected by each State, is forwarded as an advance statement to the Federal Department, thus providing a provisional national mortality in advance of regular tabulations. In Sweden, a sample birth register has been established which includes all births occurring on the 15th day of each month; it permits complex tabulations, which would otherwise be a heavy expense. Sampling also helps to overcome the hazards of incompleteness which result from resistance by doctors to 100 per cent reporting.

Sampling in vital and health statistics has its most important application in survey work. In addition to its use in censuses, the sample survey has been applied to the measurement of many important criteria of health in the community, throughout the developed and underdeveloped world (see p. 286). The method is now being widely promoted by WHO, as a means to examine vital and health statistics, and through these to improve health services.

Sampling in surveys

After Francis Galton had invented the coefficient of correlation, followed by his survey method in inheritance through studying twins, and Karl Pearson's tests of significance, including 'chi square', a new mathematical outlook eventually revolutionized all survey work. In 1912, A. L. Bowley, in his study of five towns, introduced *random sampling*.[43] Up to this time, with the exception of Smith's dietary survey,[74] all surveys had examined the whole of a group or a complete area, an enormous task, as illustrated by Booth's work in London, which took 18 years and involved the labour of many persons.

Bowley's study in Reading was based upon a sample of 1,840 households i.e., 1 in 10 of 18,000 households on the rating list. Bowley also recalculated Rowntree's results in York (see p. 271) to show that they could have been produced by a 1 in 10, or even a 1 in 50, sample at a great saving of expense, time, and effort. After World War II, and the United Nations Statistical Commission, Yates wrote his classic work *Sampling Methods*;[118] a sub-commission of statistical sampling drew up a guide to investigators, with a recommended terminology (1952).[62]

Area probability sampling provides an attractive alternative to the full census in all parts of the world. In developed countries it can be used to elucidate matters, as in relation to fertility, which cannot be conveniently handled by the full census. In the underdeveloped and developing world it provides the only practical approach to the ascertainment of basic vital rates.[40, 47, 63, 115] This has been accomplished successfully in India, where complete enumeration is not only cumbersome but in terms of accuracy impossible, since vital rates on population growth, marriage, fertility, and infant and general mortality cannot be accurately determined without special enquiries, because marriages are mostly religious and not registered, and birth and death registration is defective.

The National Sample Survey of India begun in 1950–1, completed its 22nd round between July 1967 and June 1968 (see United Nations Sample Surveys of Current Interest 19th and 20th annual reports). With a staff of 600 it operates in the form of two or more 'rounds' of surveys on a country-wide basis every year, covering both rural and urban areas. From the second to the sixth 'round', information was collected on age at marriage, interval between successive births, sex, and age of children born, and detailed economic and social data. The household, as the sample unit, is defined, on the lines of the Indian census, as a common messing unit of persons, who have lived together, and taken food from the same kitchen, during a period of sixteen days or more out of thirty days preceding the date of investigation.[72]

Many other measurements of health in the community – social, socio-medical, and medical – have been made in recent years by means of the Sample Survey,[71] for example, nutrition studies (Japan and the United Kingdom), heights and weights of children (France), the use and misuse of alcoholic liquors (Sweden), family budgets (Poland and USSR). In 1954, the British studied the problem of 'early leaving' among secondary school children, using a stratified sample of one tenth of the secondary schools in England and Wales, in order to determine the relationship, among other aspects, of the home circumstances to educational behaviour. A questionnaire asked for details of progress from entry in 1946 to leaving in 1953 or earlier. Scholastic attainment, related to father's occupation, was shown to vary greatly with the home; only 9·2 per cent of children entering school from the unskilled home sat for advanced level certificate, as compared with 48 per cent of the children of professional parents; 71 per cent of the unskilled workers' children left school without obtaining more than two passes at the ordinary level. 'The reasons for this phenomenon,' said the report, 'must be very complex and we do not claim fully to understand them . . . it is most important that further research into the problem of the effect of the home background, particularly that of the semi-skilled and unskilled worker, upon a child's education at a grammar school should be undertaken.'[16] This subject was further studied in relation to University entrants (1963).[6]

26. Methods of Collecting Data

Data can be collected from a great variety of sources – existing and specially designed; and both the sources and the methods can be classified in different ways. The following classification has been adopted for convenience of systematizing; the classes are not mutually exclusive.

Data collected by experimentation

Data collected by observation
1. Already recorded
    a. existing data { Primary sources
    b. extracted data { Secondary sources
2. Specially designed records
3. Collected in the field (surveys).

Data collection by experimentation

Experiments are planned studies designed *to provide data by measurement;* thus in medicine, preventive medicine, sociology or psychology they provide the circumstances in which the effects can be measured of subjecting the human being to differing courses of medical treatment, of social measures or of psychological devices. Experiments seek to establish relationships between varying factors by controlling all other variables. In making objective observations the greatest care has to be taken in defining the measurements themselves. Experiments are not the only means to deduce cause and effect; but they are generally speaking the most searching and the most likely to reach definite conclusions. They can be used to learn more about the nature of disease, the effects of various forms of treatment, or the success or otherwise of preventive measures; they can equally help to unravel the complexities of human behaviour and of social problems. They have a place in health education and in speeding up the rejection or acceptance of preventive measures. In disease, they can help to solve problems not only of acute and dramatic disease but also of chronic illness, of less important maladies and of the many lesser misfortunes of mankind.

The chief distinguishing characteristic of an experiment is that it takes place *in controlled circumstances.* Thus the basic requirement of most experiments, including clinical trials in medicine, is that they should have *concurrent controls,* i.e. a group acting as controls at the same time as the experiment. Experiments seek information about groups with similar characteristics differing only in a particular treatment given, i.e. the preventive, sociological or psychological measure which is imposed. Success lies very largely in *the integrity of the control sample* and in *the elimination of conflicting* variables. These two requirements for success are difficult to achieve; so that inadequate controls constitute an all too common cause of failure in experimentation. Volunteer groups (acting as controls) by their very nature of coming forward to volunteer differ from the experimental group. Thus the control group may differ not only in the treatment given but also in a number of other characteristics, e.g. the cooperation of parents, the attendances at clinics or the high proportion of only children. Those conducting experiments need highly technical skills in some particular branch of experimental sciences.

Data collected by observation

1. *Data already recorded*

Data exists in a wide range of records from newspapers, magazines, almanacs, writings, films, legends or personal documents on the one hand to a variety of official compilations on the other hand. Official compilations exist as part of a registration process, in insurance data and in a multiplicity of parts of the health service – in records of general practice, of hospitals, clinics, industrial health, maternity and child welfare, school health and various aspects of public health (see Chapter 22). They form part of services which exist for other reasons than research, although research itself may be designed to learn more about them.

Recorded data may be in the form originally collected, e.g., in the census, when it is *primary*; or it may already have been compiled into *secondary* records, e.g., data in publications by the Registrar General. In both instances it exists in a form which allows immediate study; in contrast data in writings and films needs to be extracted before it can be used. Such *extracted* data can be useful in studies of behaviour. Recorded data has the disadvantage that it permits of retrospective examination only and has therefore often to contend with lack of relevant facts.

Data from specially designed records

Designed records are maintained in such a way as to further the collection of relevant data for research purposes. Such records perform a double purpose; they provide the usual official record of a service, data for administration as well as clinical activities, and they record other data for research on a prearranged plan. The dual function is compatible with, and often beneficial to, efficiency in the operation of the service. Thus in the National Health Service in Britain, hospital records have been redesigned to provide data for research; records of the Mental Health Service in Salford were redesigned to enable an epidemiological study of the Mental Health of the whole community to be carried out.[82] The designed record is valuable for operational studies of services. Since it starts with the designing of new records rather than the use of old ones it can be *prospective* in character.

Data collected in the field (surveys)[115]

Data can be collected in the field by asking questions or doing tests, the results of which are recorded in pre-established categories. The questions are formed in such a way as to bring out certain kinds of answer. This form of data collection is known as a survey, i.e., *an individual inquiry the results of which can be statistically analysed.* The object of a survey is to obtain data with which to make comparisons between groups or within the same group at different times. It can gather *facts* or *opinions.* It must be objective and, even when dealing with opinions, feelings or reasons, it has to quantify, since ultimately it deals in numbers, adding up units to make totals and calculating percentages and rates. The data may be the result of observations, measurements or questions; or a mixture of all three. Measurements are most exact. Observations and measurements, where appropriate, are generally preferable to questions (just as facts are preferable to opinions and questions on facts preferable to those on opinions). Nevertheless, observations and questions can be standardized by grading qualitatively e.g. the state of damp in the walls of a house can be graded as much damp, damp, little damp, no damp, and grading by this means can become for the purposes of the survey an excellent effective substitute for measurement.

Surveys are subject to inconsistencies arising from human errors in observation when one observer records a different state altogether from that considered to be correct and which has been made by other observers. *Observer errors* should be distinguished from *observer variations,* which occur when a condition is being classified into one of a number of variables on a continuum – as e.g. much damp, little damp, no damp as applied to the walls of a house. There will be observer variations in degrees of dampness bordering on the lines of demarcation between damp, much damp and little damp.

The inquiry may be addressed to all members of a group or to a sample – the latter being more usual in view of the difficulties of obtaining the whole of a group, which may be too large or too inaccessible. The subject of study, or units, whether the whole of a group or a sample, must be taken, where possible, from an existing document or record which is known as *the frame.* Thus the frame provides the subject matter of the survey, the list of units to be studied. It may be found in a great variety of documents dependant upon the subject: lists of patients in a hospital ward, an electoral roll, areas on a map, food rationing files, a census or registration list, etc., etc.

Various categories of surveys can be distinguished. In our context, they may be *social, socio-medical,* or *medical.* Social surveys analyse the circumstances in which people live; socio-medical surveys relate findings to medical phenomena (biological, physiological, pathological or clinical data), e.g., sickness can be related to the facts of industrial life, syphilis to prostitution, tuberculosis to density of living; medical surveys deal with disease as a group phenomenon, its distribution in time and space, sickness in general or tuberculosis in particular, without attempting to relate the findings to social factors. They may be *multipurpose,* when a wide range of factors is examined, or *special purpose* when a single set of complex factors is under review.[102] Multi-purpose surveys, essentially socio-medical, collect information on environmental factors, health activities and services, together with general household inquiries: employment, education, housing, food, consumer goods, transport, etc. Special surveys, more medical in character, examine nutrition, mental disorder, socio-economic conditions, environmental sanitation, etc.; these latter employ professional investigators, as, e.g., a medical team examining prevalent diseases. They may constitute a *single phase* operation, when the group is examined first and last in one step; or *multiphase,* when a second or third more intense examination is made of smaller fractions of the group.

Surveys can be *national,* where the population to be studied covers the whole country, either absolutely or by means of sampling; or *local,* where the population is confined to one area, as in the case of a town studied for the extent of poverty. They can also relate to a group with a particular characteristic, as, for example, expectant mothers booking for hospital delivery, or perhaps the hospital itself.

Surveys can be distinguished as either *diagnostic or descriptive.* Diagnostic surveys seek to prove a relationship between two or more factors, when they are either analytic in the sense of being *retrospective,* or as longitudinal follow-up studies, *prospective.* When we look forward we may follow established cases in an attempt to learn their life history, or we may take a group of persons and follow them over a spell of time to determine the numbers who develop a particular condition, or the circumstances which surround its development. Prospective studies can be made satisfactorily only in groups of sufficient size to produce enough cases, which involves planning and sampling to the correct size; they have been performed in diagnostic surveys to determine the relationship of cancer of the lung to smoking,* which involved a questionnaire returned by approximately 39,000 doctors.

Surveys are of value for conditions which are relatively frequent, for example the common cold, bronchitis, or coronary thrombosis, but are not easily adapted to rarer diseases, such as von Willebrand's disease or even disseminated sclerosis. Some do not regard the follow-up of established cases as a truly prospective survey, since one is looking back as well as forward. Truly prospective studies can provide stronger evidence of causal relationship than can the retrospective inquiries, often prejudiced by failing memory or lack of relevant data.

Most of the surveys with which we are concerned in vital and health statistics, however, are *descriptive,* seeking to paint a picture of a number of different characteristics, which significantly distinguish the group. In a survey of sickness the incidence and prevalence of a variety of different diseases is measured – or, in a study of old age, the social backround. Thus they describe an existing situation. Descriptive surveys are sometimes, but not always, *exploratory* in the sense that they make a preliminary estimate of important findings, some or all of which need to be studied more intensely by diagnostic surveys.

Surveys are not new, except in their increasingly scientific management. They

* Reports were published by R. Doll & A. Bradford Hill in the *British Medical Journal* (1952) ii, 1271, and (1956) ii, 1071. See also P. Stocks & J. M. Campbell, *Brit. Med. J.* (1955) ii, 923; *Smoking and Health* (1964) U.S. Public Health Service No. 1103; Haenszel, Loveland & Sirken *Lung Cancer M.R.R.S. History.* U.S. Dep. of Hlth; Nash, Morgan & Tomkins (1968), South London lung cancer study. *Brit. Med. J.* June.

have been made in some form in every civilization. In Europe, one of the earliest was that of the Domesday, an inventory of land, people and goods in Britain (1088), obtained by questioning by a panel of twelve jurors on oath in public court in every township and manor. Surveys developed widely in the 18th century, when censuses began. John Howard, Sheriff of Bedfordshire, wrote *A Winter's Journey* in 1777, the result of a pilgrimage through the prisons of Britain and the Continent.[36] This survey was undertaken in the conviction, which came to Howard as he sat on the Bench, that prison conditions were bad for health and harmful to society. His observations, which covered the health of the prisoners, their food, living conditions, and sanitation, were embodied in a *critical analysis,* a work of imagination and scholarship, a model for all surveyors, despite his modest disclaimer that 'a person of more ability, with my knowledge of facts, would have written better'.

> Certain it is that many of those who survive long confinement are by it rendered incapable of working. Some of them by scorbutic distempers; others by their toes mortified, or quite rotted from their feet, many instances of which I have seen. . . . In order to redress these various evils, the first consideration is the prison itself. Many county gaols, and other prisons, are so decayed or ruinous, or, for other reasons, so totally unfit for the purpose, that new ones must be built in their stead.[36]

Howard may well have been the first to introduce the *critical appraisal,* 'as the means of exciting the attention of my countrymen to this important national concern'.

The nineteenth century witnessed a continued growth of surveys. *The Sanitary Condition of the Labouring Population of Britain* by Edwin Chadwick was published in 1842, and was followed almost immediately by Shattuck's survey in Massachusetts (1850). Edwin Chadwick, Secretary to the Poor Law Commission in London, believed that pauperism was caused by preventable illness and that money spent on public health would save that spent on paupers (see Chapter 14). He circularized the parish doctors in every 'union' or group of parishes appointed to give free medical care to paupers, with a questionnaire on 29th September 1829. Like Howard, Chadwick wrote his final report with imagination and keen critical ability.

Between 1858 and 1871, Sir John Simon, Chief Medical Officer to the Central Health Authority (the Privy Council) in London, conducted a variety of surveys of socio-medical and medical subjects.* Simon had a feeling for social problems and a flair for finding medical men whose particular experience had equipped them to make individual inquiries in a wide range of important subjects. In 1863 Edward Smith[74] did a dietary survey; in 1864 Julian Hunter[37] a housing survey; and in 1860–61 Edward Headlam Greenhow[22] surveyed sickness in industry.

Edward Smith, in perhaps the first dietary survey ever made, studied silk weavers, throwsters, needlewomen, kid-glovers, stocking and glove weavers, shoemakers, and the agricultural labourers throughout Britain. He introduced two indispensable aids to survey work, the *sample* and the *standard of measure-*

* Royston Lambert gives a detailed account of this period in *Sir John Simon and English Social Administration,* 1816–1904 (1963). London: MacGibbon & Kee.

ment. His study was national in the sense that he covered the whole country; but, since he was unable to visit all the households whose menfolk worked in the industries mentioned, he had to select a sufficient number from each to make his results representative of the whole. Smith chose 634 households, which, he said, he took care to make 'thoroughly typical'.[74]

In order to compare the diet of individuals or groups of individuals Smith had to find standards of measurement. He first supposed that everyone of ten years and over required the same amount and quantity of food and that two children under ten years could be regarded as equal to one adult. This was rough and arbitrary, and fairly wide of the truth, but we still have no exact means of converting children and adults of various ages into a standard unit. Smith also needed a standard of diet to be regarded as a minimum for his standard unit. He therefore postulated, on the basis of his research in physiological chemistry, a standard daily diet of 28,600 grains of carbon and 1,330 grains of nitrogen. Smith visited 553 households in England and Wales, 52 in Ireland, and 29 in Scotland, a formidable undertaking. He himself interviewed the family and made a record, by inquiry of the housewife, of the amount and cost of various foods consumed. These totals he converted into his standard diet, as shown in Table 26.1.

Table 26.1 Standard diet; results of Edward Smith's dietary survey (1863).

Class	No. of families examined	Average weekly supply of each adult	
		Carbon grains	Nitrogen grains
Silk weavers	42	27,620	1,151
Needlewomen	31	29,900	950
Kid-glovers	10	28,623	1,213
Shoemakers	21	31,700	1,332
Stocking-weavers	21	33,537	1,316

In comparison with these low levels, the diet of the agricultural workers was better; nevertheless, 'a fifth were with less than the estimated sufficiency of carbonaceous food, more than a third were with less than the estimated sufficiency of nitrogenous food' and in three counties the average diet was deficient in nitrogen.

Smith wrote his report in exemplary fashion, setting out how he came to undertake it, how he drew his sample, the difficulties he encountered, the methods he adopted, and his results. A summary of his findings for the indoor workers was as follows: no class under inquiry exhibited a high degree of health; the least healthy classes were the kid-glovers, needlewomen, and Spitalfields weavers; the average quantity of food supplied was too little for health and strength; the worst fed classes were the needlewomen, silk weavers, and kid-glovers; as a class they did not spend their money upon food economically; the instances of Macclesfield weavers and of London needlewomen show in remarkable contrast the effect of economical and wasteful expenditure of money on food. Smith's survey left little doubt that 'the degrees of scantiness of food which were to be found among the lowest fed of the examined classes' must be the cause of illness and that the associated causes of disease must be greatly strengthened by it and their hurtfulness'.[74]

During the early part of the twentieth century, the thoughts of two remarkable people, Seebohm Rowntree and Charles Booth, were centred upon poverty. Chadwick had believed, and demonstrated, that poverty could be rooted in ill-health and disease, much of it preventable. Booth and Rowntree saw poverty as part of irregularities of employment and inadequate wages, aggravated by the biological processes of family growth and old age. Booth spent seventeen years of his leisure in the East End of London to produce his *Life and Labour of the People of London*, 1883–1897. Rowntree did the same on a smaller scale for the city of York, and published his report under the title of *Poverty: A study of Town Life* in 1901. Rowntree is remarkable for having been sufficiently single-minded and long-lived to have completed two further surveys in the same town: *Poverty and Progress* (1941), and *Poverty and the Welfare State* (1951). Neither Booth nor Rowntree made any attempt to sample. They used a team of carefully briefed investigators to visit all households. Booth in addition used the records of the visitors appointed by the London School Boards. Both Booth and Rowntree used standards for comparison. Rowntree fixed minimum standards of diet and household expenditure and arranged his households in economic groups according to the wage of the chief earner. Booth made the first attempt to standardize occupation.

In recent years surveys have been undertaken in vast numbers, so great has been the advantage of learning about what has been styled the anatomy and physiology of society. Surveys, now in a sense mass-produced, have gained much from improved methods of measuring by the use of standards, as for occupation (see p. 233), for social class (see p. 235), for household densities, for diet and other attributes. Dietary standards have gone far beyond Edward Smith's early concept – they provide a measurement of the utmost national and international significance[81] (see p. 148). From the 1930s and through the Second World War, surveys by individual inquiry, some based upon sampling large populations, many through the examination of complete or nearly complete local groups or selected areas, have developed widely in many different fields of work, through the Western World and elsewhere. Opinion surveys, originally designed for market research and for political science, have been used, particularly in America, to assess the attitudes of the public to health services. Diagnostic surveys have become an indispensable research weapon.

Surveys are necessary to the development of public health (1) as experimental research to test the relationship of phenomena to circumstances under experimental conditions, e.g., dental caries to water supplies before and after fluoridation, opinions in hospital before and after a change in routine; and (2) as operational research, particularly in the form of descriptive surveys, which provide information essential to the organization and reorganization of services. By this means we learn essential details about the old, the handicapped, slum dwellers, pregnant women, to mention but few of the innumerable issues that now affect public health. Surveys now provide one of the great and indispensable public health weapons, to be used increasingly, with experts in other social sciences, as public health extends into the social and anthropological fields.

Sickness survey

Until recent years few surveys were specifically designed for sickness. William Farr suggested, in 1839, that sickness should be studied by taking '100,000 persons of given ages, indiscriminately, and observing them for one, two, three, etc., years',[20] but this idea was never taken up. The censuses in Ireland were used incidentally for sickness (1851 to 1911); as also in the USA. Life insurance made studies, e.g., The Metropolitan Life Insurance Company of New York in Montreal (1926); and many were made by public health departments in Europe and the USA. The first large scale survey of all sickness was conducted in the USA in 1936. In 1965, general morbidity surveys were made in 33 countries; and surveys in selected areas are commonplace.

Sickness surveys may seek information about a. all illnesses or b. particular diseases. They can be categorized as:

1. According to population served
   a. Whole population by household sample
   b. Selected area
      i. all households
      ii. sample of households
2. According to the information sought
   a. Information about all illness
   b. Information about particular illnesses

Combinations of these categories can be devised to meet local conditions and needs.

Sickness surveys can be by physical examination, examination of existing records, and interviewing.

Physical examinations combined with laboratory and other diagnostic tests can be made in groups large and small, either sampled or in total. These surveys achieve greater diagnostic accuracy; but they are costly, require skilled staff and encounter more resistance. They provide excellent assessments, particularly when combined with interviewing, with which to formulate public health programmes.

Records of hospitals, of institutions, of medical practitioners, of social insurance agencies, etc., can, as earlier indicated (pp. 251–258), be surveyed for morbidity data.

Interview sickness surveys may be either by simple retrospective inquiry or by short-term diary records. This method of morbidity study contends with many difficulties, not least of which for the retrospective inquiry is failing memory, although the measure of error can be calculated. One of the greatest difficulties experienced, both for interviewers and coders, is to distinguish between separate illnesses and multiple symptoms of one illness. Many are inclined to criticize the recording of medical information by lay persons, holding that errors in measuring both general sickness and also specific disease must, in consequence, be considerable. On the other hand, the Interview Survey aims to discover the extent to which people feel themselves to be ill or to have something wrong with them (see p. 4); and this can be done as competently by laymen as by doctors. Much more study of the method is needed before we can know how closely the lay records can correspond with medical diagnoses; but there is evidence to suggest that the results are reasonably accurate: certainly the incidence of diabetes and tuberculosis has been shown to approximate closely to that calculated using information from other sources.[78, 85]

Interview surveys of the whole population are most suited to developed countries, in view of the need for this purpose, among much else, of a complete population census. Information obtained provides the nearest to complete estimate of total sickness in a community so far obtained. Details vary from country to country and are clearly dependent on social patterns and the organization of health services.

The Sickness survey in England and Wales (1944–52), which arose out of the wartime need to know more about general levels of sickness, 'the consequential incapacity and calls upon the services of doctors', was the work of the Social Surveys Division of the Central Office of Information, working with the Ministry of Health and the General Register Office.[66] A stratified sample of 2,910 persons over 16 years old was drawn from 11 regions, divided into rural districts and towns of four sizes. Specific towns and districts were selected; and within each a random sample was drawn, originally from Food Office records, then from National Registration records (1944), and finally from the electoral register (1951). Thus in the North-West region, containing 15·6 per cent of the total population, there were 454 interviews, of which 43 were allotted to rural districts (9·4 per cent of the population); 74 to towns of between 40,000 and 80,000 (16·5 per cent of the population), etc. When the frame for the selection of the random sample in each area was the National Register, as in Blackpool scheduled for 53 interviews, the total block of cards for the 115,000 adults (1,240 inches long) was sampled by measurement; 1 card was picked out of every 23 inches. Interviewers visited the sample of people in their own homes, inquired about illnesses and injuries during the three previous months, and recorded on a designed schedule the illnesses mentioned by the subject and not according to the interviewer's diagnosis. The results were examined, using the measurements outlined in Appendix 7, for totals of illness, days of incapacity, and consultations, together with the appropriate rates, for consultation, incapacity, prevalence, etc. Sickness and incapacity also were related to occupation, income, and density of living.

In England and Wales the number of medical consultations in the year averaged about 4 per cent for each sex up to the age 45, and then increased to 6 at 55–65, and over 7 in advanced age; at all adult ages the average was about 5 visits annually for each sex. Yet out of 46,112 persons who had some illness during the average month of 1947, 39,904 reported no days of incapacity during that month. In other words, only one out of every seven sick people (13·5 per cent) was away from work, or confined to the house, on account of illness. Only one in four (23 per cent) of those recording an illness or injury during the month had consulted a doctor during that month. The extent to which incapacity depends upon the job, as much as upon the illness, can be seen by comparing different occupations for both prevalence and incapacity. The prevalence rates of miners did not differ greatly from those of the professional classes; but the incapacity rates were much higher. The much higher loss of working hours among miners than among professional people reflects the difficulties of the miner's life and his attitude. Such glimpses into the vast amount of information yielded by the Sickness Survey, reveal more clearly the significance of ill-health in a community: certainly more than morbidity statistics based solely upon the records of the general practitioner, industry, or the hospital; perhaps 4, 7, and 20 times more, respectively. (For sampling see p. 263.)

Interview surveys limited to selected areas, either by visiting all households or by questioning representative samples, can be used effectively in countries at all stages of development. They are economical; they link morbidity with social conditions; they define population automatically; they are flexible and easily controlled. If using a team, including a doctor, they can build up a complete picture of morbidity, and thus serve, among other purposes, to show to what extent other sources, of morbidity, for example, records of absence, of general practitioners' or hospital work, are incomplete. The whole population of an area of say 5,000–10,000 persons may be taken; or alternatively for large areas, after preparation of house lists, every nth house may be selected in proportion to the size of the area. Districts may be selected for their representative character and may need to be changed at intervals.

In countries where the state of development is least, the importance of such surveys is perhaps greatest, as 'one of the most promising methods of obtaining morbidity statistics'.[99] Medical field units have demonstrated the advantage to be gained by surveys which serve 'to identify the endemic diseases and to throw light on their relative incidence'. The survey can readily be incorporated into a campaign against a specific disease, for example, yaws. Household visiting of the whole area, or of a sample within the area, may in fact, be the only means to obtain full and reliable information of illness. This is the field which is being developed by WHO; studies by households have been conducted in Sweden, India, and Puerto Rico. Special surveys can also be combined with the decennial census in underdeveloped countries, 'to obtain information on infant mortality in areas for which no data have hitherto been available, or to rectify the register of births' (see Chapter 29).[70]

The sickness survey method requires experience of the sampling theory, unless all households are visited, and of the techniques of field surveys. Analysis of the morbidity data also presents difficulties (see 247–248). One useful expedient is to use the numbers interviewed as the denominator for the rates. The development of sickness surveys, and the necessary expert advice, should be one of the most important functions of national committees (see p. 222).

A check-list of factors bearing on the design of health interview surveys is given in WHO Technical Report Series No. 218 (1961).

27. Planning and Conducting the Survey

The survey needs a director to plan, organize, supervise and finally produce a critical appraisal of the results. His first task is to formulate the plan in detail, jointly with interviewers, advisers and statisticians; to settle the category or categories to be examined, the information to be sought, the means to collect it; the frame from which the sample is to be drawn; the questions, observations and measurements to be made and the standards to be used in classification. *All decisions in the planning sessions, agreed by all parties, should be recorded in detail.* The plan itself should be made available, in sufficient detail, to those concerned, as well as to organizations and individuals likely to be interested in the results. Agreement should be obtained from responsible persons and bodies involved.

The first step is to define the object concisely: what question it is meant to answer, in order to be certain that the study is worthwhile; that there is a community problem which commands attention; that a survey is the best way to find an answer; that the material available is enough to answer the questions; that the answer is not already known. Reading available literature – to learn what other people have done about it, to understand the difficulties, and to arrive at the best method of tackling it – is an indispensable early step.

There follow decisions on the following important matters:

1. *The categories to be covered by the survey* – population, areas, institutions. There are always some people or areas that cannot be easily reached, migrants or gipsies, for example, so-called marginal types or floating members which may have to be excluded.

2. *The nature of the information to be collected.* The details will vary greatly, but the general principles are to see that the items of information form a rounded whole; that the questions are all relevant and capable of explanation to the people interviewed; that there is nothing redundant; that the whole is practicable; that nothing vital has been omitted. The failure to record a mother's age at the birth of the child and the total children born were serious omissions in the 1921 and 1931 censuses in Britain.

3. *The methods of collecting information.* These will depend upon the subject and the type of information required. A decision has to be taken on what is to be done about those who do not respond.

4. *The frame to be used.* Frames can be inaccurate, incomplete, subject to duplication, inadequate, or out of date. In practice most frames suffer to a greater or less extent from all these defects. Most suffer from incompleteness in some respect, as, for example, where a list describes some married women as single, which makes it incomplete for single women, although complete as a

frame for women as a whole. Incompleteness of the frame is more serious than at first appears, because it is in the missing units that special characteristics are often to be found, as in mass radiography studies of tuberculosis. At the outset of the survey a careful investigation should be made of any frame it is proposed to use.

5. *The questionnaire.* The exercise of imagination is needed in order to devise questions that are able to produce the answers that are wanted. A pre-test with selected people will help to understand what the questions are yielding.

When properly designed the questionnaire provides the means of recording facts directly in the form of categorized data. Since the ultimate integrity of the research depends upon the validity of the data which the questionnaire produces, it has to be drawn up with care and forethought. All questions must be capable of definite interpretation by the respondent and for the interviewer. Questions posed without due consideration may be ambiguously worded; they can be worded in such a form as to cause bias; they can be vague or incomplete; they can embarrass and so lead to evasion; they can be too general, too unprecise; or, only too often, sadly although vital to success, they can be forgotten or omitted. Ambiguity is a frequent sinner, as examination candidates will readily agree. Of this the census carried out in 1801 for England and Wales is a nice example. To learn something about numbers employed in various occupations, the question was put 'What number of persons in your parish, township, or place, are chiefly employed in agriculture; how many in trade, manufacture, or handicraft; and how many are not comprised in any of the preceding classes?' 'Chiefly employed' was an ambiguous term, which might or might not include wives and children; in the result, the data from the question had to be completely ignored and the inquiry in this respect was null and void. Total omission of vital questions is likewise a frequent and much to be deplored hazard. Thus, in the Stockport Survey of over eighties questions were put about visits from relatives; but no questions were asked about the degree of their proximity, thus making it impossible to gauge what differences existed in visiting by relatives of various degrees of proximity in differing home-backgrounds.[5] Beware, too, of vagueness. 'How are you feeling?' can mean different things to different people.

The interviewer should record his or her own observations in a space provided; these may not lend themselves to exact analysis, but can point to relevant facts not covered by the questionnaire. The questionnaire should be pruned to remove all questions not absolutely needed. Temptation to overload questionnaires should be strenuously resisted in the interests of both economy and accuracy. There is a definite limit of usefulness of the material sought; we pass this at our peril.

Questionnaires may be *structured,* i.e. consisting of direct questions to which the answer yes or no can be given, e.g .'is your job clerical?' or where there are alternatives to be tested, e.g. 'is your job that of a clerk, farmer, shop assistant?' Or they may be *unstructured,* consisting of open-ended questions designed for answers which elaborate and may be discursive, e.g. 'what is your occupation?' Open-ended questions suffer from lack of standardization, so that replies about the same occupation, e.g. may be variously interpreted. They may be *independent*, i.e. separately interpreted or they may be *interdependant*, i.e. taken together for interpretation. A number of interdependant questions taken together can often give a better insight into behaviour than any single question. Thus in an inquiry of female patients on the list of the University Health Centre, Manchester, knowledge about cancer of the cervix was asked in six different questions (1, 3, 7, 19, 20, 22). Six replies were then ranked in order of correctness, six correct being very good, five correct good, three correct low, one correct very low. Interdependant questions also help to check accuracy. In the above study, e.g., questions about the preventability of cancer differently couched produced contradictory answers, indicating that respondents had not understood, or did not have a clear view of the meaning of 'preventability'.[4]

Extraneous factors may influence replies and so distort the truth; some in the mind of the person questioned and others involving the interviewer. Respondents may have their status in mind, as when being asked whether they drink beer, the reply is 'no, whisky', if they regard whisky drinking as socially more desirable. Desire to please may lead to answers which it is supposed the interviewer or the questionnaire, wish to record; 'do you give your husband a hot meal every day?' may get the answer yes more frequently than in fact is the case. Interviewers can ask questions with inflections, so that the same question by different interviewers gets different answers. The sequence of questions is important because of the influence which it may have on the respondent. Lack of order or sequence tends to confuse or build up resistance and questions on the same topic are better grouped. Yet lack of order is often necessary to avoid suggestion by influence, or to insert questions about the same subject more than once. Thus it is that drawing up the questionnaire can be a long, arduous and often frustrating task.

Questions may be asked by post or by interview or by both. The advantages and disadvantages of postal inquiries and personal interrogation are much debated. The choice will depend most upon the circumstances and nature of the survey. Anonymity is sometimes of greater importance than the more reliable information generally to be obtained by interview, since many who willingly tick a document are reluctant to answer questions to a person's face. An interview gives the opportunity to explain and to amplify and thus may avoid errors and inconsistencies, which would have occurred by misunderstanding or ignorance of a term or phrase, or because of latent ambiguity; when questions are answered without understanding the results are worse than no information at all. Interviews take time and cost more. They more commonly require technical knowledge, although this is not true of all survey work, in order correctly to put questions and to interpret answers. Apart from technical knowledge, generally resting in a professional qualification, there is the need for careful briefing. Even highly qualified persons must fully understand the aspects and methods of the survey if they are to discuss questions with respondents and correctly interpret replies. Interviewing imposes considerable strain, since it involves an intellectual synthesis and evaluation of a wide range of

K

replies from people of varying capacity. *All information obtained at interview should be written down in its final form at the time of the interview.*

6. *Interviewers.* The amount which each interviewer can do varies with the area to be covered, the time spent in travel, and the nature of the inquiry – perhaps seven completed questionnaires a day. Interviewers should preferably have a background knowledge of the subject, particularly in investigations of the research type. But in multi-type surveys unspecialized teams of workers can be used, provided that no observations or measurements are needed which depend on special skills, and that the interpretation of the questionnaire is well understood. Briefing is of the greatest importance, and every interviewer should understand what the survey is intended to achieve.

7. *A pilot study* can be conducted on a small but representative group, preferably, but not necessarily, out of the area covered. The results can show whether questions are being understood; whether they tend to bias the answer; whether they are ambiguous, unnecessary, vague, embarrassing; or any other deadly sins. It may help to find missing questions. It can tell something about the variables we are seeking to measure; can be used to test the questionnaire; to train staff; to assess costs; and to judge the type of sampling unit.

8. *Drawing the sample,* including the control, is an increasingly important element in a survey. Nevertheless it is not always essential; surveys can tackle the whole of a group, or in certain cases an incomplete group, in which the missing members are well documented. Apart from this, surveys can deal with any group of persons providing the findings are limited to the group in question; many excellent surveys of this kind have been done in recent years. But if a sample is drawn it must be representative of the group and free from bias. Apart from the obvious dangers of selection, there are many hidden sources of error; a group of mothers attending the welfare centre is self-selected. In case of doubt checks should be made. Stratification of the sample sometimes helps to make it more representative of the area (see p. 261) and multi-phase sampling allows of considerable precision at a small cost (see p. 262).

9. *Handling data.* Data can be analysed direct from the forms, or processed through the computer to which the various punched card systems have now almost entirely given place. Direct analysis and the use of ordinary cards for hand sorting can yield excellent results, providing there is a simple format with rigorous and continuous scrutiny of incoming forms. For small studies, or in the case of material slowly accumulating, the Cope-Chat card, with holes around the edges, for hand use can be effective; otherwise the *computer* has much to commend it, particularly for large scale studies. It is capable of storing a programme of instructions with which it can proceed step by step at very high speed. 'Programmes', initially costly in time, money and skilled professional labour, but ultimately, by repeated use both locally and through telelinkage from a distance, economical in all these respects, can be prepared for all the analyses previously discussed. Data can be fed in on tape (magnetic or paper) and on punched cards of various kinds.

The computer* can handle data of great complexity; perform statistical exercises otherwise impossible except as a 'tour de force'; keep basic files for individuals; link records relating to the same person; record in detail departures from health, operative and therapeutic data of considerable complexity; sift and scan data to detect significant relationships and unusual trends, as in the incidence of congenital malformations; check records for consistency, immediately listing unsatisfactory returns; calculate rates, standardizations and indices; store data for subsequent processing and for the preparation of indexes; perform laboratory analyses; prepare schedules of individuals or items currently in need of attention as, e.g., schedules of children to be immunized with letters issued to physicians or clinics.

Such a wide range of functions can help greatly in epidemiology and vital and health statistics. Punched cards can be discarded after input, providing care is taken to store magnetic tapes in dust and magnetic free conditions. With improving apparatus, better understanding of requirements and education of potential users, the computer will increasingly become an indispensable aid to data collection and analysis.[9, 12] There is improved random access to computer data by the use of discs.†

* An automatic sequence controlled calculator, which followed the mechanical principles evolved by Charles Babbage in the 19th century, was first successfully constructed at Harvard in 1944. The electronic calculating machine came in 1946; first using the thermionic valves, it has since improved steadily with transistors and integrated circuits in both speed and reliability.

† Personal communication Dr Abe Adelstein, O.P.C.S., London.

28. The Presentation of Data

The basic considerations in the presentation of data are those which govern its collection – namely, accuracy, consistency, and thoroughness. But there are other and more subtle attributes which arise from the inherent difficulties of expressing scientific, and indeed all philosophic, matter in words, which can be great deceivers. Words must be honestly employed, i.e., with their meaning unambiguously clear and definite; and they must be understood by the writer and be understandable by the reader in their full significance. The elimination of jargon and a clear and logical sequence of thought are among the first essentials. When simplicity has been achieved in the spoken or written presentation, the result is likely to please everyone, uninformed and informed alike.

The chief considerations governing the actual presentation of data are as follows:

1. The *basic documents,* which give the results of the analysis in full, generally in the form of gross data (the protocols), should if possible be published. Unless this is done research workers, either present or future, cannot examine the validity of the conclusions, or re-examine the material from other points of view. Copies of all the important forms used, e.g. questionnaires, should be published. These basic documents will best appear in appendices.

2. Data should be *clearly, concisely* and *precisely* set out. This is easier to prescribe than to carry out, since the three attributes are in some measure in conflict. Tables and graphs often succeed in being both concise and clear only through the *sacrifice* of detail; whereas precision too often can be achieved only through the *use* of detail. It is not easy, at one and the same time, to achieve clarity and to present material concisely without sacrificing precision; and vice versa. The publication of protocols in full, while leaving the writer free to simplify in tables and graphs, does something to answer the call for precision; but in the end only the most rigorous scrutiny can ensure that tables and graphs have not been over-simplified, or alternatively are not so detailed as to be unintelligible.

3. *Tables* should as far as possible be small and simple. They should be headed to describe their contents clearly and precisely; with similar descriptive subheadings for rows and columns. The accepted formula for such headings is to give subject, distribution, place and time in that order. The source of information can be given, where necessary, in a footnote; and footnotes are also proper for explanations of abbreviations, terms and unusual entries. The matter in the tables should be arranged to suit the convenience of the reader, generally by logical or convenient sequences and groupings. Data should be given so far as possible in whole numbers or to a single place of decimals, especially when the

reliability of the sources of information is questionable. Good tabular presentation is in consequence an art for which advice is needed from both statistician and printer. Tables can be produced, with modern tools, with great ease. Fed by means of a programme into a computer, basic data is transformed into tables in the twinkling of an eye. Any relationship can be reduced by coding and programming at the speed of thought; so that proliferation of tables itself becomes a problem. The machine will also perform all or most essential statistical calculations, *standard deviations, coefficient of correlation* and other statistical checks upon validity. Tables can thus be equipped with indices, indicating the extent to which the particular association could have occurred by chance; the *probable or standard* error to help in evaluating differences in measuring the same value in different circumstances; and the *standard deviation* to guide the reader as to the importance to be placed upon averages. Thus if the statistician has prevented the use of biased or unrepresentative samples and oversmall groups likely to give chance results, the informed reader will have everything to hand with which to reach his own conclusions about the results. It follows that the chief difficulties of presenting data begin *after tabulation* and consist for the most part of questions involving judgment and discrimination – abstract values outside the scope of mechanical instruments. Some of these difficulties, prone to result in bias, will be dealt with in the next section.

4. *Graphs,* which aim to convey information at a glance, can do much to show clearly and concisely the most important findings. They also serve to demonstrate the existence of cyclical variations, which would not otherwise easily be seen to exist, and which call for further investigation. They may be in the form of line charts, bar diagrams, maps, *pi* diagrams and correlation diagrams; as well as various ways of illustrating material by the use of pictures, sketches and quotations. Of these the most commonly used are the line charts which show variations in indices or quantities measured (on the vertical) against time in seasons, age or years (on the horizontal). *Bar diagrams,* or *histograms,* show variations in indices or quantities by means of bars proportional in length to their magnitude. The bars can be drawn horizontally from the vertical or vertical from the horizontal; they may be measured against time, place, age, etc. *Maps* can be used for the obvious purpose of showing the topographical features of a geographical area; or as another substitute for the table by showing values in terms of distinctive shading; or by the use of dots proportional to the events recorded. *Pi diagrams* are a simple device to show proportional variations by dividing a circle into sectors, each sector being proportional to the quantities (usually percentages) of the constituent categories. Finally, *correlation diagrams* use individual dots to record magnitude of individual events, measured as to size on the vertical and in terms of a specific factor on the horizontal. The correlation diagram then is basically the same as the line chart but with no attempt to connect the individual dots one to another. When the dots do tend to fall on a line, or to form a pattern, a correlation probably exists between the specific factor and the magnitude of the recorded event. Thus the dots indicating infant mortality in relation to communities living at different densities will fall upon a line with mortalities increasing with congestion of living.

Tables and graphic representations of particular aspects of the subject, as distinct from the protocols previously mentioned, should appear in the body of the report, *accompanied by an explanation in the text*. No tables should be allowed to appear without forming part of the narrative.

5. *Avoiding bias*. Our interest in classification lies in its value as a philosophic and generalizing instrument. Tabulation, graphic representation and statistical analyses aim to find *distinguishing characteristics*; and help in the search for *uniqueness* in the data which can provide at least the starting point for new knowledge. The next logical step is to distinguish characteristics and relationships which appear to be 'unique'; to try to extract their full meaning. This calls for the setting up and, if necessary, knocking down of *hypotheses*. Discussion and comment will lead on to recommendations. In presenting data there is the danger of bias, either verbal or graphic.

Verbal bias. This error of interpretation arises when the writer states or infers a causal relationship to exist, when an association has been shown without any evidence as to cause and effect. This has been styled the 'post hoc' fallacy, since 'statistically significant' relationships can be post hoc and not necessarily propter hoc; the relationship may be due to both variables being related to a third known or unknown variable. Decrease in tuberculosis in Western Europe has been correlated with increasing sugar consumption, a factor which has had no causal relationship with the decline. Both the decline and the increase of sugar consumption are related to one or more outside factors, better housing, better medical services, better diet, etc. On the other hand statistically significant correlations can be due to cause and effect (as almost certainly the case with smoking and carcinoma of the lung). Verbal bias also arises from misinterpretation and misuse of a variety of simple mathematical calculations; particularly proportions and averages. Two children possess IQs of 98 and 101 respectively, with the inference that one is necessarily that much more intelligent than the other. But the probable error in the calculation can make any such inference false; in the Binet-Simon test the error may be taken to be 3 per cent, enough to give a one in four chance that the IQs of the two children could in fact have been reversed. In the case of averages, the *median* and the *mode* can differ from each other and from the *arithmetic mean*. Failure to make it clear what kind of average you are using, or to use one sort at one moment and another kind at another moment, can literally make nonsense of any presentation of data.* The standard deviation which gives an idea of what emphasis can be placed upon any average, is too often ignored. When those attending VD clinics vary in age from 15 to 55, the mode (say age 18) conveys something important; the median (say age 22) conveys less; and the arithmetic mean (say age 28) conveys little. In the case of decimals it is possible to give a false impression by overuse. Accuracy cannot in any case transcend that of the original observations from which the calculations were made; if these were not impeccable, results given to one or more decimal places are misleading.

---

* The *arithmetic mean* is obtained by adding up all the examples and dividing by the number there are. The *median* is the example in the middle with an equal number above and below. The *mode* is the example which occurs most frequently.

Graphic bias. Distortion or manipulation of graphs, maps and other devices to present data in easily comprehensible form is by no means uncommon; although generally found in journals or advertisements which have no claim to scientific integrity, the public health worker should none the less be aware of this hazard. Maps can distort facts and give false impressions by manipulating the shading without due regard for the comparability of the areas shaded. Graphs can be truncated by chopping off the bottom, so that the line on the chart cannot be seen in relation to zero; or the proportion of either the vertical or the horizontal measurements can be altered to produce exaggerated effects. Pictures can be used to demonstrate differences in one measurement, when in fact they differ in two measurements. If, for example, two pictures are used to present an object, one can be made to vary both in height and in width and will thus have grown geometrically not arithmetically, if twice as high and twice as wide it will appear four times as large.

Writing the report. A good report will detail the nature of the inquiry in a *preface* and will have section or chapter headings that stimulate interest and arrest attention. It will give an exact description of the material, the geographic region and the categories, as well as the nature of the information collected, the method of collecting data, the sample, the date or period of time to which the data refer, the degree of accuracy, cost, an assessment of fulfilment, and the name of the responsible organization.[62] It will set out the objectives, methods, results, and conclusions, with a bibliography and list of references. Appendices can be used for tables and detailed matters which have formed the basis of the study, but which are not immediately necessary for the reading matter. Tables which are to be discussed should generally appear in the body of the report itself and be interpreted in the text. An account of previous investigations of the same or allied subjects should be set out in the preface, or in the first section or chapter.

Many of the great pioneer surveyors have achieved their end more by the skill with which they have written the report of their studies than by the work itself. These great minds have not scorned to dwell at length upon the arts and finesses of writing readable matter. For those who write in English *Plain Words* by Ernest Gowers is a useful guide to simplicity and clarity. When genius is missing, hard work and the use of plain words can do much to simulate it.

29. The Statistical Needs of Underdeveloped Countries

The need to hasten slowly

The dilemma of underdeveloped countries has to be faced. National systems of comprehensive vital and health statistics must take many decades to achieve. Indeed, since existing systems in technically advanced countries have grown by long and painful processes, dependent largely upon the particular types of culture, there is no certainty that they could be achieved in less developed countries. Western processes, greatly accelerated, may not easily be impressed upon peoples whose social pattern is based upon different cultural values.[77]

Registration is a case in point. Absence of compulsory registration has often been blamed[19] for lack of vital statistics; but even where registration exists, as in Malaya and parts of India, 'failure to enforce the law against defaulters has resulted in no material improvement being effected in such areas',[40] and in those areas where registration succeeds, at least partly, the information may be inaccurate and misleading. Registration of death is easier to enforce where permission for burial is made dependent upon it, but, as we have already seen, compulsory registration of births follows naturally only upon some need for documentary evidence as, for example, rationing in Malaya in World War II; it may have to wait upon school systems and upon other personal interests. The obstacles to the development of comprehensive systems are in fact much more fundamental. They include absence of government, particularly at the local level, and the lack of professional persons – physicians, midwives, nurses, and sanitarians. Illiteracy and indifference of large sections of the population prevent any real understanding of the part each has to play. Ignorance and poor communications hamper co-operation with officials. Local traditions and customs impede the introduction of new ideas or stultify their operation.

Despite the great need for reliable information upon which to build health services and with which to satisfy international organizations, vital and health statistics provide an instance where more haste may mean less speed. Edge has said:[17]

Any attempt to carry out specific enquiries in the interest of public health, or to introduce systems of human book-keeping among a people having no previous experience of works of this kind, should start with the intention of hastening slowly, and with the determination that so far as is humanly possible, schemes of work will follow along lines not too far removed from local custom so that their purpose may be understood. . . . Legislative measures providing for the introduction of reformative schemes may be framed with ease, but it is sometimes forgotten that unless the requirements such enactments desire to implement are likely to receive the approval of local public opinion, they may prove inoperative.

If anyone doubts the truth of what Edge wrote in 1947 and its applicability to modern times, he should refer back to Chapter 22 for the evidence that, 25 years after the formation of WHO, for half the world's population statistical data about disease and death are virtually non-existent.

The difficulties of producing worthwhile data in matters of fundamental importance to national planning are clearly great; and the means to counter these are not only elusive, but also cannot be the same in any two countries. In general the answers are to be found in the discussion of principles throughout Part Seven of this book and in a thorough study of the references; but it may serve a useful purpose to summarize the main points in terms of the under-developed and developing world.

The use of the infrastructure of health. The infrastructure of health, wher-ever sufficiently developed, should be used to validate data at ground level (see Chapter 20).

1. All non-medically certified deaths should be followed up from a health centre (see p. 191).

2. Death certificates, medical and non-medical, should be submitted first to the health centre before registration.

3. An abbreviated code of causes of death and disease should be used for certification and classification. Where a medical certificate is available from a general practitioner who attended the deceased before death, or from a public health officer, who comes to the best conclusion possible on the evidence avail-able, the List of 150 causes is probably most appropriate (Appx. 1); otherwise for laymen a List of 50 causes is best (Appx. 4). WHO is now preparing three lists for lay reporting (see p. 227).

4. The International Death Certificate should be used for both medical and non-medical certification and instruction in its use should be given to doctors and lay reporters (see p. 223). A single cause, the underlying cause, only should be entered, if the person certifying is other than a general practitioner who attended the deceased in his last illness.

5. Auxiliary statisticians should be trained to work from 'group' or 'district' levels in the infrastructure (see p. 206) for supervision of data collection and classification (see p. 227).

6. Village headmen and others reporting deaths should receive instruction 'in-service' in the use of the Abbreviated Code of Mortality and Morbidity.

7. Wherever possible data should be analysed for medically certified and non-medically certified deaths in separate tables.

The training of statistical staff. Statisticians are required at two levels. A limited number of professional statisticians, with the skills necessary to plan and supervise statistical systems, will be needed to work in the higher echelons of the infrastructure of health. These can be obtained by the adaptation of courses in the University, by sending 'fellows' for training abroad, or by sending experts to seminars and training centres organized by WHO and the United Nations. Both these bodies have collaborated with various governments in such ventures (e.g. seminars at Santiago, Chile 1950; Tokyo, 1952; training centres in Sri Lanka, 1951; Cairo, 1951; Afghanistan, 1954; Fiji, 1962; Bangkok, 1965). There is a permanent Inter-American Centre of Biostatistics at Santiago.

Auxiliary statisticians are needed in greater numbers to staff the infrastructure. The most practical means to satisfy this need is the use of Training Institutes (see p. 205).

The calculation of numerators and denominators. Comprehensive systems of census enumeration and civil registration are of fundamental importance (see p. 242); but they must be limited in scope to provide the minimum of information necessary for planning. It is better to limit the data tabulated in registration to a minimum than to overload a weak machinery.

It is essential to have an estimate of population, without which the calculation of mortality, natality and morbidity is not possible[28, 90] (see p. 242); and the interpretation of the significance of most observations in the field difficult. The minimum of selected questions should be asked, with, in some cases, special measurements for age.[69]

Internal migration is a feature of most developing countries and such movements of population can vitiate the most painstaking recording. Even the simple movements of expectant mothers to other localities for confinement, to seek better medical care or for family reasons, can introduce errors, as in mortality rates where the infant dies soon after birth. The first international conference of national committees recommended a five yearly census for age, sex, marital status and occupation.

The determination of numerators and denominators for infant mortality is subject to many errors. Although some form of birth registration, compulsory or otherwise, is relatively easy to get, nevertheless the totals obtained in this way rarely make satisfactory denominators without careful checks by midwives, registrars and others concerned with reporting; and all such persons must be aware of the standard definition of live births (see p. 230). Particular attention needs to be given to late foetal deaths if only to avoid the failure to record those dying soon after birth; this also makes it possible to calculate the ratio of live births to late foetal deaths.

One means to get worthwhile infant mortality data is to calculate rates over the first three year span. A card index of all children born, subjected to continual checks by whatever agencies are working in the field, including, where they exist, teachers, health visitors, or health assistants, provides the framework. This should result, over a period of time and with local enthusiasm, in an estimate of child survival more accurate than the standard infant mortality calculations, and one at the same time which is equally valuable as a comparative index of healthiness.[79] It is also of value to register peri-natal mortality by aggregating late foetal deaths and deaths in the first year.

The use of sampling.[108, 112, 118] Sampling provides a practical alternative to comprehensive national systems for data collection. Not only do sample surveys provide answers to immediate problems of numerators and denominators for calculation of vital statistics, but also they can be used for morbidity, fertility and other data beyond the scope of the census or civil registration: they can, e.g. determine the age of mother, duration of marriage and numbers previously born alive, information which is needed for fertility studies.

For morbidity data the main weapon in underdeveloped countries should be the survey particularly 'ad hoc' surveys seeking specific, rather than general information. Otherwise some help will be obtained where a school system exists, although rates only can be calculated for the highly selected school child population, using the school register as the denominator. Health centres, special treatment centres, and notification, will all be of value for easily recognizable diseases. Hospital data, with all their limitations (see p. 251), can provide valuable morbidity data in developing countries and efforts to simplify and improve methods of recording in hospitals can be rewarding.

Model areas

Model areas, in which registration and the development of public health practice go hand in hand, should be of general application. Each such area of approximately 40,000 to 100,000 population should operate both as a local health unit – with nurses, midwives, and sanitarians working from health centres – and as a model registration area, with the technicians trained in vital statistical methods. The area should be directed by a medical officer of health with special training in public health work. A concentration of effort with skilled staff in a relatively small area is of inestimable value in learning what are the main obstacles to be overcome in obtaining vital and health statistics, as well as in providing a valuable check for the remainder of the country. In model areas it becomes possible to obtain complete recording of live births and deaths at all ages. The card index already suggested can be maintained and the conduct of a census is relatively easy. Morbidity surveys are possible. General and specific death rates can be determined, together with data about the incidence and prevalence of the main diseases, which will serve as indices of unhealthiness in different parts of the country. The model area provides an admirable training ground for all types of staff in the significance of statistics to public health work.

Conclusion

Our world tour is over and every reader is back in his homeland – the best in the world; if a little wiser, less complacent, and more aware of the world-wide issues from which no country can now stand aloof, then these words have served their purpose.

> If a man will begin with certainties, he shall end in doubts; but if he will be content to begin with doubts, he shall end in certainties.
>
> *Bacon*[2]

Bibliography

Part One: Chapters 1 and 2

1 Allee, W. C. *et al.* (1949) *Principles of Animal Ecology*, p. 580. Philadelphia.
2 Bernard, Claude (1865) *Introduction à l'Étude de la Médecine Experimentale*. Paris.
3 Eliot, T. S. (1955) *Four Quartets*, p. 25. London.
4 Farr, W. (1839) *Vital Statistics; McCulloch's Statistical Account of the British Empire*. London.
5 Galen. (1951) *Hygiene (de Sanitate tuenda)*, trans. Green, R. M. Springfield, Ill.: Thomas.
6 Huxley, A. (1921) *Chrome Yellow*, p. 148. London.
7 Lack, D. (1954) *The Natural Regulation of Animal Numbers*. Oxford.
8 Meadower, P. B. (1957) *The Uniqueness of the Individual*. London.
9 Perkins, J. E. (1950) *To-morrow's Horizon in Public Health*. New York.
10 Scheele, L. A. (1953) Public health, 1852–1952. *Journal of the Mount Sinai Hospital*. Symposium on medicine and society. pp. 76–89. Baltimore.
11 Selye, H. (1950) *The Physiology and Pathology of Exposure to Stress*. Montreal.
12 Stieglitz, E. S. (1949) *Social Medicine, its Derivatives and Objectives*, pp. 76–89. New York.
13 WHO. (1946) *Constitution of the World Health Organization*. New York.
14 WHO. (1952) *Expert Committee on Public Health Administration: First Report. Tech. Rep. Ser.* 55.
15 Winslow, C. E. A. (1923) *Evolution and Significance of the Modern Public Health Campaign*. London.

Part Two: Chapters 3 and 4

1 Berman, C. (1955) Nutritional states in the causation of primary liver cancer. *Intern. Soc. of Geographical Pathology: Transactions of the Fifth Meeting*, 1954. Basel.
2 Brockington, C. F. (1965) *The Health of the Community*, ch. 12. London.
3 Burgess, R. C. (1956) *Proc. of Nutr. Soc.*, **15**, No. 1, 13.
4 Cockburn, W. C. & Assaad, F. (1973) Some observations on the communicable diseases as public health problems. *Bull. Wld Hlth Org.*
5 Comfort, A. (1956) The biology of ageing. *Lancet, ii*, pp. 772–8.
6 Davies, J. N. P. (1955) Nutritional states as causal factors of cancer. *Intern. Soc. of Geographical Pathology: Transactions of the Fifth Meeting*, 1954. Basel.
7 Demographic Year Book. (1972). United Nations. New York.
8 FAO. (Food and Agriculture Organization). (1946) *Proposals for a World Food Board and World Food Survey*. Washington.
9 FAO. (1952) *Second World Food Survey*. Rome.
10 FAO. (1964) *Third World Food Survey*, 2nd edn. Rome.
11 Khanolkar, V. R. (1955) Habits and customs as causal factors in cancer. *Intern. Soc. of Geographical Pathology: Transactions of the Fifth Meeting, 1964*. Basel.
12 Meadower, P. B. (1957) *The Uniqueness of the Individual*. London.
13 Muir, C. S. (1973) *Geographical Differences in Cancer Patterns*. Lyon: International Agency for Research on Cancer.
14 Oberling, C. (1955) What can experimentation teach us with regard to geographical distribution of cancer? *Intern. Soc. of Geographical Pathology: Transactions of the Fifth Meeting, 1954*. Basel.
15 Simmons, J. S. *et al.* (1944–54) *Global Epidemiology: A Geography of Disease and Sanitation*, 3 vols. Philadelphia.

16 Steiner, P. E. (1955). World distribution of cancer. *Intern. Soc. of Geographical Pathology: Transactions of the Fifth Meeting, 1954.* Basel.
17 Swaroop, S. (1954) *Demographic and Health Statistics relating to Urban and Rural Areas.* World Health Organization. Geneva: unpublished.
18 UNICEF. (1974) *Facts behind the World Child Emergency.* PI/4/74.
19 UNICEF. (1974) *General Progress Report.* E/ICEF/632.
20 WHO. (1965) *Activities in Nutrition,* 1948–1964.
21 WHO. (1970) *Hypovitaminosis A in the Americas.* PAHO.
22 WHO. (1973/74) *World Health Statistics 1970.* Geneva.
23 WHO. (1974) *Development of the Antimalarial Programme.* A 27/WP/5.
24 *World Atlas of Epidemic Diseases,* 3 vols. (1952) Hamburg.
25 Woytinsky, W. S. & E. S. (1953) *World Population and Production.* New York.

Part Three: Chapter 5

1 Brockington, C. F. (1944) Trace elements in relation to health. *Public Health,* **58**, No. 2, p. 19.
2 Hippocrates trans. Jones, W. H. S. (1923) *Hippocrates,* vol. 1: Airs Waters Places. London: Loeb Classical Library.
3 Huntington, E. (1924) *Civilization and Climate,* 3rd edn. New Haven.
4 Markham, S. F. (1944) *Climate and the Energy of Nations.* Oxford.
5 May, J. M. (1950) Medical geography: its objectives and methods. *Geographical Review,* **40**, 9–41.
6 Simmons, J. S. *et al.* (1944–54) *Global Epidemiology: A Geography of Disease and Sanitation,* 3 vols. Philadelphia.
7 Stern, B. J. (1941) *Society and Medical Progress.* Princeton.

Part Three: Chapter 6

1 Benedict, R. (1952) *Patterns of Culture,* fifth impression, p. 66. London.
2 Bridgman, R. F. (1955) The rural hospital: its structure and organization. *World Health Organization Monograph No. 21.* Geneva.
3 Burgess, R. C. & Musa, L. B. A. (1950) Diet . . . in Malaya: *Institute of Medical Research, Report 13,* p. 26. Malaya.
4 Caudill, W. (1952) Applied anthropology in medicine. In *International Symposium on Anthropology.* New York; and (1953) *Anthropology To-day,* pp. 771–806. Edited by A. L. Kroeber. Chicago.
5 Conant, J. B. (1948) The role of science in our unique society. *Science,* **107**, pp. 77–83.
6 Experience with human factors in agricultural areas of the world, (1949). *Conference on Extension Experiences Around the World.* Washington.
7 Firth, R. (1956) *Acculturation in Relation to Concepts of Health and Disease.* New York: unpublished.
8 Foster, G. (1951) *A Cross-cultural Anthropological Analysis of a Technical Aid Program.* Washington.
9 Hsu, F. L. K. (1951) *Religion, Science and Human Crises.* London.
10 Brockington, C. F. ed. (1957) Mental health and the world community. *World Federation for Mental Health.* London.
11 Paul, B. D. & Miller, W. B. (1955) *Health, Culture and Community.* New York.
12 Read, M. (1956) *Social and Cultural Backgrounds for Planning Public Health Programmes in Africa.* Geneva: WHO, unpublished.
13 Rosen, G. (1954) The community and the health officer: a working team. *Amer. J. Publ. Hlth,* **44**, pp. 14–17.
14 Ryle, J. A. (1948) *Changing Disciplines: Lectures on the History, Method and Motives of Social Pathology,* p. 21. Oxford.

15 Sigerist, H. E. (1956) *Landmarks in the History of Hygiene.* Oxford.
16 Simey, T. S. (1946) *Welfare and Planning in the West Indies.* Oxford.
17 Valentin, P. E. (1894) *Les Religions Orientales Considérées dans leurs Rapport avec l'Hygiène et la Prophylaxie des Maladies Contagieuses.* Paris.
18 World Federation for Mental Health. Cultural Patterns and Technical Change (1953) Edited by M. Mead. Paris.

Part Three: Chapter 7

1 Booth, C. (1889–97) *Life and Labour of the People in London.* London.
2 Bowlby, J. (1951) Maternal care and mental health. *WHO Monograph No. 2.* See also (1962) Deprivation of maternal care. A re-assessment of its effects. *Public Health Papers No. 14.* WHO.
3 Brockington, C. F. (1966) *A Short History of Public Health.* 2nd ed, ch. 4.
4 Burgess, A. (1957) Traditional systems of child care. *Health Education Journal,* 15, p. 105.
5 Burton, J. (1957) Soap and education. *Health Education Journal,* 15, p. 72.
6 Dicks, H. V. (1954) *Experiences with Marital Tensions in the Psychological Clinic.* 5th International Congress on Mental Health.
7 Ferguson, T. & Pettigrew, M. G. (1954) *Glasgow Medical Journal,* 35, pp. 183–201.
8 Firth, R. (1953) The child and its relationship to the community. *International Child Welfare Review,* 9, pp. 123–136. Geneva.
9 Hargreaves, G. R. (1954) *The Mental Hygiene Aspects of Pregnancy and Childbirth.* Paper read at International Congress of Obstetrics. Geneva. See also *Lancet,* 1955, *i,* 39.
10 Hoggart, R. (1957) *The Uses of Literacy.* London.
11 Jeffreys, M. (1957) Social class and health promotion. *Health Education Journal,* 15, 109–117.
12 Lewis, H. (1954) *Deprived Children.* Oxford.
13 Mayhew, H. (1851) *London Labour and the London Poor.* London.
14 Mead, M. (1970) *Male and Female.* Penguin.
15 Report to the Ministry of Education. (1954) *Early Leaving.* London: HMSO.
16 Robb, J. H. (1953) *Brit. J. of Med. Psych.* 26, p. 215.
17 Sheldon, J. H. (1954) The social philosophy of old age. *Lancet, ii,* pp. 151–5.
18 Stocks, P. (1949) *Studies on Medical and Population Subjects, No. 2.* London: HMSO.
19 Williams, C. D. (1955) *Focus on Child Health in the Tropics,* p. 54. London (Royal Sanitary Institute): 62nd Health Congress.
20 Young, M. & Willmott, P. (1957) *Family and Kinship in East London.* London.

Part Three: Chapter 8

1 Carr-Saunders, A. M. (1936) *World Population: Past Growth and Present Trends,* 2nd impression, 1964. Oxford.
2 Chandrasekhar. (1967) *Discussion of Health Aspects of Population Dynamics.* WHO, Twentieth World Health Assembly.
3 Dandekar, V. M. & Dandekar, K. (1953) *Gokhale Institute of Politics and Economics, Publication No. 27.* Poona.
4 Darwin, C. (1953) *The Next Million Years.* Garden City, New York.
5 Demographic Yearbook. (1972) New York: United Nations.
6 Hertzler, J. O. (1956) *The Crisis in World Population.* Lincoln (Neb.)
7 Malthus, T. R. (1798) *An Essay on the Principles of Population.* London.
8 Notestein, F. W. (1954) *The Reduction of Human Fertility ... The Inter-relations of Demographic, Economic and Social Problems.* New York: Milbank Memorial Fund.
9 Paul, B. D. & Miller, W. B. (1955) *Health, Culture and Community.* New York: Russell Sage Foundation.
10 Taeuber, I. B. (1954) *Demographic Transition in Japan.* New York: Milbank Memorial Fund.

11 The determinants and consequences of population trends. *Population Studies*, No. 17. (1953) New York: United Nations.
12 WHO. (1964) Biology of human reproduction. *Tech. Rep. Ser.* No. 280.
13 WHO. (1965) Mechanism of action of sex hormones and analogous substances. *Tech. Rep. Ser.* No. 303.
14 WHO. (1966) Clinical aspects of oral oestrogens. *Tech. Rep. Ser.* No. 326.
15 WHO. (1966) Basic and clinical aspects of intra-uterine devices. *Tech. Rep. Ser.* No. 332.
16 WHO. (1967) Biology of fertility control by periodic abstinence. *Tech. Rep. Ser.* No. 360.
17 WHO. (1968) Hormonal steroids in contraception. *Tech. Rep. Ser.* No. 386.
18 WHO. (1968) Intra-uterine devices: physiological and clinical aspects. *Tech. Rep. Ser.* No. 397.
19 WHO. (1969) Developments in fertility control. *Tech. Rep. Ser.* No. 424.
20 WHO. (1971) Endocrine Regulation of human gestation. *Tech. Rep. Ser.* No. 471.
21 WHO. (1971) Methods of fertility regulation: advances in research and clinical experience. *Tech. Rep. Ser.* No. 473.
22 WHO. (1973) Advances in methods of fertility. *Tech. Rep. Ser.* No. 527.
23 WHO. (1973) Agents stimulating gonadal function in the human. *Tech. Rep. Ser.* No. 514.
24 WHO. (1973) Reproductive function in the human male. *Tech. Rep. Ser.* No. 520.
25 World Population Conference (Bucharest). 1974. New York: United Nations.
26 Woytinsky, W. S. & E. S. (1953) *World Population and Production*. New York.

Part Three: Chapter 9

1 Brockington, C. F. (1965) *The Health of the Community*, Ch 17 and Appendix 5. London.
2 Delmege, J. A. (1931) *Towards National Health*. London.
3 Greenhow, E. H. (1858) *Papers Relating to the Sanitary State of the People of England*. Reprinted in Gregg's *Pioneers of Demography* (1973).
4 Greenhow, E. H. (1860) *Third Report of the Medical Officer of the Privy Council*, pp. 102–194. London.
5 Guy, A. (1862) *Fifth Report of the Medical Officer of the Privy Council*, pp. 126–162. London.
6 Hunter, D. (1964) *The Diseases of Occupation*, 3rd edn. London.
7 Legge, T. M. (1934) *Industrial Maladies*. Oxford.
8 M'Cready, B. W. (1836–7) On the influence of trades, professions, and occupations in the United States, in the production of disease. *Transactions of the Medical Society of the State of New York*, pp. 91–150.
9 Ministry of Pensions and National Insurance. *Digest of Statistics Analysing Certificates of Incapacity, 1958–1961*.
10 Patissier, P. (1822) *Traité des Maladies des Artisans*. Paris.
11 Ramazzini, B. (1700) *De Morbis artificum diatriba*. Modena.
12 Schilling, R. S. F. (1956) Byssinosis in cotton and textile workers. *Lancet*, ii, pp. 261–265 & 319–325.
13 Thackrah, C. T. (1831) *The Effects of Arts, Trades and Professions and of Civic States and Habits of Living on Health and Longevity*. London.
14 The determinants and consequences of population trends. *Population Studies*, No. 17 (1953) p. 62. New York: United Nations.

Part Three: Chapter 10

1 Census, 1971. Great Britain. *Housing Summary and Housing Tables*, Pt. 111. London: HMSO.
2 Chamberlayne, E. (1669) *The Present State of England*. London.
3 Cleland, J. (1820) *The Rise and Progress of the City of Glasgow*. Glasgow.
4 Delmege, J. A. (1931) *Towards National Health*. London.

5 Demographic Yearbook, 1972. New York: United Nations.
6 Graunt, J. (1662) *Natural and Political Observations upon the Bills of Mortality*. London.
7 Hammond, J. L. & B. (1949) *The Town Labourer (1760–1832)*, **1**, p. 48. London: Guild Books.
8 Hoffman, F. & Ramazzini, B. (1750) *On those Distempers which arise from Particular Climates, Situations and Methods of Life*. London.
9 Khairallah, A. A. (1946) *Outline of Arabic Contributions to Medicine*. Beirut.
10 M'Cready, B. W. (1836–7) On the influence of trades, professions and occupations in the United States, in the production of disease. *Transactions of the Medical Society of New York*, pp. 91–150.
11 Mumford, L. (1938) *The Culture of Cities*, p. 50. London.
12 Patissier, P. (1822) *Traité des Maladies des Artisans*. Paris.
13 Poore, G. V. (1889) *London (Ancient and Modern)*, p. 26. London.
14 Ramazzini, B. (1700) *De Morbis artificum diatriba*. Modena.
15 *Royal Commission on Population Report* (1949) Cmd. 7695, London.
16 Royal Commission into the State of Large Towns and Populous Districts in England and Wales (1845) *General Report*, vol. 1, p. 4. London.
17 Shattuck, L. *et al.* (1850) *Report of the Sanitary Commission of Massachusetts*, 1850, reprinted Cambridge, Mass., 1948.
18 Simon, J. (1887) *Public Health Reports*, **1**, p. 48. London.
19 Swaroop, S. (1954) *Demographic and Health Statistics Relating to Urban and Rural Areas*. Geneva: WHO, unpublished.
20 The determinants and consequences of population trends. *Population Studies*, No. 17, p. 62. (1953) New York: United Nations.
21 Woytinsky, W. S. & E. S. (1953) *World Population and Production*, p. 112. New York.

Part Three: Chapter 11

1 Abel-Smith, B. & Titmuss, R. M. (1956) *The Cost of the National Health Service in England and Wales*. Appendix H: The hospital population, pp. 139–152. Cambridge.
2 Bowlby, J. (1952) Maternal care and mental health, 2nd edn, *World Health Organization Monograph* No. 2. Geneva.
3 Bridgman, R. F. (1955) The rural hospital. *World Health Organization Monograph* No. 21. Geneva.
4 Brockington, C. F. (1949) The nurse in Great Britain, *Can. J. Publ. Hlth*, **40**, pp. 292–301.
5 Brockington, C. F. (1965) *The Health of the Community*, pp. 115–122. London.
6 Brockington, C. F. & Lempert, S. (1965) *The Social Needs of the Over-eighties*. Manchester University Press.
7 Burdett, H. C. (1891–93) *Hospitals and Asylums of the World*, vol. 3, p. 26. London.
8 Daley, A. (1953) The place of the hospital in a National Health Service. *Brit. Med. J.*, **ii**, pp. 163–170 & 243–250.
9 Elgood, C. (1951) *A Medical History of Persia and the Eastern Caliphate from the Earliest Times until the Year A.D. 1932*, p. 183. Cambridge.
10 Great Britain. (1957) *Royal Commission on the Law Relating to Mental Illness and Mental Deficiency. Report, 1954–1952*, p. 207. London: HMSO. (Cmnd 169).
11 Haggard, H. W. (1929) Quoted in *Devils, Drugs and Doctors*, p. 33. London.
12 Khairallah, A. A. (1946) *Outline of Arabic Contributions to Medicine*, p. 62. Beirut.
13 Montefiore Hospital for Chronic Diseases. (1949) *Home Care; Origin, Organization and Present States of the Extramural Program of Montefiore Hospital*. New York.
14 Mumford, L. E. (1938) *The Culture of Cities*, p. 49. London.
15 Nightingale, F. (1860). *Notes on Nursing*, p. 5. London.
16 *Odyssey*, iv, 231 f.
17 Papyros Ebers. (1875) *Das Hermetische Buch über die Arzneimittel der alten Aegypter in hieratischer Schrift*, 2 vols. Edited by Georg Ebers. Leipzig.
18 Paul H. (1964) *The Control of Communicable Diseases*, 2nd edn. London.
19 Sigerist, H. E. (1951) *A History of Medicine*, vol. 1, p. 425. New York.
20 Tenon, J. R. (1788) *Mémoires sur les Hôpitaux de Paris*. Paris.

21 Watkins, A. G. & Lewis-Fanning, E. (1949) Incidence of cross-infection in children's wards. *Brit. Med. J. ii*, pp. 616–619.
22 West Riding. *County Medical Officer of Health: Annual Reports. Wakefield, 1947–1951.*
23 WHO. (1954) Expert Committee on Public Health Administration. Second Report. Methodology of planning an integrated health programme for rural areas. *Tech. Rep. Ser.*, No. 83.
24 WHO. (1954) Public health problems in rural areas. *Technical Discussions*. A7 Technical Discussions/1–8. Seventh World Health Assembly, unpublished working papers.
25 WHO. (1957) *Expert Committee on Organization of Medical Care. First Report*. Role of hospitals in programmes of community health protection. *Tech. Rep. Ser.*, No. 122. Geneva.

Part Three: Chapter 12

1 Bengoa, S. M. (1966) *Priorities in Public Health Nutrition Disorders*. WHO International Congress on Nutrition.
2 Brockington, C. F. (1952) *The Principles of Nutrition for Practitioners and Students*. London.
3 Burgess, R. C. (1956) WHO and nutrition. *Proc Nutr. Soc.* 15, No. 1, p. 13; also unpublished report (1957). Geneva.
4 Burgess, R. C. & Musa, L. B. A. (1950) Diet . . . in Malaya. *Institute of Medical Research, Report* No. 13, p. 26. Malaya.
5 Domestic food consumption and expenditure. (1953) *Annual Report of the National Food Survey Committee, 1955*, also 1972, published 1974. London: HMSO.
6 Drummond, J. C. (1940) Food in relation to health in Great Britain during the past two hundred years. *The Nation's Larder*. London.
7 FAO. (1963) *Third World Food Survey*. Rome.
8 Hertzler, J. O. (1956) *The Crisis in World Population*. Lincoln.
9 Hopkins, F. G. (1906) *The Analyst*, 31, 395.
10 Horder, D. *et al.* (1954) *Bread*. London.
11 Joint FAO/WHO Expert Committee on Nutrition. (1953) WHO *Tech. Rep. Ser.* No. 72. Geneva.
12 Lind, J. (1753) *A Treatise on the Scurvy*. Edinburgh.
13 McCarrison, R. (1936) Nutrition and health. In *Cantor Lectures*. Republished by Faber, 1944, 3rd edn., 1961.
14 McCarrison, R. (1940) *The Nation's Larder*. London.
15 Orr, J. B. (1936) *Food, Health and Income*. London.
16 Rowntree, S. B. (1901) *Poverty: a Study of Town Life*. London.
17 Russell, E. J. (1949–50) *Food Resources in the Modern World*. University of Nottingham, Montague Burton International Relations Lecture.
18 UNICEF. (1956) *Proc. Nutr. Soc.*, 15, No. 1, p. 27.
19 UNICEF. (1963) *Children of Developing Countries*.
20 UNICEF. (1974) *General Progress Report*, E/ICEF/632.
21 WHO. (1965) *Activities in Nutrition. 1948–1964.*
22 WHO. (1972) A Review of the WHO Programme. 1965–1971. *Nutrition.*

Part Three: Chapter 13

1 Ginsburg, E. L. (1950) *Public Health is People*. New York: Commonwealth Fund.
2 Hammond, J. L. (1925) *The Rise of Modern Industry*, 9th edn., 1966. London.
3 *Social Implications of Industrialization and Urbanization in Africa, South of the Sahara*. (1956) Paris: UNESCO.
4 Ling, T. M. (ed.) (1954) *Mental Health and Human Relations in Industry*. London.
5 Mayo, E. (1949) *The Social Problems of an Industrial Civilization*. London.
6 Mayo, E. (1952) *The Human Problems of an Industrial Civilization*, 2nd edn. London.
7 Mead, M. (ed.) (1953) *Cultural Patterns and Technical Change*. Paris: UNESCO.

8 *Interrelations between the Social Environment and Psychiatric Disorders.* (1953) New York: Milbank Memorial Fund.
9 *The Interrelations of Demographic, Economic and Social Problems in Selected Underdeveloped Areas.* (1954) New York: Milbank Memorial Fund.
10 Moore, W. E. (1951) *Industrialization and Labor.* New York: Ithaca.
11 Romero, H. (1957) *Chile at the Cross Roads,* ch. 4, part 4, 33, p. 378. London: World Federation for Mental Health.
12 Spicer, E. H. (ed.) (1952) *Human Problems in Technological Change.* New York: Russell Sage Foundation.

Part Four: Chapters 14, 15 and 16

1 Banning, C. (1950) *Co-ordination between the Public Health Service and Private Enterprise in Holland; its Results.* London.
2 Barthelemy, J. (1924) *Le Gouvernment de la France.* Paris.
3 Bowditch, H. I. (1876) Address on hygiene and preventive medicine. Reprint from *Transactions of the International Medical Congress,* p. 11. Philadelphia.
4 Bridgman, R. F. (1955) The rural hospital; its structure and organization. *World Health Organization Monograph* No. 21. Geneva.
5 Brockington, C. F. (1955) *Turkey.* Geneva: WHO, unpublished report. Also (1969) Copenhagen: WHO.
6 Brockington, C. F. (1955) *Yugoslavia.* Geneva: WHO, unpublished report.
7 Brockington, C. F. (1956) Medical education in the U.S.S.R. *Publ. Hlth,* 69, pp. 149–151.
8 Brockington, C. F. (1956) Public health in Russia. *Lancet, ii,* pp. 138–141.
9 Brockington, C. F. (1958) Public health in Siam. *Publ. Hlth,* 78, No. 5.
10 Brockington, C. F. (1965) *The Health of the Community.* London.
11 Brockington, C. F. (1965) *Public Health in the Nineteenth Century.* Edinburgh.
12 Brockington, C. F. (1966) *A Short History of Public Health,* 2nd edn. London.
13 Brockington, C. F. (1967) *Rapport sur l'organisation de santé en Espagne.* 0030 Copenhagen: WHO.
14 Calcutta: All-India Institute of Hygiene and Public Health, Singur Health Unit. (1945) *The Rural Community Controlled Practice Field of the All-India Institute of Hygiene and Public Health, Calcutta.* Government of India Press.
15 Emerson, H. (1945) *Local Health Units for the Nation.* New York: Commonwealth Fund.
16 Emerson, H. (1948) *Local Units the Basis of the Nation's Health.* Address to National Health Assembly, May 1. Quoted by Wyatt, in *Intergovernmental Relations in Public Health,* p. 4.
17 Fox, T. F. (1954) Russia revisited. Impressions of Soviet Medicine. *Lancet, ii,* pp. 748–753 & 803–807.
18 France (1952) Ministère de la Santé Publique et de la Population. *Public Health Services in France.* Geneva: WHO.
19 Frandsen, J. (1955) On health systems, 2. The Danish system. *Danish med. Bull.,* 2, p. 224.
20 Frank, J. P. (1790) The people's misery: mother of diseases. An address delivered by J. P. Frank, translated from the Latin with an introduction by H. E. Sigerist. In *Bull. Hist. Med.* (1941) 9, pp. 81–100.
21 Gale, G. W. (1950) *Health Services in Three Continents.* Pretoria.
22 Galen (1951) trans. Green, R. M. *Hygiene (de Sanitate tuenda),* p. 51. Springfield, Ill.
23 Galen. *Hygiene (de Sanitate tuenda), vi,* 309. Quoted by Sigerist, H. E. in *Landmarks in the History of Hygiene,* p. 4. (1956) Oxford.
24 Grant, J. B. (1947) The health department and medical care; certain trends. *Amer. J. publ. Hlth,* 37, pp. 269–275.
25 Great Britain. Consultative Council on Medical and Allied Services (1920) *Interim Report on the Future Provision of Medical and Allied Services.* London: HMSO.
26 Hanlon, J. J. (1969) *Principles of Public Health Administration,* 5th edn. St. Louis.
27 India. (1946) *Health Survey and Development Committee: Report.* Delhi.
28 India. (1954) *Evaluation Report on First Year's Working of Community Projects,* pp. 33–34. Delhi: Planning Commission, Programme Evaluation Organization.
29 International Bank for Reconstruction and Development (1951) *The Economy of Turkey,* 178–193. Washington.

30 Japan. (1956) *A Brief Report on Public Health Administration in Japan*. Tokyo: Ministry of Health and Welfare.
31 Leimena, J. (1956) *Public Health in Indonesia; Problems and Planning*. The Hague.
32 *Public Health in the People's Republic of China* (1973) New York: Macy Foundation Conference.
33 *Report of the Sanitary Commission of Massachusetts, 1849*. (1850) Massachusetts Sanitary Commission. Reprinted Cambridge Mass. 1948. Boston.
34 Mead, R. (1744) *Discourse on the Plague*, 9th edn. London.
35 Brockington, C. F. (ed.) (1957) *Mental Health and the World Community*, ch. 5. London: World Federation for Mental Health, and Wickremesinghe, W. G. *Health Units in Ceylon*.
36 Murray, D. S. (1943) *Health for All*. London.
37 Newsholme, A. (1931) *International Studies on the Relation between the Private and Official Practice of Medicine with Special Reference to the Prevention of Disease*. London: Milbank Memorial Fund.
38 Nightingale, F. (1870) *Proposals for a Uniform Plan of Hospital Statistics*. London. 4th Int. Stat. Conf.
39 Pan-American Sanitary Bureau. *Summary of Reports on the Health Conditions in the Americas, 1950–53*. (1956) Washington.
40 Péquignot, H. (1954) *Eléments de politique et d'administration sanitaires*, p. 149. Paris.
41 Péquinot, H. (1954) *Eléments de politique et d'administration sanitaires*, p. 85. Paris.
42 Péquinot, H. (1954) *Eléments de politique et d'administration sanitaires*, p. 164. Paris.
43 Richardson, B. W. (1887) *The Health of Nations: a review of the works of Edwin Chadwick*, vol. 2. pp. 100–102. London.
44 Rosen, J. (1953) Cameralism and the concept of medical police. *Bull. Hist. Med.*, **27**, pp. 21–42.
45 Scheele, L. A. (1953) Public Health, 1852–1952. *Journal of the Mount Sinai Hospital: Symposium on Medicine and Society*, pp. 764–789. Baltimore.
46 Silva, D. M. de. (1956) *Health Progress in Ceylon: a Survey*. Colombo.
47 Smillie, W. G. (1955) *Public Health: its Promise jor the Future*, p. 76. New York.
48 *Soviet Medical Bulletin* (1957) **4**, No. 2. London: Society for Cultural Relations.
49 Toha, Dean of the Medical Faculty, Sourabaya. Quoted in Leimena, *Public Health in Indonesia*, p. 69.
50 Turkey. *The Organization and Legislation concerning Health and Social Assistance in Turkey*. (1956) Ankara: Ministry of Health and Social Assistance.
51 U.S. War Department. *Medical and Sanitary Data on Turkey*. (1944) Washington.
52 Uttar Pradesh. Planning and Development Department (1953) *Community Projects in Uttar Pradesh 1952–53*. Lucknow.
53 Weir, J. M. *et al.* (1952) An evaluation of health and sanitation in Egyptian villages. *J. Egypt. publ. Hlth Ass.*, 27, pp. 55–114.
54 Williams, H. (1956) The influence of Edwin Chadwick on American Public Health. *Med. Offr.*, **95**, p. 275.
55 WHO. (1952–54) *Expert Committees on Public Health Administration 1st-2nd reports Tech. Rep. Ser.* **55, 83**.
56 WHO. (1954) Seventh World Health Assembly. *Technical Discussions*. (A7/Technical Discussions/1–8). Geneva: unpublished working papers.
57 WHO. Brockington, C. F. (1963) *Mass Campaigns and General Public Health*. Geneva: WHO, unpublished paper.
58 WHO. Gonzalez, C. L. (1965) Mass campaigns and general health services. *Public Health Papers No. 29*.
59 WHO. Integration of mass campaigns against specific diseases into general public health services. (1965) *Tech. Rep. Ser.* **294**.
60 Wyatt, L. R. (1951) *Intergovernmental Relations in Public Health*. Minneapolis.

Part Five: Chapters 17, 18 and 19

1 Berkov, R. (1957) *The World Health Organization: a Study in Decentralized International Administration*. Geneva.
2 Biraud, Y. (1950) The international control of epidemics. *Brit. Med. J.*, i, pp. 1046–1050.
3 Brockington, C. F. (1958) Public health in Siam. *Publ. Hlth*, **72**, No. 5.

4 Brockington, C. F. (1969) *Evaluation of Auxiliary Training in Saudi Arabia*. EM/Ed. Tr./163. 3.
5 Brockington, C. F. (1969) *Report on the Organization of Public Health Services in Turkey*. 0500 Copenhagen: WHO.
6 Brockington, F. & Stahlie, D. T. (1970) *Report on a Visit to Greece*. Copenhagen: WHO Greece 0025.
7 Burgess, R. C. (1956) WHO and nutrition. *Proc. Nutr. Soc.*, **15**, No. 1, pp. 14–16.
8 Calder, R. (1957) *Ten Steps Forward, 1948–1957*, p. 6. WHO.
9 Candau, M. G. (1956) Some aspects of WHO's work in 1955. *S. Afr. Med. J.*, **30**, pp. 75–78.
10 Chisholm, B. (1950) The World Health Organization. *Brit. Med. J.*, **i**, pp. 1021–1027.
11 Erasmus, C. J. (1954) An anthropologist views technical assistance. *Scientific Monthly*, **78**, p. 147. Washington.
12 *European Conference on Rural Hygiene, Geneva, 1931: Recommendations, Minutes*, 2 vols. Geneva: League of Nations.
13 Gear, H. S. & Deutschman, Z. (1956) *Disease Control and International Travel: A Review of the International Sanitary Regulations*. Geneva: WHO.
14 Gowers, E. (1948) *Plain Words: A guide to the use of English*. London: HMSO.
15 Guthe, T. & Willcox, R. R. (1954) *Treponematoses; a World Problem*. Geneva: WHO.
16 *Inter-Governmental Conference of Far Eastern Countries on Rural Hygiene, Bandoeng*. (*1937*) *Report*. Geneva: League of Nations.
17 Jackson, R. G. A. (1969) *A Study of the Capacity of the United Nations Development System*, vol. 1. Geneva: United Nations.
18 Jungalwalla, N. (1961) *A Brief Note on the Singur Health Centre, India*. WHO/Res. PHA/9. 1961.
19 Kinglake, A. W. (1844) *Eothen*. London.
20 Gonzalez, C. L. (1965) Mass campaigns and general health services. *Public Health Papers* No. 29.
21 Goodman, N. M. (1952) *International Health Organizations and their Work*. London.
22 League of Nations (1936) *The Problem of Nutrition*. 2. Report on the physiological bases of nutrition drawn up by the Technical Commission of the Health Committee. Geneva.
23 Lind, J. A. (1753) *A Treatise on the Scurvey*. Edinburgh.
24 Mead, R. (1720) *A Short Discourse concerning Pestilential Contagion and the Methods to be used to Prevent It*, 2nd edn. London.
25 Nightingale, F. (1870) *Proposals for a uniform Plan of Hospital Statistics*. London: 4th Int. Stat. Conf.
26 *Off. Rec. Wld Hlth Org. 1947*, **1**, p. 39.
27 *Off. Rec. Wld Hlth No. 213, 1974*. Also personal communication, T. Lepes, Geneva.
28 Pampana, E. J. & Russell, P. F. (1955) *Malaria; a World Problem*. Geneva: WHO.
29 Proust, A. (1896) *L'Orentation nouvelle de la politique sanitaire*. Paris.
30 Self-help—its uses and limitations in the field of health. In *Health Information Digest for Hot Countries*, **11**, *ii*, No. 1. London: Central Council for Health Education.
31 *Seminar on Training of Medical Officers in Rural Areas*. SEA/PHA/106. 1972.
32 Simon, J. (1849) *1st Annual Report to City of London*.
33 Snow, J. (1849) *On the Mode of Communication of Cholera*.
34 UNICEF/WHO. Joint Committee on Health Policy. (1965) *Basic Health Services*. JC 14/2. 65.
35 WHO. (1961) *Expert Committee on Malaria, Tech. Rep. Ser.* **205**.
36 WHO. (1962) *Working Paper*. I/Conf. 39/F.38. Geneva.
37 WHO. *Tech. Rep. Ser.* 1952 (No. 55), 1954 (No. 83), 1960 (No. 194), 1961 (No. 215), 1967 (No. 350), 1970 (No. 456).
38 WHO. Brockington, C. F. (1963) *Mass Campaigns and General Public Health*. Geneva: WHO, unpublished paper.
39 WHO. Integration of mass campaigns against specific diseases into general Public Health Services. (1965) *Tech. Rep. Ser.*, **294**.
40 WHO. Supplement to MoF/369, 1962.
41 WHO. *Development of Malaria Eradication Programme, 1967*. A20/P. and B/1.
42 WHO. *Development of the Antimalarial Programme 1974*. A27/WP/5.
43 WHO. (1968) Immunology of malaria. *Tech. Rep. Ser.*, **396**. Geneva.
44 Wortley, B. A. (1957) *The United Nations; the First Ten Years*. To be reprinted by Greenwood Press, Connecticut.

Part Six: Chapter 20

1 Arnold, V. A. & Brockington, C. F. (1972) *Report on a Visit to Turkey.* 4001 Copenhagen: WHO, Turkey.
2 Brockington, C. F. (1966) *A Short History of Public Health,* 2nd edn. London.
3 Brockington, C. F. (1967) *Administration of the Health Services in the Hashemite Kingdom of Jordan,* EM/PHA/118. Alexandria: WHO.
4 Brockington, C. F. (1967) *Rapport sur l'Organisation de Santé en Espagne.* 0030 Copenhagen: WHO.
5 Brockington, C. F. (1969) *Report on the Organization of Public Health Services in Turkey.* 0500 Copenhagen: WHO.
6 Brockington, C. F. (1969) *Evaluation of Auxiliary Training in Four Countries.* EM/Ed. Tr./163. Alexandria: WHO.
7 Brockington, C. F. (1969) *Evaluation of Auxiliary Training in Ethiopia.* EM/Ed. Tr./163. 1. Alexandria: WHO.
8 Brockington, C. F. (1969) *Evaluation of Auxiliary Training in Somalia.* EM/Ed/ Tr./163. 2. Alexandria: WHO.
9 Brockington, C. F. (1969) *Manpower Development Institute Peoples' Republic of Southern Yemen.* EM/PHA/124. Alexandria: WHO.
10 Brockington, C. F. (1969) *Evaluation of Auxiliary Training in Saudi Arabia.* EM/Ed. Tr./163. 3.
11 Brockington, C. F. *Report on the Training of Auxiliaries and Multipurpose Workers in the Hashamite Kingdom of Jordan.* EM/Ed. Tr./106. Alexandria: WHO.
12 Brockington, C. F. & Stahlie, D. T. (1970) *Report on a Visit to Greece.* Copenhagen: WHO.
13 Cockburn, W. C. & Assaad, F. (1973) Some observations on the communicable diseases as public health problems. *Bull. Wld Hlth Org.*
14 Emerson, H. (1948) *Local Units: the Basis of the Nation's Health.* Address to National Health Assembly, May 1. Quoted by Wyatt, in *Intergovernmental Relations in Public Health,* p. 4.
15 Grant, J. B. (1947) The Health Department and Medical Care; Certain trends. *Amer. J. Publ. Hlth,* **37,** pp. 269–275.
16 Great Britain. Consultative Council on Medical and Allied Services. (1920) *Interim Report on the Future Provision of Medical and Allied Services.* London: HMSO.
17 Hanlon, J. J. (1969) *Principles of Public Health Administration,* 5th edn. St. Louis.
18 India. (1954) *Evaluation Report on First Year's Working of Community Projects,* pp. 33–34. Delhi: Planning Commission, Programme Evaluation Organization.
19 UNICEF/WHO. 1965, JC14/2. 65.
20 Weir, J. M. *et al.* (1952) An evaluation of health and sanitation in Egyptian villages. *J. Egypt. publ. Hlth Ass.,* 27, pp. 55–114.
21 WHO. (1952–54) *Expert Committees on Public Health Administration, 1st-2nd Reports. Tech. Rep. Ser.* **55, 83.**
22 WHO. (1961) *Tech. Rep. Ser.* **205.**
23 WHO. (1963) EM/PHA/109. Alexandria.
24 WHO. Brockington, C. F. (1963) *Mass Campaigns and General Public Health.* Geneva:
25 WHO. (1965) Integration of mass campaigns against specific diseases into general public health services. *Tech. Rep. Ser.* **294.**
26 WHO. Gonzalez, C. L. (1965) *Mass Campaigns and General Public Health,* Papers No. 29.
27 WHO. (1966) AID/NESA/182. Alexandria.
28 WHO. (1966) *Expert Committee on National Health Planning: Background Paper.* NHP/WP/66/1.
29 WHO. (1966) *The Speedy Training of a Large Number of Auxiliaries.* WPR/Educ/6. Geneva.
30 WHO. (1967) National Health Planning in Developing Countries. *Tech. Rep. Ser.* **350.** Also (1970) *Tech. Rep. Ser.* **456.**
31 WHO. (1970) AFR/RC20/TD/2.
32 WHO. (1972) *Higher Education in Nursing Symposium.* Euro 4408. Copenhagen.
33 WHO. (1974) *Development of the Antimalarial Programme.* A27/WP/5.
34 WHO. (1962) *Expert Committee on Malaria,* 9th Report. *Tech. Rep. Ser.* **243.**
35 WHO/WPRO. (1966) *Report of the First Regional Seminar on Education and Training.* Manila.

Part Seven: Chapters 21 to 29

1 Amplification of Medical Certification of causes of death. (1953) *Bull. Wld Hlth Org.*, Suppl. 5.
2 Bacon, F. (1605) *Proficience and Advancement of Learning*. London.
3 Baird, D. *et al.* (1953) *J. Obstet. and Gynaec. of Br. Emp.*, **60**, p. 17.
4 Baric, L. (1966) Personal communication.
5 Brockington, C. F. & Lempert, S. (1965) *The Social Needs of the Over-eighties*. Manchester University Press.
6 Brockington, C. F. & Stein, Z. (1963) Admission, achievement and social class. *Universities Quarterly*, Dec.
7 *Bull. Wld Hlth Org.* (1966) **35**, 783–784.
8 Cancer registration in England and Wales. *Studies on Medical and Population Subjects*, No. 3 and Supplement. (1950–2) London: HMSO.
9 Carpenter, R. G. *A Review of Developed and Developing Routine Computer Applications in Medicine*. HS/ADP/66.1. WHO.
10 Census, 1951. *Classification of Occupations*. (1956) London: HMSO. See also *Classification of Occupations* (1960). HMSO.
11 Census, 1951. England and Wales. *Preliminary Report*, p. iii (1951) London: HMSO.
12 *Chronicle of World Health Organization*, **21**, 100 (1967).
13 *Conf. Econ. Stats.* WG/6/81, (1959).
14 Demographic Yearbook. (1972) New York: United Nations.
15 Dunn, H. (1954) Objectives underlying future patterns of work of national committees on vital statistics. *Bull. Wld Hlth Org.* **11**, p. 148.
16 *Early Leaving*. A report of the Central Advisory Council for Education, p. 35. (1954) London: HMSO.
17 Edge, P. G. (1947) *Vital Statistics and Public Health Work in the Tropics*. London.
18 Fales, W. T. (1953) *Health and Vital Statistics in South-East Asia*. WHO, unpublished Report.
19 Fales, W. T. (1954) *Bull. Wld Hlth Org.* **11**, p. 132.
20 Farr, W. Vital statistics. In McCulloch (1839) *Statistical Account of the British Empire*.
21 Graunt, J. (1662) *Natural and Political Observations upon the Bills of Mortality*. London.
22 Greenhow, E. H. (1860, 1861) *Report of the Medical Officer of the Privy Council*. London.
23 *Guides to Official Sources*. No. 2. Census reports of Great Britain, 1801–1931, p. 104. (1951) London: HMSO.
24 General Practitioners' Records . . . April 1953–1954. (1954) *Studies on Medical and Population Subjects*, No. 9. London: HMSO.
25 General Practitioners' Records . . . April 1951–March 1952. (1953) *Studies on Medical Population Subjects*, No. 7. London: HMSO.
26 Glass, D. V. (1931) A note on the occupational grouping used in tabulating the 1939 births. In *Registrar General's Decennial Supplement, England and Wales*, 1931, Part iiB, Appendix 7.
27 Hall & Jones, C. (1950) The social grading of occupations. *British Journal of Sociology*, **1**, p. 31.
28 *Handbook of Vital Statistics Methods*. (1955) New York: United Nations.
29 *Handbook of Population Census Methods*. (1954) New York: United Nations. See also (1958) Series F, No. 5, Rev. 1 and 1967.
30 Harris, F. F. (1954) The use of sampling methods for ascertaining the total morbidity in the Canadian sickness survey, 1950–1. *Bull. Wld Hlth Org.*, **11**, p. 27.
31 Hauser, P. M. (1954) The use of sampling for vital registration and statistics. *Bull. Wld Hlth Org.*, **11**, p. 14.
32 Heady, J. A. *et al.* (1961) Coronary heart disease in London busmen. *Brit. J. prev. and soc. Med.*, **15**, 143.
33 Heady, J. A. & Morris, J. N. (1956) *Brit. J. prev. and soc. Med.*, **10**, pp. 97–106.
34 *Health in Industry*. (1956) British Transport Commission: London.
35 HMSO. (1957) *The Registrar General's Statistical Review of England and Wales for the Year 1952*. Supplement on cancer. London.
36 Howard, J. (1792) *The State of the Prisons*, 4th edn. London.
37 Hunter, J. (1864) *Report of the Medical Officer of the Privy Council*, pp. 126–302. London.
38 I.L.O. (1968) *International Standard Classification of Occupations*.

39 *Index to the International Standard Industrial Classification of all Economic Activities.* (1956) New York: United Nations.
40 India, Health Survey and Development Committee. (1946) Report. Delhi.
41 International Union Against Cancer. (1966) *Cancer Incidence in Five Continents.*
42 Jones, A. F. (1957) Clinical and social problems of peptic ulcer. *Brit. Med. J. i*, pp. 719–723 and 786–792.
43 Jones, D. C. (1949) *Social Surveys.* London.
44 Knowelden, J. (1966) The collection and use of health statistics in national and local health services. *Tech. Disc.* WHO.
45 Logan, W. P. D. (1954) Instruction of medical practitioners in death certification in England and Wales. *Bull. Wld Hlth Org.*, **11**, pp. 258–261.
46 Logan, W. P. D. (1958) *Morbidity Statistics from General Practice.* Studies on death and population subjects. No. 14. London: HMSO.
47 Mahalonobis, P. C. & Gupta, A. D. (1954) *World Population Conference, vi*, pp. 363–383.
48 Malthus, T. R. (1803) *An Essay on the Principles of Population*, 2nd edn, book I chii, p. 16. London.
49 *Manual of the International Statistical Classification of Diseases, Injuries, and Causes of Death, (1948–9)*, 8th edn. (1966) Geneva: WHO.
50 Meade, T. W. *et al.* (1968) Recent history of ischaemic heart disease and duodenal ulcer in doctors. *Brit. Med. J., iii*, 701–4.
51 Measurement of morbidity. In *Studies on Medical and Population Subjects*, No. 8 (1954). London: HMSO.
52 Medical certification of causes of death: instructions to physicians. *Bull. Wld Hlth Org.* Suppl. 3. (1952).
53 Ministry of Pensions and National Insurance. (1969–70) *Digest of Statistics Analysing Certificates of Incapacity.*
54 Moriyama, I. M. (1958) Personal communication.
55 Moriyama, I. M. & Shapiro, S. (1954) Birth and Death Statistics in the USA. *Bull. Wld Hlth Org.*, **11**, p. 286.
56 Morris, J. N. (1975) *Uses of Epidemiology*, 3rd edn. Edinburgh.
57 Morris, J. N. *et al.* (1966) Incidence and prediction of ischaemic heart disease in London busmen. *Lancet, P.* 553
58 Morris, J. N. & Dale, R. A. (1955) *Proc. Roy. Soc. Med.* **48**, p. 667.
59 Morris, J. N. & Raffle, P. A. B. (1954) *British Journal of Industrial Medicine*, **11**, p. 260.
60 Nielson, J. (1973) *Availability of Data in Vital and Health Statistics Global Developments since 1950.* Copenhagen: Second International Conference of National Committees.
61 Nightingale, F. (1870) *Proposals for a Uniform Plan of Hospital Statistics.* London: Fourth Intern. Statistical Congress.
62 *Preparation of Sampling Reports.* (1950) New York: United Nations.
63 *Principles for a Vital Statistics System.* (1953 and 1973) New York: United Nations.
64 *Record of the Eleventh International Conference of Labour Statisticians* (1967). Geneva: ILO. Also eighth conference 1955.
65 *Registrar General's Statistical Review of England and Wales, 1949*: Supplement on Hospital in-patient statistics, p. vii. (1954) London: HMSO.
66 *Registrar General's Statistical Review of England and Wales, 1949.* Supplement on general morbidity, cancer and mental health. (1953) London: HMSO.
67 Reid, D. D. (1957) *Absenteeism in Industry*, p. 93. Royal Soc. Health, 64th Congress.
68 Reid, D. D. (1956) *Proc. Roy. Soc. Med.*, **49**, p. 767.
69 *Report of African Seminar on Vital Statistics.* No. HS 85. (1956) Geneva: WHO, unpublished.
70 Romero, H. & Vildosola, J. (1954) Needs of vital and health statistics in Latin America. *Bull. Wld Hlth Org.* **11**, pp. 272–277.
71 *Sample Registration of Births and Deaths in India. An Experimental Study (Rural 1964–65).* (1968) New Delhi: M. Home Affairs.
72 *Sample Surveys of Current Interest.* 12th Report (1973) New York: United Nations.
73 Shaul, J. R. H. (1955) Vital statistics of Africans living in Southern Rhodesia. *Cent. Afr. J. of Med.*, **1**, pp. 83–85, 120–4, 145–50, 246–9, 307–11.
74 Smith E. (1863) *Report to the Medical Officer of the Privy Council*, pp. 216–329. London.
75 Some important health statistics available in various countries. *Bull. Wld Hlth Org.* **11**, pp. 201–228.
76 Spratling, F. H. (1957) *Absenteeism in Industry*, p. 88. 64th Health Congress, Folkestone, Royal Society of Health.

77 Stocks, P. (1947) Regional and local differences in cancer death rates. *Studies on Medical and Population Subjects*, No. 1. London: HMSO.
78 Stocks, P. (1949) Sickness in the population of England and Wales in 1944–47. *Studies on Medical and Population Subjects*, No. 2. London: HMSO.
79 Stocks, P. (1954) Needs in vital and health statistics. *Bull. Wld Hlth Org.* **11**, pp. 131–145.
80 *Supplement to the Thirty-Fifth Annual Report of the Registrar-General.* (1875).
81 Survey Committee (National Food) (1951) *Domestic Food Consumption and Expenditure* London: HMSO. See also 1952, 53, 55, 72.
82 Susser & Kushlick (1961) *A Report on the Mental Health Services of the City of Salford.* 1960. Salford Hlth Dept.
83 *The Determinants and Consequences of Population Trends* (1953) New York: United Nations.
84 Titmuss, R. M. & Abel-Smith, B. (1956) *The Cost of the National Health Service in England and Wales.* Cambridge.
85 Trends in the study of morbidity and mortality. *Public Health Paper* No. 27. (1965) WHO.
86 Types of vital statistics available in different countries. *Bull. Wld Hlth Org.* **11**, pp. 177–99, (1954).
87 UNICEF/WHO. (1965) *Basic Health Service.* JC14/UNICEF/WHO 2. 65. Joint Committee on Health Policy.
88 United Kingdom. (1951) *The Colonial Territories* (1950–1). London.
89 United Nations. *Report on International Definition and Measurement of Standards and Levels of Living,* (1954) New York.
90 United Nations. *Seminar on Evaluation and Utilization of Population Census Data in Latin America (Santiago, Chile, 1959).* (1960) New York.
91 United Nations. Document E/CN3/52.
92 United Nations. *Demographic Year Book,* 1972.
93 United Nations (1963) *The Economic Value of Preventive Medicine and Organized Health Services.* 2/Conf. 39/F/145.
94 Warner, W. L. *et al.* (1960) *Social Class in America.* New York.
95 Warner, W. L. (1952) *Structure of American Life.* Edinburgh.
96 Whitehead, F. E. (1971) Trends in Certificated Sickness Absence. *Social Trends* No. 2.
97 WHO. (1948) *Regulations regarding Nomenclature (including the Compilation and Publication of Statistics) with respect to Diseases and Causes of Death.* Amended 1965.
98 WHO. Expert Committee on Health Statistics: Report on Second Session. *Tech. Rep,* *Ser.* No. **25**, 1950.
99 WHO. Expert Committee on Health Statistics: Third Report. *Tech. Rep. Ser.* No. **53**. 1952.
100 WHO. First International Conference of National Committees on Vital and Health Statistics. *Tech. Rep. Ser.* No. **85**, 1954. Second Conference, Copenhagen, 1973. DHSS/C/73. 5.
101 WHO. (1957) Expert Committee on Health Statistics: Fifth report. *Tech. Rep. Ser.* No. **133**.
102 WHO. (1957) Measurement of levels of health. *Tech. Rep. Ser.* No. **137**.
103 WHO. (1959) Expert Committee on Health Statistics: Sixth report. *Tech. Rep. Ser.* No. **164**.
104 WHO. (1961) Expert Committee on Health Statistics: Seventh report. *Tech. Rep. Ser.* No. **214**.
105 WHO. (1963) Expert Committee on Health Statistics: Eighth report. *Tech. Rep. Ser.* No. **261**.
106 WHO. (1963) Paying for health services. *Public Health Paper No. 17.*
107 WHO. (1965) National Committee on Vital and Health Statistics. HS/8 Rev. Conf. 6. 65.
108 WHO. (1966) Sampling methods in morbidity surveys and public health investigations. *Tech. Rep. Ser.* No. **336**.
109 WHO. (1966) de Bernis, J. Expert Committee on National Health Planning in Developing *Countries,* Background Paper. WHP/WP/66. 2.
110 WHO. (1967) Smith, A. *Expert Committee on Health Statistics, Background Paper.* HS/WP/66. 1.
111 WHO. (1967) Dougherty, W. & Taylor, I. *Expert Committee on Health Statistics.* Background Paper. HS/WPP/66. 2.
112 WHO. (1968) Expert committee on morbidity statistics. *Tech. Rep. Ser.,* No. **389**.
113 WHO. (1969) Statistics of health services and of their activities. *Tech. Rep. Ser.,* No. **429**.

114 WHO. (1971) Statistical indicators for the planning and evaluation of public health programmes. *Tech. Rep. Ser.*, No. **472.**
115 WHO. (1972) Statistical principles in public health field studies. *Tech. Rep. Ser.*, No. **510.**
116 Winslow, C. & E. A. (1951) The cost of sickness and the price of health. *Monograph* No. 7.
117 Woytinsky, W. S. & E. S. (1953) *World Population and Production.* New York.
118 Yates, F. (1960) *Sampling Methods for Censuses and Surveys,* 3rd edn. London.

Appendixes

Introduction

The establishment of health services and their maintenance at the highest level of efficiency in terms of money available, depends ultimately upon accurate assessments of the extent and distribution of disease in the community; and this in turn upon the common use of standards. The following appendices are included for easy reference. Appendices 1–6 are abbreviations to be used in tabulating mortality and morbidity in circumstances where the full *international statistical classification of disease injuries and causes of death* is too detailed. Appendix 7 gives standards for measurement of morbidity; Appendix 8 is the *international standard classification of occupations.*

APPENDIX 1

List of 150 *Causes for Tabulation of Morbidity and Mortality* (A)

			Detailed List Numbers
A	1	Cholera	000
A	2	Typhoid fever	001
A	3	Paratyphoid fever and other Salmonella infections	002, 003
A	4	Bacillary dysentery and amoebiasis	004, 006
A	5	Enteritis and other diarrhoeal diseases	008, 009
A	6	Tuberculosis of respiratory system	010–012
A	7	Tuberculosis of meninges and central nervous system	013
A	8	Tuberculosis of intestines, peritoneum and mesenteric glands	014
A	9	Tuberculosis of bones and joints	015
A	10	Other tuberculosis, including late effects	016–019
A	11	Plague	020
A	12	Anthrax	022
A	13	Brucellosis	023
A	14	Leprosy	030
A	15	Diphtheria	032
A	16	Whooping cough	033
A	17	Streptococcal sore throat and scarlet fever	034
A	18	Erysipelas	035
A	19	Meningococcal infection	036
A	20	Tetanus	037
A	21	Other bacterial diseases	005, 007, 021 024–027, 031 038, 039
A	22	Acute poliomyelitis	040–043
A	23	Late effects of acute poliomyelitis	044
A	24	Smallpox	050
A	25	Measles	055
A	26	Yellow fever	060
A	27	Viral encephalitis	062–065
A	28	Infectious hepatitis	070
A	29	Other viral diseases	045, 046, 051–054 056, 057, 061 066–068, 071–079
A	30	Typhus and other rickettsioses	080–083
A	31	Malaria	084
A	32	Trypanosomiasis	086, 087
A	33	Relapsing fever	088
A	34	Congenital syphilis	090
A	35	Early syphilis, symptomatic	091
A	36	Syphilis of central nervous system	094
A	37	Other syphilis	092, 093 095–097
A	38	Gonococcal infections	098
A	39	Schistosomiasis	120
A	40	Hydatidosis	122

L

AE139 Other transport accidents $\left.\begin{array}{l}\text{E800–807} \\ \text{825–845}\end{array}\right\}$

AE140 Accidental poisoning E850–877
AE141 Accidental falls E880–887
AE142 Accidents caused by fires E890–899
AE143 Accidental drowning and submersion E910
AE144 Accident caused by firearms weapons E922
AE145 Accidents mainly of industrial type $\left.\begin{array}{l}\text{E916–921} \\ \text{923–928}\end{array}\right\}$

AE146 All other accidental causes $\left.\begin{array}{l}\text{E900–909} \\ \text{911–915, 929} \\ \text{930–936, 940–949}\end{array}\right\}$

AE147 Suicide and self-inflicted injury E950–959
AE148 Homicide and injury purposely inflicted by other persons:
  legal intervention E960–979
AE149 Injury undetermined whether accidentally or purposely inflicted E980–989
AE150 Injury resulting from operations of war E990–999
AN138 Fracture of skull N800–804
AN139 Fracture of spine and trunk N805–809
AN140 Fracture of limbs N810–829
AN141 Dislocation without fracture N830–839
AN142 Sprains and strains of joints and adjacent muscle N840–848
AN143 Intracranial injury (excluding those with skull fracture) N850–854
AN144 Internal injury of chest, abdomen and pelvis N860–869
AN145 Laceration and open wound N870–908
AN146 Superficial injury, contusion and crushing with intact skin surface N910–929
AN147 Foreign body entering through orifice N930–939
AN148 Burns N940–949
AN149 Adverse effects of chemical substances N960–989
AN150 All other unspecified effects of external causes $\left.\begin{array}{l}\text{N950–959} \\ \text{990–999}\end{array}\right\}$

APPENDIX 2

List of 50 Causes for Tabulation of Mortality (**B**) (1965 revision)

B 1	Cholera	000
B 2	Typhoid fever	001
B 3	Bacillary dysentery and amoebiasis	004, 006
B 4	Enteritis and other diarrhoeal diseases	008, 009
B 5	Tuberculosis of respiratory system	010–012
B 6	Tuberculosis, other forms, including late effects	013–019
B 7	Plague	020
B 8	Diphtheria	032
B 9	Whooping cough	033
B10	Streptococcal sore throat and scarlet fever	034
B11	Meningococcal infection	036
B12	Acute poliomyelitis	040–043
B13	Smallpox	050
B14	Measles	055
B15	Typhus and other rickettsioses	080–083
B16	Malaria	084
B17	Syphilis and its sequelae	090–097
B18	All other infective and parasitic diseases	Rest of 000–136
B19	Malignant neoplasms, including neoplasms of lymphatic and haematopoietic tissues	140–209
B20	Benign neoplasms and neoplasms of unspecified nature	210–239
B21	Diabetes mellitus	250
B22	Avitaminoses and other nutritional deficiency	260–269
B23	Anaemias	280–285

B24	Meningitis	320
B25	Active rheumatic fever	390–392
B26	Chronic rheumatic heart disease	393–398
B27	Hypertensive disease	400–404
B28	Ischaemic heart disease	410–414
B29	Other forms of heart disease	420–429
B30	Cerebrovascular disease	430–438
B31	Influenza	470–474
B32	Pneumonia	480–486
B33	Bronchitis, emphysema and asthma	490–493
B34	Peptic ulcer	531–533
B35	Appendicitis	540–543
B36	Intestinal obstruction and hernia	550–553, 560
B37	Cirrhosis of liver	571
B38	Nephritis and nephrosis	580–584
B39	Hyperplasia of prostate	600
B40	Abortion	640–645
B41	Other complications of pregnancy, child-birth and the puerperium. Delivery without mention of complication	630–639, 650–678
B42	Congenital anomalies	740–759
B43	Birth injury, difficult labour and other anoxic and hypoxic conditions	764–768, 772 776
B44	Other causes of perinatal mortality	760–763, 769–771 773–775, 777–779
B45	Senility without mention of psychosis, ill-defined and unknown causes	780–796
B46	All other diseases	Rest of 000–779
BE47	Motor vehicle accidents	E810–E823
BE48	All other accidents	E800–E807 E825–E949
BE49	Suicide and self-inflicted injuries	E950–E959
BE50	All other external causes	E960–N999
BN47	Fractures, intracranial and internal injuries	N800–N829 N850–N854 N860–N869
BN48	Burns	N940–N949
BN49	Adverse effects of chemical substances	N960–N989
BN50	All other injuries	Rest of N800–N999

APPENDIX 3

List of 70 *Causes for Tabulation of Morbidity* (C)

C 1	Typhoid, paratyphoid fever, other salmonella infections	001–003
C 2	Bacillary dysentery and amoebiasis	004, 006
C 3	Enteritis and other diarrhoeal diseases	008, 009
C 4	Tuberculosis of respiratory system	010–012
C 5	Tuberculosis, other forms, including late effects	013–019
C 6	Brucellosis	023
C 7	Diphtheria	032
C 8	Whooping cough	033
C 9	Streptococcal sore throat and scarlet fever	034
C10	Smallpox	050
C11	Measles	055
C12	Viral encephalitis	062–065
C13	Infectious hepatitis	070
C14	Typhus and other rickettsioses	080–083
C15	Malaria	084
C16	Syphilis and its sequelae	090–097
C17	Gonococcal infections	098

c18 Helminthiasis   120–129

c19 All other infective and parasitic diseases
      000, 005, 007
      020–022, 024–027
      030, 031, 035–039
      040–046, 051–054
      056, 057, 060, 061
      066–068, 070–079
      085–089, 099
      100–104, 110–117
      130–136

c20 Malignant neoplasms, including neoplasms of lymphatic and haematopoietic tissues   140–209

c21 Benign neoplasms and neoplasms of unspecified nature   210–239

c22 Thyrotoxicosis with or without goitre   242

c23 Diabetes mellitus   250

c24 Avitaminosis and other nutritional deficiency   260–269

c25 Other endocrine disorders; other metabolic diseases   240, 241, 243–246
      251–258, 270–279

c26 Anaemias   280–285

c27 Psychoses and non-psychotic mental disorders   290–309

c28 Inflammatory diseases of eye   360–369

c29 Cataract   374

c30 Otitis media and mastoiditis   381–383

c31 Other diseases of nervous system and sense organs   320–324, 330–333
      340–349, 350–358
      370–373, 375–379
      380, 384–389

c32 Active rheumatic fever   390–392

c33 Chronic rheumatic heart disease   393–398

c34 Hypertensive disease   400–404

c35 Ischaemic heart disease   410–414

c36 Cerebrovascular disease   430–438

c37 Venous thrombosis and embolism   450–453

c38 Other diseases of circulatory system   420–429, 440–447
      454–458

c39 Acute respiratory infections   460–466

c40 Influenza   470–474

c41 Pneumonia   480–486

c42 Bronchitis, emphysema and asthma   490–493

c43 Hypertrophy of tonsils and adenoids   500

c44 Pneumoconioses and related diseases   515, 516

c45 Other respiratory diseases   501–508, 510–514
      517–519

c46 Diseases of teeth and supporting structures   520–525

c47 Peptic ulcer   531–533

c48 Appendicitis   540–543

c49 Intestinal obstruction and hernia   550–553, 560

c50 Cholelithiasis and cholecystitis   574, 575

c51 Other diseases of digestive system   526–529, 530
      534–537, 561–569
      570–573, 576–577

c52 Nephritis and nephrosis   580–584

c53 Calculi of urinary system   592, 594

c54 Hyperplasia of prostate   600

c55 Other diseases of genito-urinary system   590, 591, 593
      595–599, 601–607
      610–616, 620–629

c56 Abortion   640–645

c57 Other complications of pregnancy, child-birth and the puerperium   630–639, 651–678

c58 Delivery without mention of complication   650

c59 Infections of skin and subcutaneous tissue   680–686

c60 Other diseases of skin and subcutaneous tissue   690–709

c61 Arthritis and spondylitis   710–715
c62 Other diseases of musculo-skeletal system and connective tissue   } 716–718, 720–729
                                                                             730–738
c63 Congenital anomalies   740–759
c64 Certain causes of perinatal morbidity   760–779
c65 Other specified and ill-defined diseases   } 286–289, 310–315
                                                                           780–796
ce66 Road transport accidents   e810–819, 825–827
ce67 Other accidents   } e800–807, 820–823
                                                                          830–949
ce68 Attempted suicide and self-inflicted injuries   e950–959
ce69 Attempted homicide and injury purposely inflicted by
           other person; legal intervention   e960–979
ce70 All other external causes   e980–999
cn66 Fractures   n800–829
cn67 Intracranial and internal injuries   n850–854, 860–869
cn68 Burns   n940–949
cn69 Adverse effects of chemical substances   n960–989
cn70 All other injuries   } n830–848, 870–939
                                                                          950–959, 990–999

APPENDIX 4

List of 300 *Causes for Tabulation of Hospital Morbidity* (D)

d	1 Cholera	000
d	2 Typhoid fever	001
d	3 Paratyphoid fever and other Salmonella infections	002, 003
d	4 Bacillary dysentery	004
d	5 Amoebiasis	006
d	6 Enteritis and diarrhoeal diseases	008, 009
d	7 Other intestinal infectious diseases	005, 007
d	8 Silicotuberculosis	010
d	9 Pulmonary tuberculosis	011
d	10 Tuberculosis pleurisy	012.1, 012.2
d	11 Tuberculosis laryngitis	012.3
d	12 Other respiratory tuberculosis	012.0, 012.9
d	13 Tuberculosis of meninges and central nervous system	013
d	14 Tuberculosis of intestines, peritoneum and mesenteric glands	014
d	15 Tuberculosis of bones and joints	015
d	16 Tuberculosis of genito-urinary system	016
d	17 Other tuberculosis	017–019
d	18 Plague	020
d	19 Brucellosis	023
d	20 Leprosy	030
d	21 Diphtheria	032
d	22 Whooping cough	033
d	23 Streptococcal sore throat and scarlet fever	034
d	24 Erysipelas	035
d	25 Meningococcal infection	036
d	26 Tetanus	037
d	27 Septicaemia	038
d	28 Other bacterial diseases	021, 022, 024–027 031, 039
d	29 Acute poliomyelitis	040–043
d	30 Late effects of acute poliomyelitis	044
d	31 Smallpox	050
d	32 Chickenpox	052
d	33 Measles	055
d	34 Rubella	056

D 35	Yellow fever	060
D 36	Viral encephalitis	062–065
D 37	Arthropod-borne haemorrhagic fever	067
D 38	Infectious hepatitis	070
D 39	Rabies	071
D 40	Mumps	072
D 41	Other viral diseases	045, 046, 051, 053 054, 057, 061, 066 068, 073–079
D 42	Typhus and other rickettsioses	080–083
D 43	Malaria	084
D 44	Leishmaniasis	085
D 45	Trypanosomiasis	086, 087
D 46	Relapsing fever	088
D 47	Early syphilis, symptomatic	091
D 48	Cardiovascular syphilis	093
D 49	Syphilis of central nervous system	094
D 50	Other syphilis	090, 092, 095–097
D 51	Gonococcal infections	098
D 52	Schistosomiasis	120
D 53	Hydatidosis	122
D 54	Ancylostomiasis	126
D 55	Other helminthiasis	121, 123–125 127–129
D 56	Other infective and parasitic diseases	089, 099, 100–104 110–117, 130–136
D 57	Malignant neoplasm of buccal cavity and pharynx	140–149
D 58	Malignant neoplasm of stomach	151
D 59	Malignant neoplasm of intestine, except rectum	152, 153
D 60	Malignant neoplasm of rectum and rectosigmoid junction	154
D 61	Malignant neoplasm of other digestive organs and peritoneum	150, 155–159
D 62	Malignant neoplasm of larynx	161
D 63	Malignant neoplasm of trachea, bronchus and lung	162
D 64	Malignant neoplasm of other and unspecified respiratory organs	160, 163
D 65	Malignant neoplasm of bone	170
D 66	Malignant neoplasm of skin	172, 173
D 67	Malignant neoplasm of breast	174
D 68	Malignant neoplasm of cervix uteri	180
D 69	Chorionepithelioma	181
D 70	Other malignant neoplasm of uterus	182
D 71	Malignant neoplasm of ovary	183.0
D 72	Malignant neoplasm of other and unspecified female genital organs	183.1, 183.9, 184
D 73	Malignant neoplasm of prostate	185
D 74	Malignant neoplasm of testis	186
D 75	Malignant neoplasm of bladder	188
D 76	Malignant neoplasm of other genito-urinary organs	187, 189
D 77	Malignant neoplasm of brain	191
D 78	Malignant neoplasm of other specified sites	171, 190, 192–195
D 79	Secondary and unspecified malignant neoplasm of lymph nodes	196
D 80	Secondary malignant neoplasm of other sites and malignant neoplasm of unspecified site	197–199
D 81	Hodgkin's disease	201
D 82	Leukaemia	204–207
D 83	Other neoplasms of lymphatic and haematopoietic tissue	200, 202, 203 208, 209
D 84	Benign neoplasm of skin	216
D 85	Uterine fibromyoma	218
D 86	Other benign neoplasm of uterus	219
D 87	Benign neoplasm of ovary	220
D 88	Benign neoplasm of kidney and other urinary organs	223
D 89	Benign neoplasm of brain and other parts of nervous system	225

D 90	Other benign neoplasm	210–215, 217, 221 222, 224, 226–228
D 91	Carcinoma *in situ* of cervix uteri	234.0
D 92	Other neoplasm of unspecified nature	230–233, 234.1 234.9, 235–239
D 93	Non-toxic goitre	240, 241
D 94	Thyrotoxicosis with or without goitre	242
D 95	Other diseases of thyroid gland	243–246
D 96	Diabetes mellitus	250
D 97	Avitaminoses and other nutritional deficiency	260–269
D 98	Other endocrine and metabolic diseases	251–258, 270–279
D 99	Iron deficiency anaemias	280
D100	Vitamin B12 deficiency anaemia	281.0, 281.1
D101	Other deficiency anaemias	281.2–281.9
D102	Other diseases of blood and blood-forming organs	282–289
D103	Alcoholic psychosis	291
D104	Schizophrenia	295
D105	Affective psychoses	296
D106	Other psychoses	290, 292–204 297–299
D107	Neuroses	300
D108	Alcoholism	303
D109	Other non-psychotic mental disorders	301, 302, 304–309
D110	Mental retardation	310–315
D111	Meningitis	320
D112	Other inflammatory diseases of central nervous system	321–324
D113	Hereditary and familial diseases of nervous system	330–333
D114	Multiple sclerosis	340
D115	Paralysis agitans	342
D116	Epilepsy	345
D117	Other diseases of central nervous system	341, 343, 344 346–349
D118	Sciatica	353
D119	Other diseases of nerves and peripheral ganglia	350–352, 354–358
D120	Keratitis with ulceration	363.0
D121	Iritis, choroiditis and other inflammation of uveal tract	364–366
D122	Inflammation of lachrymal glands and ducts	368
D123	Other inflammatory diseases of eye	360–362, 363.9 367, 369
D124	Strabismus	373
D125	Cataract	374
D126	Glaucoma	375
D127	Detachment of retina	376
D128	Other diseases of eye	370–372, 377–379
D129	Otitis media without mention of mastoiditis	381
D130	Mastoiditis with or without otitis media	382, 383
D131	Other diseases of ear and mastoid process	380, 384–389
D132	Active rheumatic fever	390–392
D133	Chronic rheumatic heart disease	393–398
D134	Essential benign hypertension	401
D135	Hypertensive heart disease	402, 404
D136	Other hypertensive disease	400, 403
D137	Acute myocardial infarction	410
D138	Other ischaemic heart disease	411–414
D139	Symptomatic heart disease	427
D140	Other disease of heart	420–426, 428, 429
D141	Cerebral haemorrhage	431
D142	Cerebral infarction	432–434
D143	Acute but ill-defined cerebrovascular disease	436
D144	Other cerebrovascular disease	430, 435, 437, 438
D145	Arteriosclerosis	440
D146	Other peripheral vascular disease	443

D206	Other diseases of ovary, Fallopian tube and parametrium	615, 616
D207	Infective disease of cervix uteri	620
D208	Infective disease of uterus (except cervix), vagina and vulva	622
D209	Uterovaginal prolapse	623
D210	Malposition of uterus	624
D211	Disorders of menstruation	626
D212	Sterility, female	628
D213	Other diseases of female genital organs	621, 625, 627, 629
D214	Infections of genito-urinary tract during pregnancy and the puerperium	630, 635
D215	Threatened abortion	632.3
D216	Other haemorrhage of pregnancy	632.0–632.2 632.4, 632.5
D217	Pregnancy with malposition of foetus in uterus	634.0
D218	Toxaemias of pregnancy and the puerperium	636–639
D219	Other complications of pregnancy	631, 633, 634.1 634.9
D220	Abortion induced for legal indications	640, 641
D221	Other and unspecified abortion	642–645
D222	Delivery without mention of complication	650
D223	Delivery complicated by placenta praevia or ante-partum haemorrhage	651
D224	Delivery complicated by retained placenta or other post-partum haemorrhage	652, 653
D225	Delivery complicated by abnormality of bony pelvis, disproportion, malpresentation or other prolonged labour	654–657
D226	Delivery with other complications, including anaesthetic death	658–662
D227	Complications of the puerperium	670–678
D228	Infections of skin and subcutaneous tissues	680–686
D229	Other inflammatory conditions of skin and subcutaneous tissues	690–698
D230	Other diseases of skin and subcutaneous tissues	700–709
D231	Rheumatoid arthritis and allied conditions	712
D232	Osteo-arthritis and allied conditions	713
D233	Other and unspecified arthritis	710, 711, 714, 715
D234	Non-articular rheumatism and rheumatism unspecified	716–718
D235	Osteomyelitis and periostitis	720
D236	Other diseases of bone	721–723
D237	Internal derangement of joint	724
D238	Displacement of intervertebral disc	725
D239	Vertebrogenic pain syndromes	728
D240	Other diseases of joint	726, 727, 729
D241	Synovitis, bursitis and tenosynovitis	731
D242	Hallux valgus and varus	737
D243	Other diseases of musculoskeletal system	730, 732–736, 738
D244	Spina bifida and congenital hydrocephalus	741, 742
D245	Congenital anomalies of circulatory system	746, 747
D246	Cleft palate and cleft lip	749
D247	Congenital pyloric stenosis	750.1
D248	Other congenital anomalies of digestive system	750.0, 750.2–750.9 751
D249	Undescended testicle	752.1
D250	Other congenital anomalies of genito-urinary system	752.0, 752.2–752.9 753
D251	Congenital clubfoot	754
D252	Congenital dislocation of hip	755.7
D253	Other congenital anomalies of musculoskeletal system	755.0–755.6, 755.8 755.9, 756
D254	Other and unspecified congenital anomalies	740, 743–745, 748 757–759
D255	Birth injury	764–768 with 4th digits .0–.3, 772
D256	Asphyxia, anoxia or hypoxia	764–768 with 4th digit .4, 776
D257	Haemolytic disease of newborn	774, 775

M

D258 Immaturity, unspecified   777
D259 Other causes of perinatal morbidity and mortality   ⎫ 760–763, 764–768
                                                                  ⎬ 4th digit .9, 769, 770
                                                                  ⎭ 771, 773, 778, 779
D260 Acute heart failure, undefined   782.4
D261 Haematemesis   784.5
D262 Abdominal pain   785.5
D263 Pain referable to urinary system   786.0
D264 Retention of urine   786.1
D265 Incontinence of urine   786.2

                                                                  ⎫ 780, 781
                                                                  ⎪ 782.0–782.3
                                                                  ⎪ 782.5–782.9, 783
                                                                  ⎪ 784.0–784.4
                                                                  ⎬ 784.6–784.8
                                                                  ⎪ 785.0–785.4
                                                                  ⎪ 785.6–785.9
                                                                  ⎪ 786.3–786.7
                                                                  ⎭ 787–789
D266 Other symptoms
D267 Senility without mention of psychosis   794
D268 Other ill-defined conditions   790–793, 795, 796
DY269 Normal pregnancy   Y60.0
DY270 Live births in hospital   Y80–Y89
                                                                  ⎫ Y00–Y59
DY271 Other special admissions or consultations   ⎬ Y60.1–Y60.9
                                                                  ⎭ Y61–Y79
DE272 Railway accidents   E800–E807
DE273 Motor vehicle accident to occupant of motor vehicle   ⎱ E810–E823 with
                                                                  ⎰ 4th digits .0–.3
DE274 Motor vehicle accident to pedal cyclist   ⎱ 810–823 with 4th
                                                                  ⎰ digit .6
DE275 Motor vehicle accident to pedestrian   ⎱ E810–E823 with
                                                                  ⎰ 4th digit .7
                                                                  ⎫ E810–E823 with
DE276 Motor vehicle accident to other and unspecified person   ⎬ 4th digits .4, .5,
                                                                  ⎭ .8, .9
DE277 Other road vehicle accidents   E825–E827
DE278 Water transport accidents   E830–E838
DE279 Air and space transport accidents   E840–E845
DE280 Accidental poisoning by drugs and medicaments   E850–E859
DE281 Accidental poisoning by other solid and liquid substances   E860–E869
DE282 Accidental poisoning by gases and vapours   E870–E877
DE283 Accidental fall on or from stairs, steps, ladders or scaffolding E880–E881
DE284 Other fall from one level to another   E882–E884
DE285 Fall on same level   E885, E886
DE286 Unspecified fall   E887
DE287 Conflagrations   E890–E892
DE288 Ignition of clothing or inflammable material   E893, E894
DE289 Accidents from controlled fires   E895–E897
DE290 Other and unspecified fires   898, E899
DE291 Drowning and submersion   910
DE292 Accident caused by firearms weapons   E922
DE293 Surgical and medical complications and misadventures   E930–E936
                                                                  ⎧ E900–E909
DE294 Other and unspecified accidents, including late effects   ⎨ E911–E921
                                                                  ⎪ E923–E929
                                                                  ⎩ E940–E949
DE295 Suicide and self-inflicted injury by poisoning by solid or
        liquid substances   E950

DE296	Suicide and self-inflicted injury by poisoning by gases in domestic use	E951
DE297	Suicide and self-inflicted injury by other and unspecified means, including late effects	E952–E954 / E955–E959
DE298	Homicide and injury purposely inflicted by other persons; legal intervention	E960–E969 / E970–E979
DE299	Injury undetermined whether accidentally or purposely inflicted	E980–E989
DE300	Injury resulting from operations of war	E990–E999
DN272	Fracture of face bones	N802
DN273	Other fracture of skull	N800, N801 / N803, N804
DN274	Fracture of spine and trunk	N805–N809
DN275	Fracture of humerus, radius and ulna	N812, N813
DN276	Fracture of phalanges and metacarpal bones	N815–N817
DN277	Fracture of neck of femur	N820
DN278	Fracture of other and unspecified parts of femur	N821
DN279	Fracture of tibia, fibula and ankle	N823, N824
DN280	Other fractures of limbs	N810, N811 / N814, N818 / N819, N822 / N825–N829
DN281	Dislocation without fracture; sprains and strains of joints and adjacent muscles	N830–N848
DN282	Intracranial injury (excluding skull fracture)	N850–N854
DN283	Internal injury of chest, abdomen and pelvis	N860–N869
DN284	Laceration, open wound, superficial injury, contusion and crushing, affecting eye	N870, N871 / N921
DN285	Laceration, open wound, superficial injury, contusion and crushing, affecting hand and fingers	N882, N883 / N885–N887 / N903, N914 / N915, N925 / N926
DN286	Laceration, open wound, superficial injury, contusion and crushing, affecting other and unspecified site	N872–N879 / N880, N881, N884 / N890–N897 / N900–N902 / N904–N908 / N910–N913 / N916–N918 / N920, N922–N924 / N927–N929
DN287	Foreign body in eye and adnexa	N930
DN288	Foreign body entering through other orifice	N931–N939
DN289	Burn confined to eye	N940
DN290	Burn of other and unspecified site	N941–N949
DN291	Adverse effects of salicylates and congeners	N965.1
DN292	Adverse effects of barbiturates	N967.0
DN293	Adverse effects of other medicinal agents	N960–N964, N965.0 / N965.2–N965.9 / N966 / N967.1–N967.9 / N968–N979
DN294	Toxic effect of carbon monoxide	N986
DN295	Toxic effect of other substances chiefly non-medicinal as to source	N980–N985 / N987–N989
DN296	Drowning and non-fatal submersion	N994.1
DN297	Asphyxiation and strangulation	N995.5
DN298	Injury, other and unspecified	N997
DN299	Complications of surgical procedures and other medical care	N998 / N999

DN300 Other effects of external causes

$$\left\{\begin{array}{l} \text{N950–N959} \\ \text{N990–N993} \\ \text{N994.0} \\ \text{N994.2–N994.9} \\ \text{N995.0–N995.4} \\ \text{N995.6–N995.9} \\ \text{N996} \end{array}\right.$$

APPENDIX 5

List of 100 *Causes for Tabulation of Perinatal Morbidity and Mortality* (P)

CHRONIC CIRCULATORY AND GENITO-URINARY DISEASE IN MOTHER (1–4)

P 1	Chronic rheumatic heart disease	760.0
P 2	Chronic hypertension	760.2
P 3	Other chronic disease of circulatory system	760.1, 760.3
P 4	Chronic disease of genito-urinary system	760.4, 760.5

OTHER MATERNAL CONDITIONS UNRELATED TO PREGNANCY (5–11)

P 5	Syphilis	761.0
P 6	Diabetes mellitus	761.1
P 7	Rubella	761.3
P 8	Injury to mother	761.5
P 9	Operation of mother	761.6
P 10	Chemical substances transmitted through placenta	761.7
P 11	Other maternal conditions	761.2, 761.4, 761.9

TOXAEMIAS OF PREGNANCY (12–17)

P 12	Renal disease arising during pregnancy	762.0
P 13	Pre-eclampsia of pregnancy	762.1
P 14	Eclampsia of pregnancy	762.2
P 15	Toxaemia unspecified	762.3
P 16	Hyperemesis gravidarum	762.4
P 17	Other toxaemia of pregnancy	762.5, 762.9

MATERNAL ANTE- AND INTRA-PARTUM INFECTION (18–20)

P 18	Pyelitis and pyelonephritis of pregnancy	763.0
P 19	Other infections of genito-urinary tract during pregnancy	763.1
P 20	Other	763.9

DIFFICULT LABOUR WITH ABNORMALITY OF BONES, ORGANS OR TISSUES OF PELVIS (21–23)

P 21	With birth injury to brain or spinal cord	760.4, 764.1
P 22	With other or unspecified birth injury	764.2, 764.3
P 23	Without mention of birth injury	764.4, 764.9

DIFFICULT LABOUR WITH DISPROPORTION (24–26)

P 24	With birth injury to brain or spinal cord	765.0, 765.1
P 25	With other or unspecified birth injury	765.2, 765.3
P 26	Without mention of birth injury	765.4, 765.9

DIFFICULT LABOUR WITH MALPOSITION OF FOETUS (27–29)

P 27	With birth injury to brain or spinal cord	766.0, 766.1
P 28	With other or unspecified birth injury	766.2, 766.3
P 29	Without mention of birth injury	766.4, 766.9

DIFFICULT LABOUR WITH ABNORMALITY OF FORCES OF LABOUR (30–32)

P 30	With birth injury to brain or spinal cord	757.0, 767.1
P 31	With other or unspecified birth injury	767.2, 767.3
P 32	Without mention of birth injury	767.4, 767.9

DIFFICULT LABOUR WITH OTHER AND UNSPECIFIED COMPLICATIONS (33–35)

P 33	With birth injury to brain or spinal cord	768.0, 768.1
P 34	With other or unspecified birth injury	768.2, 768.3
P 35	Without mention of birth injury	768.4, 768.9

OTHER COMPLICATIONS OF PREGNANCY AND CHILD-BIRTH (36–41)

P 36	Incompetent cervix	769.0
P 37	Premature rupture of membranes	769.1
P 38	Hydramnios	769.2
P 39	Ectopic pregnancy	769.3

P 40 Multiple pregnancy	769.4
P 41 Other complications of pregnancy or child-birth	769.5, 769.9

CONDITIONS OF PLACENTA (42–46)

P 42 Placenta praevia	770.0
P 43 Premature separation of placenta	770.1
P 44 Placental infarction	770.2
P 45 Other conditions of placenta	770.8
P 46 Placental insufficiency, unspecified	770.9

CONDITIONS OF UMBILICAL CORD (47–49)

P 47 Compression of cord	771.0
P 48 Prolapse of cord without mention of compression	771.1
P 49 Other	771.9

BIRTH INJURY WITHOUT MENTION OF CAUSE (50–52)

P 50 To brain or spinal cord	772.0, 772.1
P 51 Other or unspecified birth injury	772.2, 772.9
P 52 Termination of pregnancy without mention of cause	773

HAEMOLYTIC DISEASE OF NEWBORN (53–56)

P 53 With Rh incompatibility	774.0, 775.0
P 54 With ABO incompatibility	774.1, 775.1
P 55 With other or unspecified blood incompatibility	774.2, 775.2
P 56 Without mention of cause	774.9, 775.9

ANOXIC AND HYPOXIC CONDITIONS NOT ELSEWHERE CLASSIFIED (57–60)

P 57 Hyaline membrane disease and respiratory distress syndrome	776.1, 776.2
P 58 Intra uterine anoxia	776.4
P 59 Asphyxia of newborn, unspecified	776.9
P 60 Other anoxic and hypoxic conditions not elsewhere classified	776.0, 776.3

OTHER CONDITIONS OF FOETUS AND NEWBORN (61–68)

P 61 Immaturity unspecified	777
P 62 Foetal blood loss before birth	778.0
P 63 Chorio-amnionitis	778.1
P 64 Post maturity	778.2
P 65 Haemorrhagic disease of newborn	778.3
P 66 Other conditions of foetus	778.4, 778.9
P 67 Maceration foetal death or unknown cause	779.0
P 68 Other	779.9

CONGENITAL ANOMALIES (69–80)

P 69 Anencephalus	740
P 70 Spina bifida	741
P 71 Congenital hydrocephalus	742
P 72 Other congenital anomalies of central nervous system and eye	743, 744
P 73 Congenital anomalies of circulatory system	746, 747
P 74 Congenital anomalies of respiratory system	748
P 75 Congenital anomalies of digestive system	749, 751
P 76 Congenital anomalies of genito-urinary system	752, 753
P 77 Congenital anomalies of musculo-skeletal system	754–756
P 78 Down's syndrome congenital syndromes affecting multiple systems	759.3
P 79 Other	{ 759.0–759.2 759.4–759.9
P 80 Other and unspecified congenital anomalies	745, 757, 758

INFECTIONS OF FOETUS AND NEWBORN (81–88)

P 81 Diarrhoeal disease	009
P 82 Listeriosis	027.0
P 83 Tetanus	037
P 84 Septicaemia	038
P 85 Viral diseases	040–079
P 86 Congenital syphilis	090
P 87 Toxoplasmosis	130
P 88 Other infective and parasitic diseases	Rest of 000–136

OTHER DISEASES OF FOETUS AND NEWBORN (89–94)

P 89 Diseases of thyroid gland	240–246
P 90 Cystic fibrosis (mucoviscidosis)	273.0
P 91 Diseases of blood and blood-forming organs	280–289

P 92 Pneumonia   480–486
P 93 Other specified conditions   Rest of 140–738
P 94 Symptoms and ill-defined conditions   780–796
ACCIDENTS AND VIOLENCE TO NEWBORN (95–100)
P 95 Excessive heat   E900
P 96 Excessive cold   E901
P 97 Hunger, thirst, exposure and neglect   E904
P 98 Inhalation and ingestion of food causing obstruction or suffocation   E911
P 99 Accidental mechanical suffocation   E913
P100 Other violence   Rest of E800–E999

APPENDIX 6

Standardization of Causes of Death. List of 51 Causes for Tabulation of Mortality and Morbidity for use of Medical Auxiliary Personnel[69]

1. Syphilis
2. Gonorrhoea
3. Other veneral diseases
4. Whooping cough
5. Cerebrospinal meningitis
6. Plague
7. Leprosy
8. Tetanus
9. Yaws
10. Smallpox
11. Measles
12. Chickenpox
13. Mumps
14. Malaria
15. Blackwater fever
16. Trypanosomiasis
17. Bilharziasis (vesical)
18. Guinea worm
19. Elephantiasis
20. Intestinal worms
21. Scabies
22. Goitre
23. Mental disorders
24. Epilepsy
25. Blindness
26. Conjunctivitis
27. Other conditions of the eyes and eyelids
28. Diseases of the ear
29. Deafness
30. Heart diseases
31. Common cold
32. Sore throat
33. Bronchitis
34. Pneumonia
35. Diseases of the mouth and teeth
36. Nausea and vomiting
37. Stomach ache
38. Constipation
39. Diarrhoea
40. Diarrhoea with blood
41. Diseases of the genito-urinary system (excluding syphilis, yaws, gonorrhoea, and other veneral diseases)
42. Normal deliveries
43. Complications of pregnancy and delivery
44. Abortions and stillbirths
45. Chronic ulcer (of the skin)
46. Diseases of the skin and soft tissues (excluding scabies)
47. Diseases of the bones and joints
48. Other diseases and conditions not mentioned above
49. Injuries to the soft tissues
50. Injuries to the bones and joints
51. Other injuries

APPENDIX 7

Measurement of Morbidity: Rates of Inception and Prevalence[51, 107]

RATES RELATING TO INCEPTION

1, Rate of Inception of spells *of sickness*

'The number of **spells** *of sickness* which **start** during a d:fined period divided by the average number of persons exposed to risk during that period.'

Short title: 'Inception rate (spells).'

NOTES:

(a) Several 'spells' begun by any one person during the defined period of observation must each be counted separately.

(b) The relevant 'spells' in the numerator comprise only:
   (i) Spells beginning and ending in the period,
   (ii) Spells beginning in the period and still continuing at the end of the period.

(c) If some 'spells' relate to more than one disease (i.e. concurrent or consecutive diseases within the same spell) and if, in using the rates in relation to individual diseases, such spells are counted for each of the diseases separately, then the rates for individual diseases cannot be aggregated to give the equivalent rate for all diseases combined.

(d) When first 'spells' due to a particular disease can be distinguished from subsequent 'spells' for the same disease, this definition may be adapted to relate to the first 'spells' only.

(e) In many studies of morbidity the full frequency distribution, showing numbers of persons who begin different numbers of spells, will be required; such information is valuable in studying variations in people's individual tendency towards repeated sickness.

(f) It may sometimes be easier to derive a **rate of termination** of spells from the available records instead of a **rate of inception,** The uses of such a rate would be similar and, when the duration of sickness is short in relation to the period of observation, the two rates would, in effect, be interchangeable.

2. Proportion of persons who start a spell *of sickness* during a period

'The number of **persons** who **start** at least one spell *of sickness* during a defined period divided by the average number of persons exposed to risk during that period.'

Short title: 'Inception rate (persons).'

NOTES:

(a) Persons who begin more than one 'spell' during the period of observation must be counted **once** only.

(b) The relevant persons in the numerator comprise only those with:
   (i) Spells beginning and ending in the period,
   (ii) Spells beginning in the period and still continuing at the end of the period.

(c) If some persons are sick from more than one disease (i.e. at the same time or on successive occasions within the period of observation) and if, in using the rate in relation to individual diseases, such persons are counted for each of the diseases separately, then the rates for individual diseases cannot be aggregated to give the equivalent rate for all diseases combined.

RATES RELATING TO PREVALENCE

3(A). Rate of Prevalence of spells *of sickness* in a period

'The number of **spells** *of sickness* which are **current at some time** during a defined period divided by the average number of persons exposed to risk during that period.'

Short title: 'Period Prevalence rate (spells).'

NOTES:

(a) Several 'spells' experienced by any one person during the defined period of observation must each be counted separately.

(b) The relevant 'spells' in the numerator comprise:
   (i) Spells beginning and ending in the period,
   (ii) Spells beginning in the period and still continuing at the end of the period,
   (iii) Spells beginning before and ending in the period,
   (iv) Spells beginning before the period and still continuing at the end of the period.

(c) If some 'spells' relate to more than one disease (i.e. concurrent or consecutive diseases within the same spell) and if, in using the rate in relation to individual diseases, such spells are counted for each of the diseases separately, then the rate for individual diseases cannot be aggregated to give the equivalent rate for all diseases combined.

(d) In many studies of morbidity the full frequency distribution, showing numbers of person who experienced different numbers of spells, will be required; such information is valuable in studying variations in people's individual tendency towards repeated sickness.

3(B). Rate of Prevalence of spells *of sickness* at a point of time

'The number of **spells** *of sickness* which are current **at a given time** divided by the number of persons exposed to risk at that time.'

Short title: 'Point Prevalence rate.'

NOTES:

(a) The rate will be numerically the same as rate 4(B) below.

(*b*)   The number of spells may be based on an actual count at a specific point of time or may be an average calculated for a specific point of time.

(*c*)   If some 'spells' relate to more than one disease current at the given time and if, in using the rate in relation to individual diseases, such spells are counted for each of the diseases separately, then the rates for individual diseases cannot be aggregated to give the equivalent rate for all diseases combined.

4(A). Proportion of persons *sick* in a period

'The number of **persons** who *are sick* **some time** during a defined period divided by the average number of persons exposed to risk during that period.'

Short title: 'Period Prevalence rate (persons).'

NOTES:

(*a*)   The complement of this rate may be useful, i.e. the proportion of persons who were never sick during the period.

(*b*)   Persons who experience more than one 'spell' during the period of observation must be counted **once** only.

(*c*)   The relevant persons in the numerator comprise those with:
    (i) Spells beginning and ending in the period,
    (ii) Spells beginning in the period and still continuing at end of the period,
    (iii) Spells beginning before and ending in the period,
    (iv) Spells beginning before the period and still continuing at the end of the period.

(*d*)   If some persons are sick from more than one disease (i.e. at the same time or on successive occasions within the period of observation) and if, in using the rate in relation to individual diseases, such persons are counted for each of the diseases separately, then the rates for individual diseases cannot be aggregated to give the equivalent rate for all diseases combined.

4(B). Proportion of persons *sick* at a point of time

'The number of **persons** who *are sick* at a **given time** divided by the number of persons exposed to risk at that time.'

Short title: 'Point Prevalence rate.'

NOTES:

(*a*)   The rate will be numerically the same as rate 3(B) above.

(*b*)   The number of persons may be based on an actual count at a specific point of time or may be an average calculated for a specific point of time.

(*c*)   If some persons are sick from more than one disease at the given time and if, in using the rate in relation to individual diseases, such persons are counted for each of the diseases separately, then the rates for individual diseases cannot be aggregated to give the equivalent rate for all diseases combined.

APPENDIX 8

The International Standard Classification of Occupations (1968) *Major, Minor and Unit Groups*
MAJOR GROUP 0/1: PROFESSIONAL, TECHNICAL AND RELATED WORKERS
0–1 Physical Scientists and Related Technicians
       0–11 Chemists
       0–12 Physicists
       0–13 Physical scientists not elsewhere classified
       0–14 Physical science technicians
0–2/0–3 Architects, Engineers and Related Technicians
       0–21 Architects and town planners
       0–22 Civil engineers
       0–23 Electrical and electronics engineers
       0–24 Mechanical engineers
       0–25 Chemical engineers
       0–26 Metallurgists
       0–27 Mining engineers
       0–28 Industrial engineers
       0–29 Engineers not elsewhere classified
       0–31 Surveyors

0–32 Draughtsmen
0–33 Civil engineering technicians
0–34 Electrical and electronic engineering technicians
0–35 Mechanical engineering technicians
0–36 Chemical engineering technicians
0–37 Metallurgical technicians
0–38 Mining technicians
0–39 Engineering technicians not elsewhere classified
0–4 Aircraft and Ships' Officers
    0–41 Aircraft pilots, navigators and flight engineers
    0–42 Ships' deck officers and pilots
    0–43 Ships' engineers
0–5 Life Scientists and Related Technicians
    0–51 Biologists, zoologists and related scientists
    0–52 Bacteriologists, pharmacologists and related scientists
    0–53 Agronomists and related scientists
    0–54 Life sciences technicians
0–6/0–7 Medical, Dental, Veterinary and Related Workers
    0–61 Medical doctors
    0–62 Medical assistants
    0–63 Dentists
    0–64 Dental assistants
    0–65 Veterinarians
    0–66 Veterinary assistants
    0–67 Pharmacists
    0 68 Pharmaceutical assistants
    0–69 Dieticians and Public Health Nutritionists
    0–71 Professional nurses
    0–72 Nursing personnel, not elsewhere classified
    0–73 Professional midwives
    0–74 Midwifery personnel, not elsewhere classified
    0–75 Optometrists and opticians
    0–76 Physiotherapists and occupational therapists
    0–77 Medical X-ray technicians
    0–79 Medical, dental, veterinary and related workers not elsewhere classified
0–8 Statisticians, Mathematicians, Systems Analysts and Related Technicians
    0–81 Statisticians
    0–82 Mathematicians and actuaries
    0–83 Systems analysts
    0–84 Statistical and mathematical technicians
0–9 Economists
    0–90 Economists
1–1 Accountants
    1–10 Accountants
1–2 Jurists
    1–21 Lawyers
    1–22 Judges
    1–29 Jurists not elsewhere classified
1–3 Teachers
    1–31 University and higher education teachers
    1–32 Secondary education teachers
    1–33 Primary education teachers
    1–34 Pre-primary education teachers
    1–35 Special education teachers
    1–39 Teachers not elsewhere classified
1–4 Workers in Religion
    1–41 Ministers of religion and related members of religious orders
    1–49 Workers in religion not elsewhere classified
1–5 Authors, Journalists and Related Writers
    1–51 Authors and critics
    1–59 Authors, journalists and related writers not elsewhere classified
1–6 Sculptors, Painters, Photographers and Related Creative Artists

1-61 Sculptors, painters and related artists
1-62 Commercial artists and designers
1-63 Photographers and cameramen
1-7 Composers and Performing Artists
    1-71 Composers, musicians and singers
    1-72 Choreographers and dancers
    1-73 Actors and stage directors
    1-74 Producers performing arts
    1-75 Circus performers
    1-79 Performing artists not elsewhere classified
1-8 Athletes, Sportsmen and Related Workers
    1-80 Athletes, sportsmen and related workers
1-9 Professional and Technical Workers not Elsewhere Classified
    1-91 Librarians, archivists and curators
    1-92 Sociologists, anthropologists and related scientists
    1-93 Social workers
    1-94 Personnel and occupational specialists
    1-95 Philologists, translators and interpreters
    1-99 Other professional and technical workers
MAJOR GROUP 2: ADMINISTRATIVE AND MANAGERIAL WORKERS
2-0 Legislative Officials and Government Administrators
    2-01 Legislative officials
    2-02 Government administrators
2-1 Managers
    2-11 General managers
    2-12 Production managers (except farm)
    2-19 Managers not elsewhere classified
MAJOR GROUP 3: CLERICAL AND RELATED WORKERS
3-0 Clerical Supervisors
    3-00 Clerical supervisors
3-1 Government, Executive Officials
    3-10 Government executive officials
3-2 Stenographers, Typists and Card- and Tape-Punching Machine Operators
    3-21 Stenographers, typists and teletypists
    3-22 Card- and tape-punching machine operators
3-3 Bookkeepers, Cashiers and Related Workers
    3-31 Bookkeepers and cashiers
    3-39 Bookkeepers, cashiers and related workers not elsewhere classified
3-4 Computing Machine Operators
    3-41 Bookkeeping and calculating machine operators
    3-42 Automatic data-processing machine operators
3-5 Transport and Communications Supervisors
    3-51 Railway station masters
    3-52 Postmasters
    3-59 Transport and communications supervisors not elsewhere classified
3-6 Transport Conductors
    3-60 Transport conductors
3-7 Mail Distribution Clerks
    3-70 Mail distribution clerks
3-8 Telephone and Telegraph Operators
    3-80 Telephone and telegraph operators
3-9 Clerical and Related Workers not elsewhere classified
    3-91 Stock clerks
    3-92 Material and production planning clerks
    3-93 Correspondence and reporting clerks
    3-94 Receptionists and travel agency clerks
    3-95 Library and filing clerks
    3-99 Clerks not elsewhere classified
MAJOR GROUP 4: SALES WORKERS
4-0 Managers (Wholesale and Retail Trade)
    4-00 Managers (wholesale and retail trade)
4-1 Working Proprietors (Wholesale and Retail Trade)

4–10 Working Proprietors (wholesale and retail trade)
4–2 Sales Supervisors and Buyers
    4–11 Sales supervisors
    4–12 Buyers
4–3 Technical Salesmen, Commercial Travellers and Manufacturers' Agents
    4–31 Technical salesmen and service advisers
    4–32 Commercial travellers and manufacturers' agents
4–4 Insurance, Real Estate, Securities and Business Services, Salesmen and Auctioneers
    4–41 Insurance, real estate and securities salesmen
    4–42 Business services salesmen
    4–43 Auctioneers
4–5 Salesmen, Shop Assistants and Related Workers
    4–51 Salesmen, shop assistants and demonstrators
    4–52 Street vendors, canvassers and newsvendors
4–9 Sales Workers not elsewhere classified
    4–90 Sales Workers not elsewhere classified
MAJOR GROUP 5: SERVICE WORKERS
5–0 Managers (Catering and Lodging Services)
    5–00 Managers (catering and lodging services)
5–1 Working Proprietors (Catering and Lodging Services)
    5–10 Working Proprietors (catering and lodging services)
5–2 Housekeeping and Related Service Supervisors
    5–20 Housekeeping and related service supervisors
5–3 Cooks, Waiters, Bartenders and Related Workers
    5–31 Cooks
    5–32 Waiters, bartenders and related workers
5–4 Maids and Related Housekeeping Service Workers not elsewhere classified
    5–40 Maids and related housekeeping service workers not elsewhere classified
5–5 Building Caretakers, Charworkers, Cleaners and Related Workers
    5–51 Building caretakers
    5–52 Charworkers, cleaners and related workers
5–6 Launderers, Dry-Cleaners and Pressers
    5–60 Launderers, dry-cleaners and pressers
5–7 Hairdressers, Barbers, Beauticians and Related Workers
    5–70 Hairdressers, barbers, beauticians and related workers
5–8 Protective Service Workers
    5–81 Fire fighters
    5–82 Policemen and detectives
    5–89 Protective service workers not elsewhere classified
5–9 Service Workers not elsewhere classified
    5–91 Guides
    5–92 Undertakers and embalmers
    5–99 Other service workers
MAJOR GROUP 6: AGRICULTURAL, ANIMAL HUSBANDRY AND
        FORESTRY WORKERS, FISHERMEN AND HUNTERS
6–0 Farm Managers and Supervisors
    6–00 Farm managers and supervisors
6–1 Farmers
    6–11 General farmers
    6–12 Specialised farmers
6–2 Agricultural and Animal Husbandry Workers
    6–21 General farm workers
    6–22 Field crop and vegetable growing workers
    6–23 Orchard, vineyard and related tree and shrub crop workers
    6–24 Livestock workers
    6–25 Dairy farm workers
    6–26 Poultry farm workers
    6–27 Nursery workers and gardeners
    6–28 Farm machinery operators
    6–29 Agricultural and animal husbandry workers not elsewhere classified
6–3 Forestry Workers
    6–31 Loggers

6–32 Forestry workers (except logging)
6–4 Fishermen, Hunters and Related Workers
    6–41 Fishermen
    6–49 Fishermen, hunters and related workers not elsewhere classified

MAJOR GROUP 7/8/9: PRODUCTION AND RELATED WORKERS,
TRANSPORT EQUIPMENT OPERATORS AND LABOURERS

7–0 Production Supervisors and General Foremen
    7–00 Production supervisors and general foremen
7–1 Miners, Quarrymen, Well Drillers and Related Workers
    7–11 Miners and quarrymen
    7–12 Mineral and stone treaters
    7–13 Well drillers, borers and related workers
7–2 Metal Processors
    7–21 Metal smelting, converting and refining furnacemen
    7–22 Metal rolling mill workers
    7–23 Metal melters and reheaters
    7–24 Metal casters
    7–25 Metal moulders and coremakers
    7–26 Metal annealers, temperers and case hardeners
    7–27 Metal drawers and extruders
    7–28 Metal platers and coaters
    7–29 Metal processors not elsewhere classified
7–3 Wood Preparation Workers and Paper Makers
    7–31 Wood treaters
    7–32 Sawyers, plywood makers and related wood processing workers
    7–33 Paper pulp preparers
    7–34 Paper makers
7–4 Chemical Processers and Related Workers
    7–41 Crushers, grinders and mixers
    7–42 Cookers, roasters and related heat treaters
    7–43 Filter and separator operators
    7–44 Still and reactor operators
    7–45 Petroleum refining workers
    7–49 Chemical processers and related workers not elsewhere classified
7–5 Spinners, Weavers, Knitters, Dyers and Related Workers
    7–51 Fibre preparers
    7–52 Spinners and winders
    7–53 Weaving and knitting machine setters and patterncard preparers
    7–54 Weavers and related workers
    7–55 Knitters
    7–56 Bleachers, dyers and textile product finishers
    7–59 Spinners, weavers, knitters, dyers and related workers not elsewhere classified
7–6 Tanners, Fellmongers and Pelt Dressers
    7–61 Tanners and fellmongers
    7–62 Pelt dressers
7–7 Food and Beverage Processers
    7–71 Grain millers and related workers
    7–72 Sugar processers and refiners
    7–73 Butchers and meat preparers
    7–74 Food preservers
    7–75 Dairy product processers
    7–76 Bakers, pastry cooks and confectionery makers
    7–77 Tea, coffee and cocoa preparers
    7–78 Brewers, wine and beverage makers
    7–79 Food and beverage processers not elsewhere classified
7–8 Tobacco Preparers and Tobacco Product Makers
    7–81 Tobacco preparers
    7–82 Cigar makers
    7–83 Cigarette makers
    7–89 Tobacco preparers and tobacco product makers not elsewhere classified
7–9 Tailors, Dressmakers, Sewers, Upholsterers and Related Workers
    7–91 Tailors and dressmakers

7–92 Fur tailors and related workers
7–93 Milliners and hatmakers
7–94 Patternmakers and cutters
7–95 Sewers and embroiderers
7–96 Upholsterers and related workers
7–99 Tailors, dressmakers, sewers, upholsterers and related workers not elsewhere classified

8–0 Shoemakers and Leather Goods Makers
  8–01 Shoemakers and shoe repairers
  8–02 Shoe cutters, lasters, sewers and related workers
  8–03 Leather goods makers
8–1 Cabinetmakers and Related Woodworkers
  8–11 Cabinetmakers
  8–12 Woodworking-machine operators
  8–19 Cabinetmakers and related woodworkers not elsewhere classified
8–2 Stone Cutters and Carvers
  8–20 Stone cutters and carvers
8–3 Blacksmiths, Toolmakers and Machine Tool Operators
  8–31 Blacksmiths, hammersmiths and forging-press operators
  8–32 Toolmakers, metal pattern makers and metal markers
  8–33 Machine-tool setter-operators
  8–34 Machine-tool operators
  8–35 Metal grinders, polishers and tool sharpeners
  8–39 Blacksmiths, toolmakers and machine-tool operators not elsewhere classified
8–4 Machinery Fitters, Machine Assemblers and Precision Instrument Makers
        (except Electrical)
  8–41 Machinery fitters and machine assemblers
  8–42 Watch, clock and precision instrument makers
  8–43 Motor vehicle mechanics
  8–44 Aircraft engine mechanics
  8–49 Machinery fitters, machine assemblers and precision instrument makers (except electrical) not elsewhere classified
8–5 Electrical Fitters and Related Electrical and Electronics Workers
  8–51 Electrical fitters
  8–52 Electronics fitters
  8–53 Electrical and electronic equipment assemblers
  8–54 Radio and television repairmen
  8–55 Electrical wiremen
  8–56 Telephone and telegraph installers
  8–57 Electric linemen and cable jointers
  8–59 Electrical fitters and related electrical and electronics workers not elsewhere classified
8–6 Broadcasting Station and Sound Equipment Operators and Cinema Projectionists
  8–61 Broadcasting station operators
  8–62 Sound equipment operators and cinema projectionists
8–7 Plumbers, Welders, Sheet Metal and Structural Metal Preparers and Erectors
  8–71 Plumbers and pipe fitters
  8–72 Welders and flame cutters
  8–73 Sheet metal workers
  8–74 Structural metal preparers and erectors
8–8 Jewellery and Precious Metal Workers
  8–80 Jewellery and precious metal workers
8–9 Glass Formers, Potters and Related Workers
  8–91 Glass formers, cutters, grinders and finishers
  8–92 Potters and related clay and abrasive formers
  8–93 Glass and ceramics kilnmen
  8–94 Glass engravers and etchers
  8–95 Glass and ceramics painters and decorators
  8–99 Glass formers, potters and related workers not elsewhere classified
9–0 Rubber and Plastics Product Makers
  9–01 Rubber and plastics product makers (except tyre makers and tyre vulcanisers)
  9–02 Tyre makers and vulcanisers

9–1 Paper and Paperboard Products Makers
    9–10 Paper and paperboard products makers
9–2 Printers and Related Workers
    9–21 Compositors, typesetters and phototype-setters
    9–22 Printing pressmen
    9–23 Stereotypers and electrotypers
    9–24 Printing engravers (except photo-engravers)
    9–25 Photo-engravers
    9–26 Bookbinders and related workers
    9–27 Photographic darkroom workers
    9–29 Printers and related workers not elsewhere classified
9–3 Painters
    9–31 Painters, construction
    9–39 Painters not elsewhere classified
9–4 Production and Related Workers not elsewhere classified
    9–41 Musical instrument makers and tuners
    9–42 Basketry weavers and brush makers
    9–43 Non-metallic mineral product makers
    9–49 Other production and related workers
9–5 Bricklayers, Carpenters and Other Construction Workers
    9–51 Bricklayers, stonemasons and tile setters
    9–52 Reinforced-concreters, cement finishers and terrazzo workers
    9–53 Roofers
    9–54 Carpenters, joiners and parquetry workers
    9–55 Plasterers
    9–56 Insulators
    9–57 Glaziers
    9–59 Construction workers not elsewhere classified
9–6 Stationary Engines and Related Equipment Operators
    9–61 Power-generating machinery operators
    9–69 Stationary engine and related equipment operators not elsewhere classified
9–7 Material-Handling and Related Equipment Operators, Dockers and Freight Handlers
    9–71 Dockers and freight handlers
    9–72 Riggers and cable splicers
    9–73 Crane and hoist operators
    9–74 Earth-moving and related machinery operators
    9–79 Material-handling equipment operators not elsewhere classified
9–8 Transport Equipment Operators
    9–81 Ships' deck ratings, barge crews and boatmen
    9–82 Ships' engine room ratings
    9–83 Railway engine drivers and firemen
    9–84 Railway brakemen, signalmen and shunters
    9–85 Motor vehicle drivers
    9–86 Animal and animal-drawn vehicle drivers
    9–89 Transport equipment operators not elsewhere classified
9–9 Labourers not elsewhere classified
    9–99 Labourers not elsewhere classified
MAJOR GROUP X: WORKERS NOT CLASSIFIABLE BY OCCUPATION
X–1 New Workers Seeking Employment
    X–10 New workers seeking employment
X–2 Workers Reporting Occupations Unidentifiable or Inadequately Described
    X–20 Workers reporting occupations unidentifiable or inadequately described
X–3 Workers NOT Reporting Any Occupation
    X–30 Workers not reporting any occupation
ARMED FORCES MEMBERS OF THE ARMED FORCES

Index

Printed in Great Britain by
Willmer Brothers Limited, Birkenhead

Smallpox epidemiological assessment, 1967 & 1974. (By Courtesy of the World He

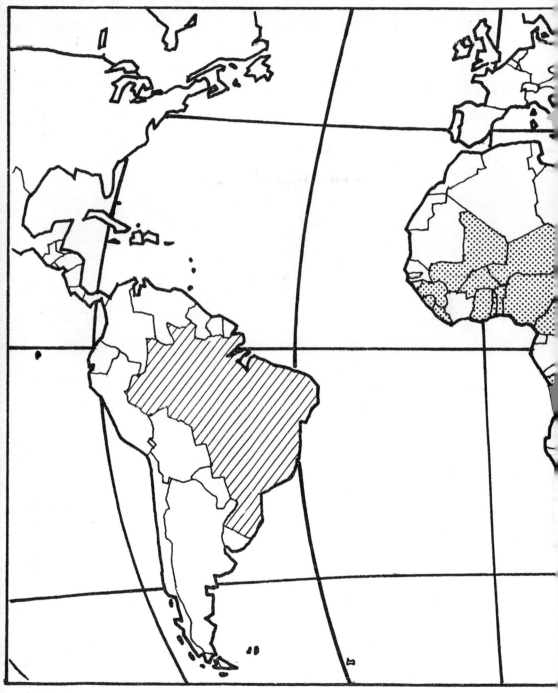

■ 1974 (May)